SELF ASSESSMENT IN RADIOLOGY & IMAGING 4

Orthopaedics

Dennis J. Stoker

MB BS, FRCP, FRCR
Consultant Radiologist
Royal National Orthopaedic Hospital, London
Director of Radiological Studies
Institute of Orthopaedics, London

Elisabeth A. Tilley

MB BS, BSc, MRCP, FRCR
Senior Registrar in Diagnostic Radiology
St. George's Hospital, London

Wolfe Medical Publications Ltd

This book is one of a series of radiology
and imaging self assessment question and
answer books. For a full list of Atlases in
the series, plus details of our other
Atlases, please write to
Wolfe Medical Publications Ltd,
Brook House, 2-16 Torrington Place,
London WC1E 7LT, England.

Some other subjects of titles in the series
Ear, Nose & Throat Radiology
Gastro-Intestinal Radiology
Mammography
Nuclear Medicine
Paediatric Radiology
Neuroradiology
Cardio-Thoracic Radiology
Urological Radiology

Acknowledgements

We wish to express our thanks to all those who have provided assistance in the compilation of this book. The radiographs are from the Film Library of the Institute of Orthopaedics, the Royal National Orthopaedic Hospital, St. George's Hospital and Atkinson Morley's Hospital, London.

We acknowledge the photographic skills of Uta Boundy and Dirk de Camp, of the Medical Photographic Department of the Institute of Orthopaedics, London, in the photographic reproduction of the radiographs.

Last, but by no means least, we thank Veronika Aurens for her invaluable secretarial assistance and for keeping the project in order throughout its gestation.

Preface

This book offers an opportunity for self assessment in Orthopaedic Radiology, which forms a major part of the work of any general radiologist.

Stress is laid on the appearances of the plain film, as this is—and will continue to be for the foreseeable future—the major primary method of imaging bone and the main means of diagnosis. Often, the reader will be invited to suggest the next step in the radiological management of the case—further projections, other methods of imaging—on the basis of the interpretation of the initial film and the history provided.

Each question is independent and the order of the cases is random. The short clinical histories are essentially those provided by the patient at the time of presentation. They are therefore what might be expected in clinical practice, usually, but not always, relevant. We believe that the book will be of value to medical students, house officers, and in the early years of radiological training. It also should prove helpful to those undergoing orthopaedic training.

In the provision of 97 cases, it is neither possible, nor intentional, to cover the whole range of bone and joint disorders. We hope that this book will serve as an introduction to the subject and as a stimulus to further reading. A short list of suggested texts is provided in Further Reading.

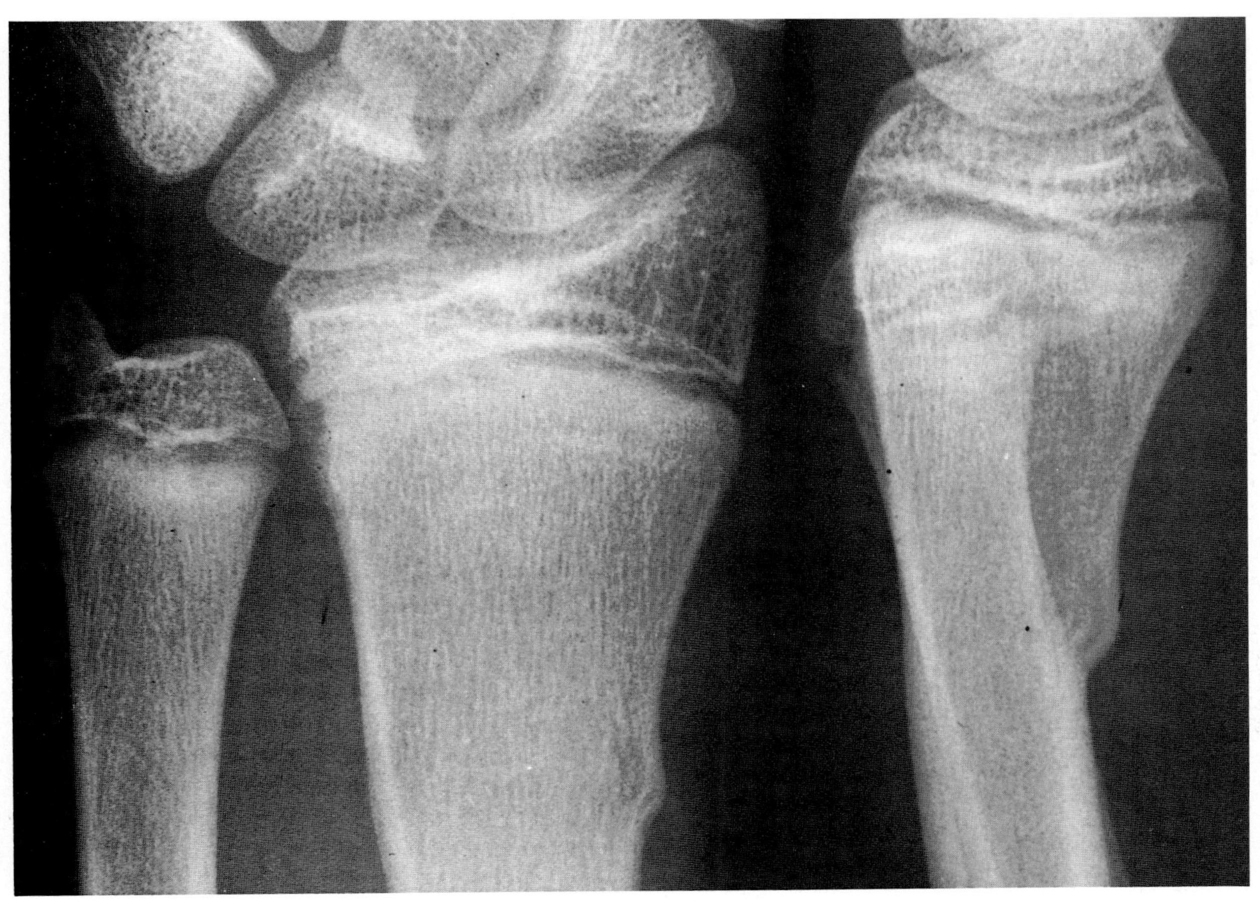

This child presented with a painful wrist following a fall.

- What is the diagnosis?

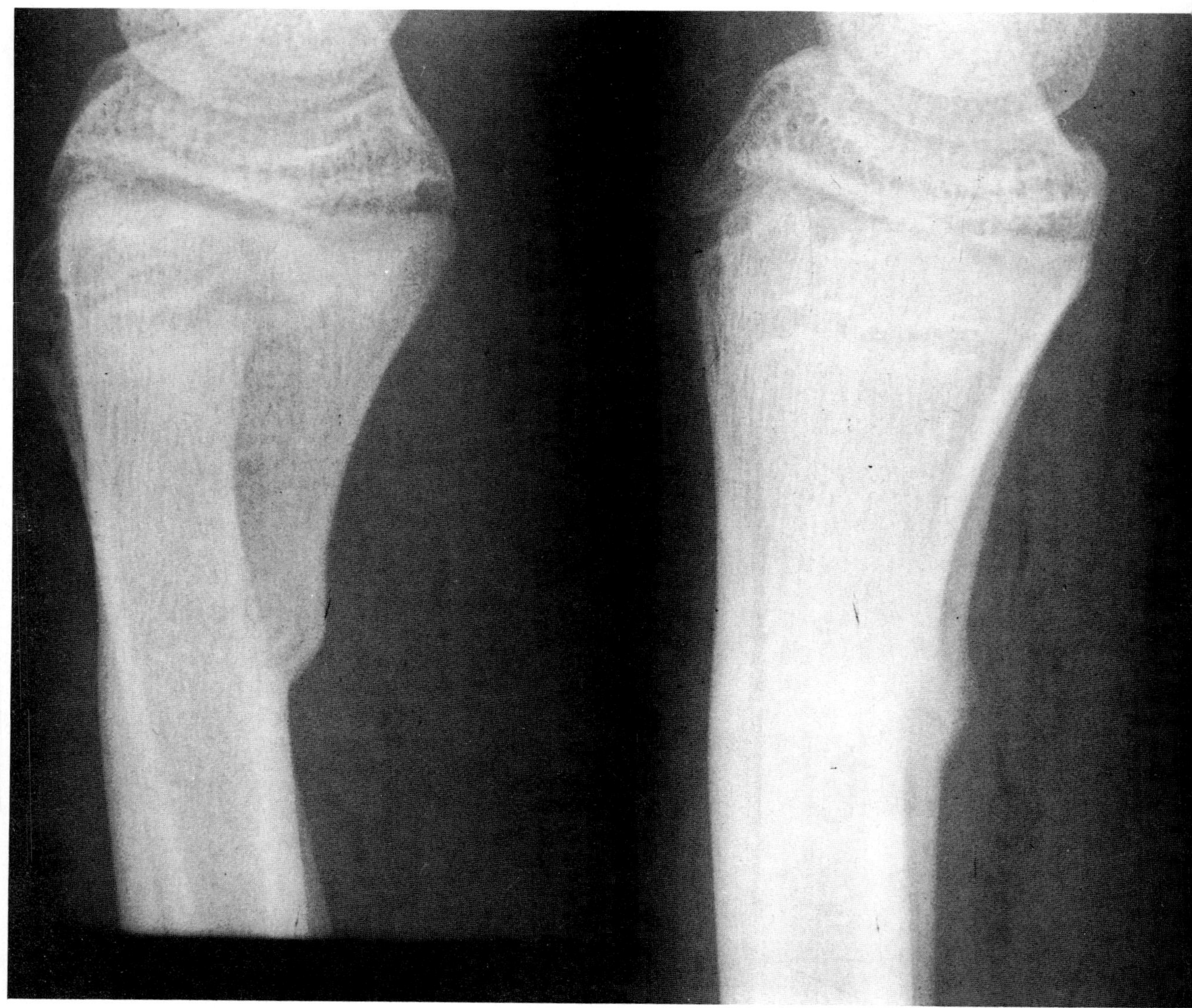

Wrinkling of the anteromedial cortex is seen in the diametaphysis of the radius.

This is a 'wrinkle' or torus fracture (Latin *torus* = protuberance or round swelling) which results from injury of insufficient force to displace the cortex. The periosteum remains intact so that healing occurs without the production of significant callus. The two lateral radiographs (see above) show the appearances at presentation (left) and after three weeks of healing when minimal callus has formed. Strictly speaking, this fracture is not the same as a greenstick injury, where one cortex splits while the other maintains its continuity.

It is a common injury in the distal forearm in the 6-10 age group.

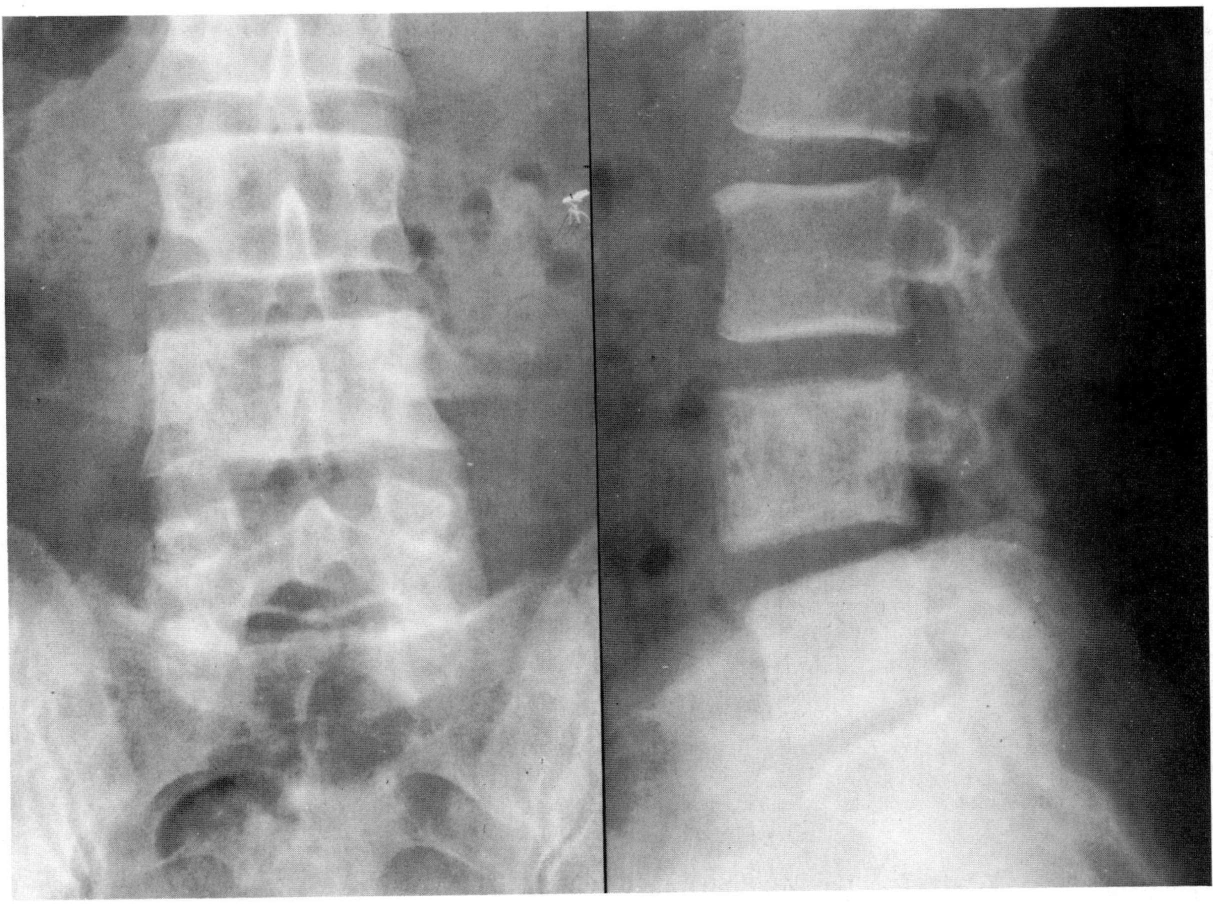

This middle-aged woman complained of low back pain.

- What is the likely cause of her pain?

- What other abnormality is seen?

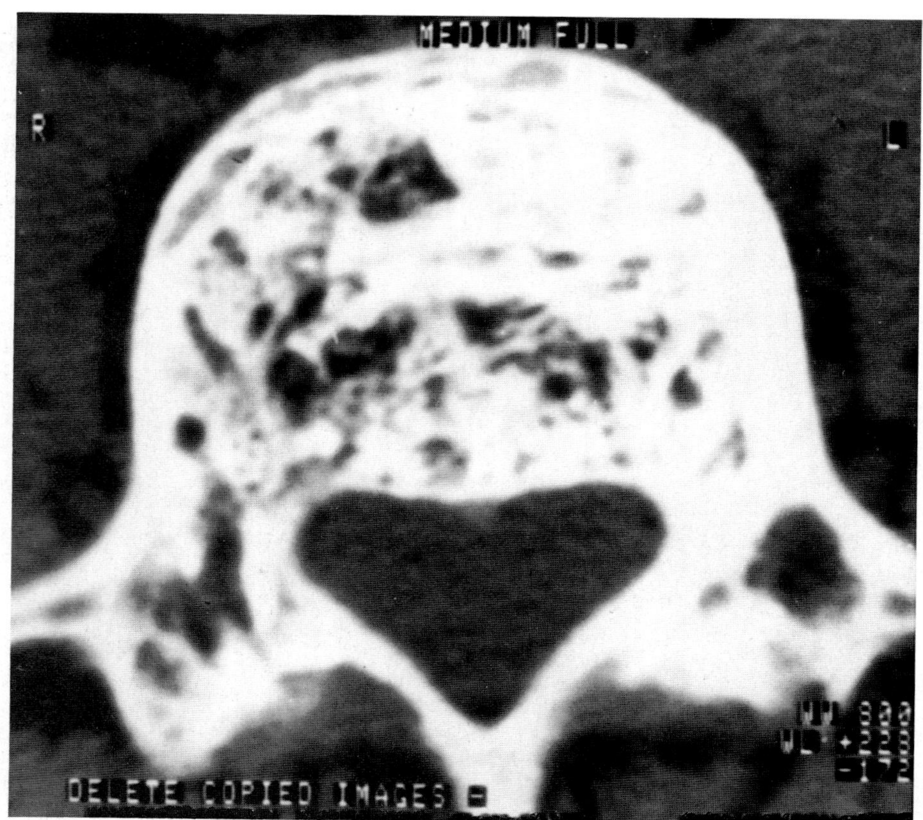

The body and pedicles of L4 are expanded slightly and the vertebral body shows coarse vertical trabeculation; this appearance is characteristic of a haemangioma.

In addition, narrowing of the disc space, marginal sclerosis and bony lipping are present at the lumbosacral junction. Haemangiomas are usually asymptomatic and this patient's pain was attributed to the degenerative intervertebral disc at the lumbosacral level.

Haemangiomas are benign tumours which occur most frequently in the vertebral bodies, particularly those in the thoracolumbar region and in the skull. They may be cavernous, capillary or venous in nature, the vascular structures replacing the medullary bone. Any remaining trabeculae thicken to produce vertical striations and the orientation is probably mediated by stress of weight-bearing.

A CT scan was performed in this patient to assess any nerve root compression at the lumbosacral junction and also to exclude any encroachment on the neural canal by the haemangioma. The scan through L4 shows not only the vascular spaces and thickened trabeculae of the haemangioma but also the characteristic lack of cortical involvement. The haemangioma extends into the pedicles but has not reduced the size of the neural canal.

The main differential diagnosis of haemangioma on the plain radiograph is Paget's disease, which also causes alteration of trabecular pattern. It is sometimes maintained that Paget's disease can be differentiated by its universal finding of enlargement of the affected bone. Such enlargement is usually absent in a vertebra affected by haemangioma, but not in this case; any enlargement that occurs is, however, almost always minor in degree.

Vertebral angiomas are usually incidental findings but may occasionally be symptomatic.

Reference

Mohan, V., Gupta, S. K., Tuli, S. M. and Sanyal, B. (1980) Symptomatic vertebral haemangiomas. *Clin. Radiol.*, **31**, 575-579.

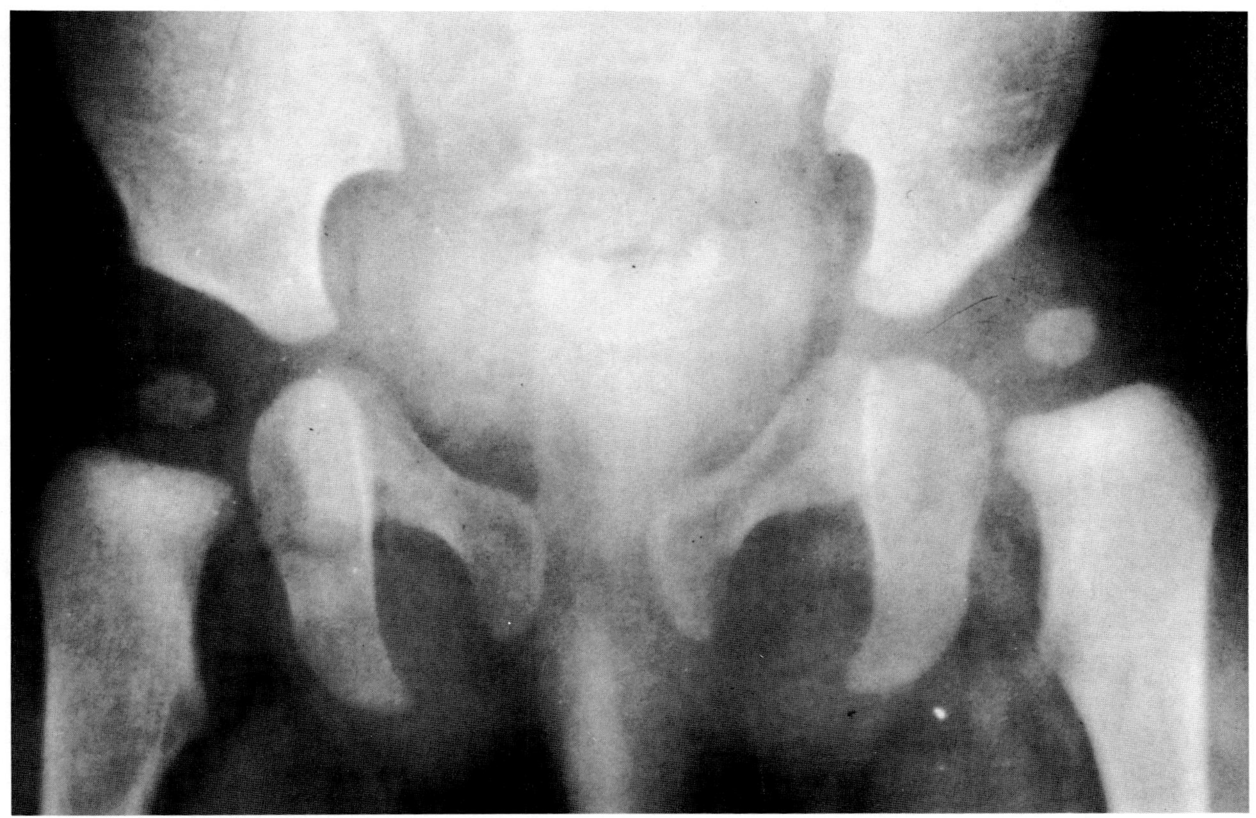

An infant under observation for reduced abduction of the left hip.

- What is the abnormality?

- What might have been done to prevent it?

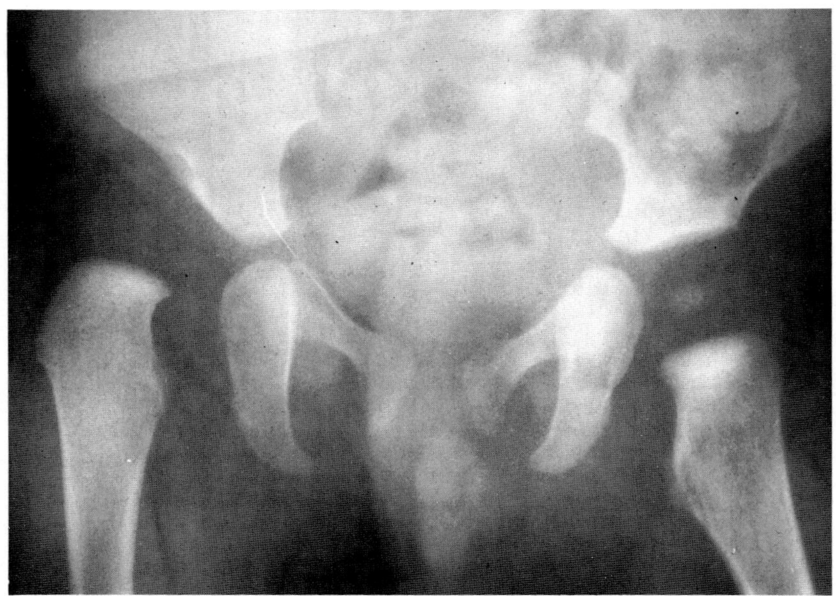

The right hip is normal; the left acetabular roof is sloping resulting in a shallow acetabulum. Consequently, the femoral capital epiphysis is at a higher level and more lateral to the Y-shaped cartilage on the left than on the right.

Congenital dislocation of the hip (CDH) can, potentially, be prevented. For many years clinical examination has been recommended for all newborn infants to identify the dislocatable femoral head. In the neonate the examination consists of the performance of the Ortolani-Barlow test by an expert in this manoeuvre. The test involves the displacing or relocating of the femoral head within the acetabulum; this is associated with a characteristic palpable 'clunk'. Unfortunately, in most centres, clinical examination fails to identify all infants with unstable hips who may present later with reduced abduction in flexion, or later still with a disorder of gait at the time of first walking.

Ultrasonography is being used increasingly in the diagnosis, particularly in patients at risk:

- those with a family history of CDH
- history of oligohydramnios
- breech deliveries (Caesarian section for unknown cause)
- any associated abnormality, such as club foot

The disorder is, of course, also more frequent in female infants.

Ultrasonography in expert hands can identify the normal and the shallow acetabulum, so that unnecessary splinting of normal hips is reduced.

The plain film (see above) shows another case with CDH of the right hip. On this occasion, delay in ossification of the femoral capital epiphysis is also present.

References

Berman, L. and Klenerman, L. (1986) Ultrasound screening for hip abnormalities; preliminary findings in 1001 neonates. *Brit. Med. J.*, **293**, 719-722.

Noble, T. C., Pullan, C. R., Craft, A. W. and Leonard, M. A. (1978) Difficulties in diagnosing and managing congenital dislocation of the hip. *Brit. Med. J.*, **2**, 620-623.

Standing Medical Advisory Committee and Standing Nursing and Midwifery Advisory Committee for the Secretaries of State for Social Services. *Screening for the detection of congenital dislocation of the hip*. London, Department of Health & Social Security, 1986.

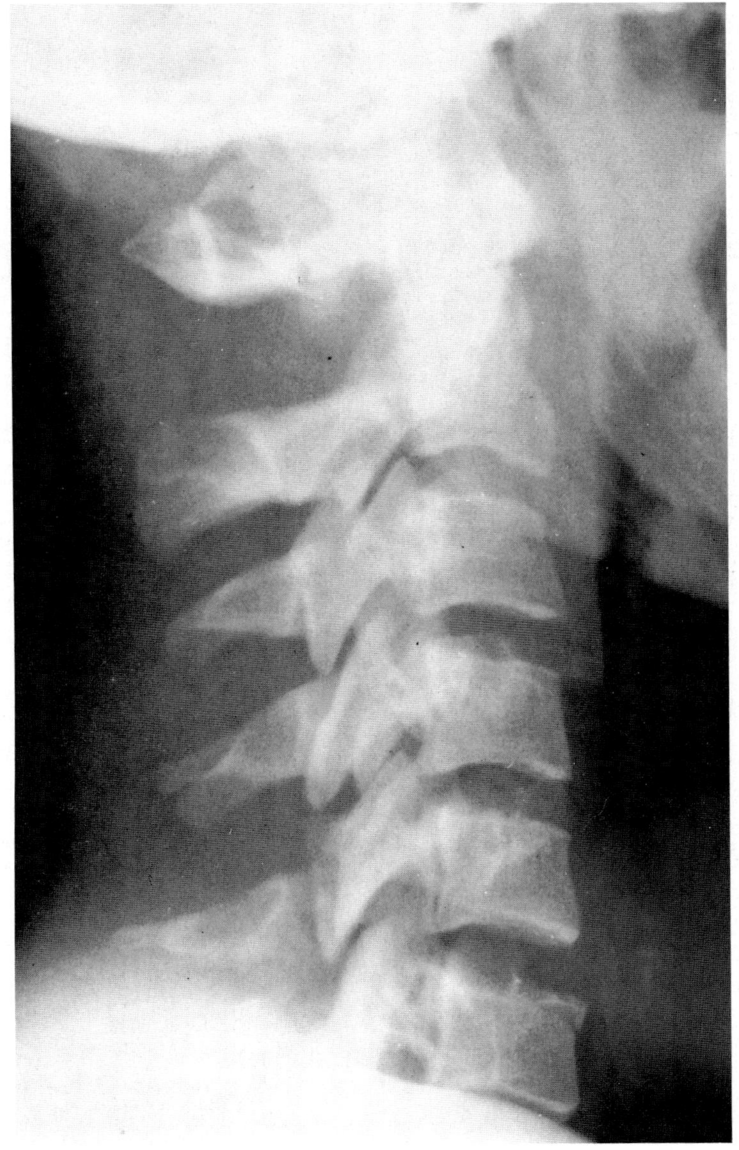

This patient sustained injuries in a road traffic accident.

- Comment on the radiograph.
- What would you do next?

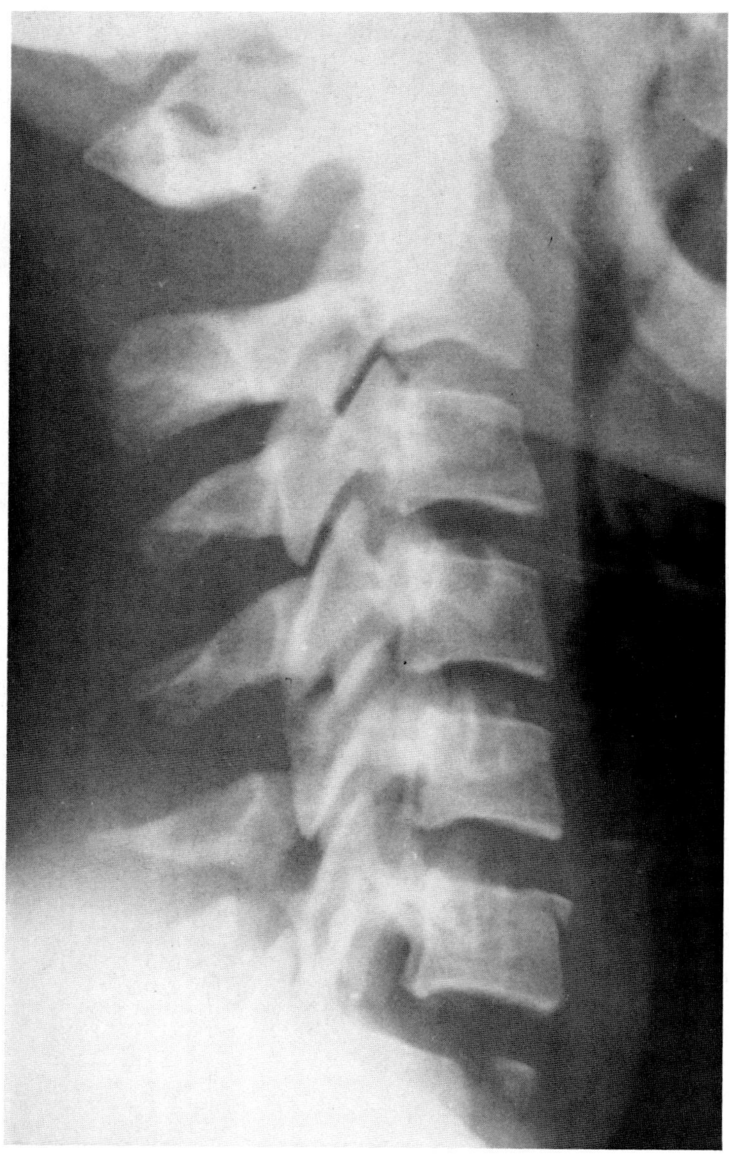

The only injury seen in this lateral view of the cervical spine is a fracture through the anterosuperior part of the body of C6, but it is crucial to note that C7 has not been included on the radiograph. The examination of the cervical spine is therefore incomplete. A repeat film with the patient's shoulders pulled down reveals forward slip of the body of C6 on C7, bilateral facet dislocation and a teardrop fracture of C7. These are the result of a severe hyper-flexion injury.

In a patient with a suspected cervical spine injury, the initial radiograph should be a horizontal beam lateral view. If this shows no significant injury it is permissible to proceed with other routine projections, without seeking expert advice. C7 must always be demonstrated, if necessary with a 'swimmer's' lateral projection or tomography. Oblique views may often be helpful.

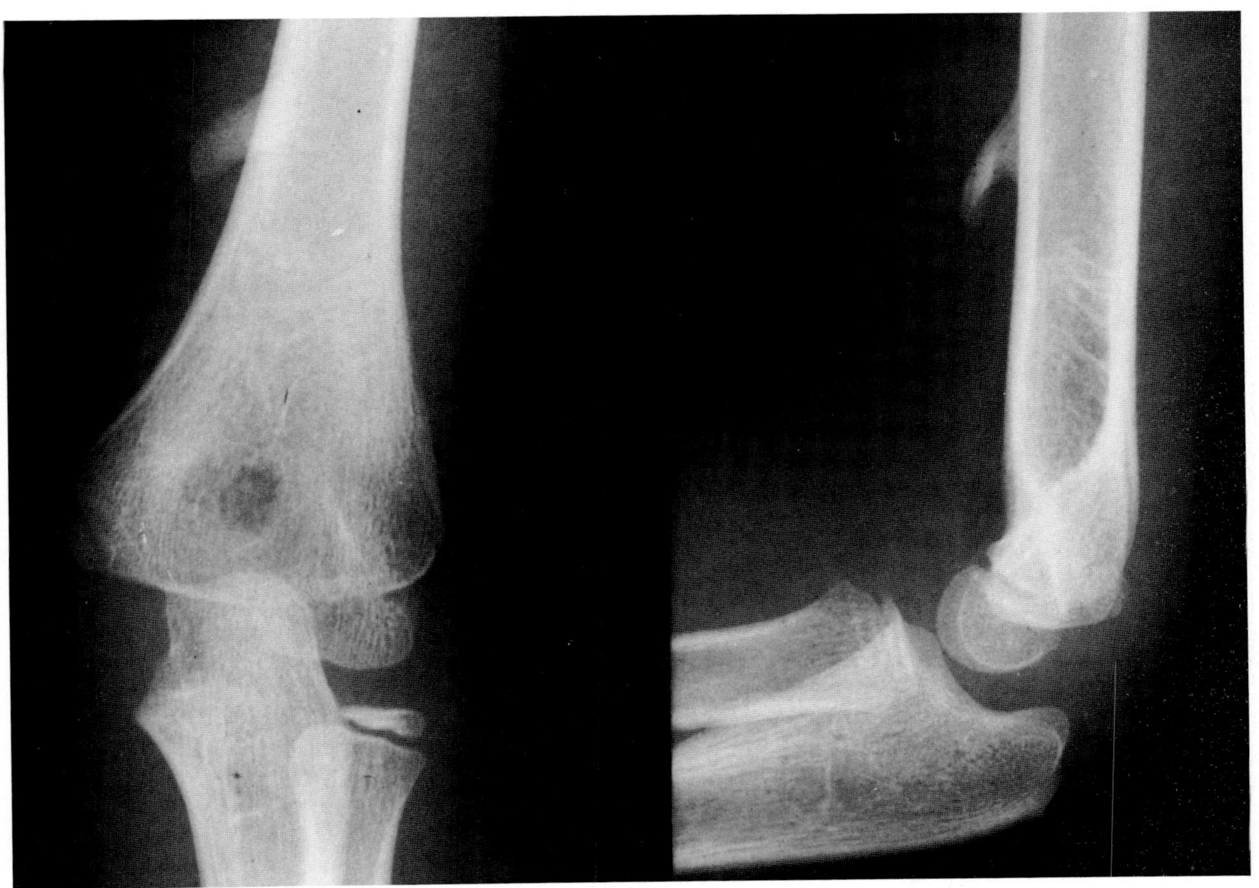

This child was examined because his mother noticed a bony lump above his elbow.

- What is the prognosis?

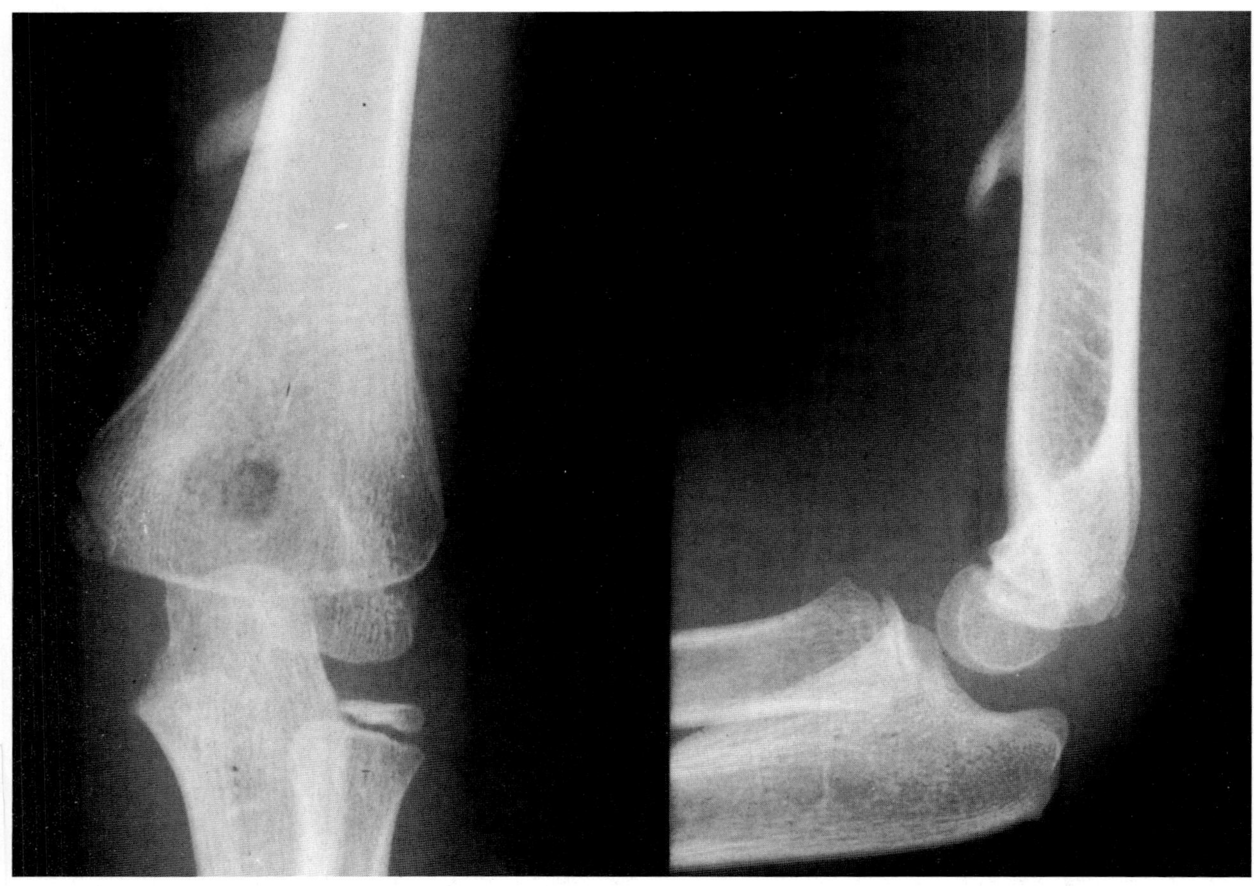

The bony excrescence arising from the anteromedial aspect of the humeral shaft is a supracondylar spur. It is a normal variant due to partial ossification in a ligament which attaches distally to the medial epicondyle. The median nerve lies deep to the ligament and is vulnerable to compression. The spur also provides an attachment for the pronator teres muscle. It should not be mistaken for an osteochondroma.

The 'supracondyloid process' was described in 1848 by John Struthers, whose name has been given to the attached ligament. It is an atavistic remnant, forming a foramen in cats and other lower animals. It is probably the lower part of the tendon of a vestigial muscle—the latissimo-condyloideus—present in climbing mammals. It is important in surgical anatomy as, in about one-third of cases, the brachial artery divides above it; one of the trunks passes medially, the other follows the usual course.

Sir John Struthers (1823-1899) graduated from Edinburgh University and became Professor of Anatomy at the University of Aberdeen.

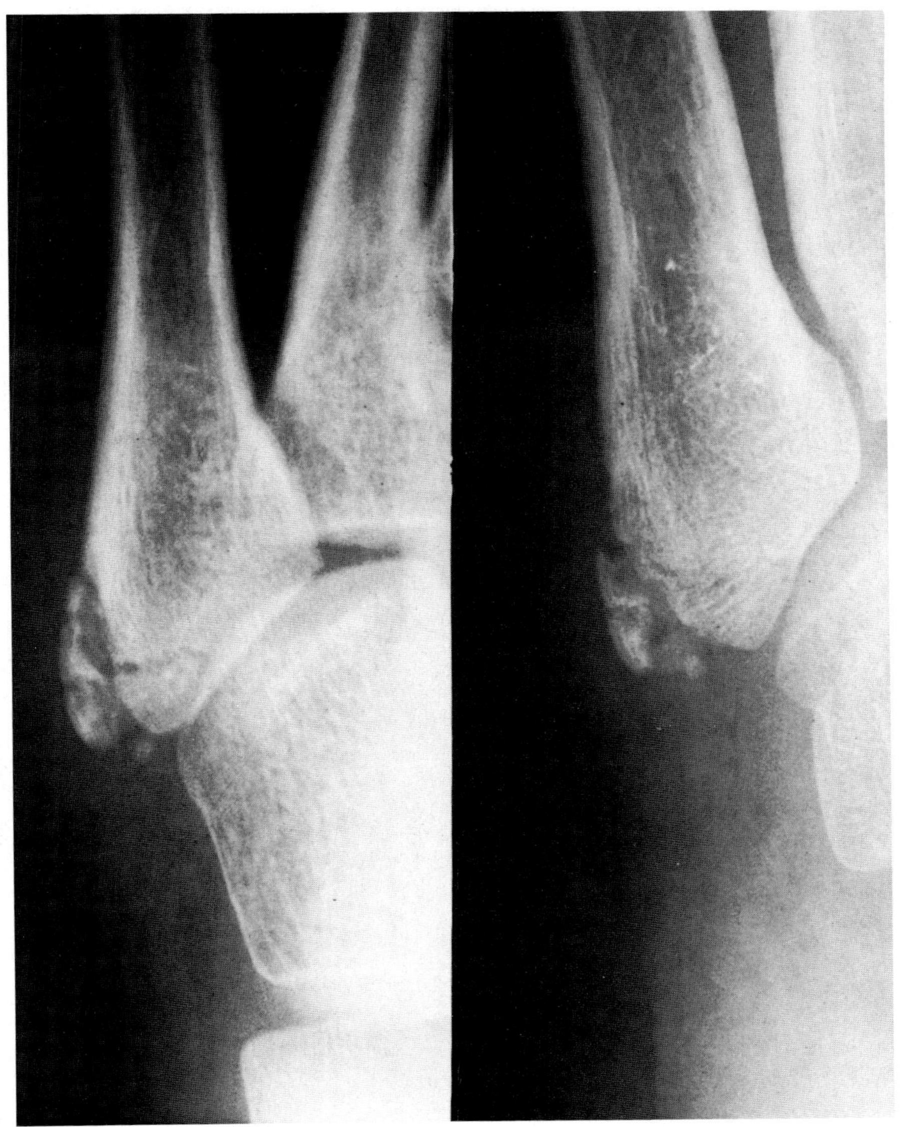

This 13-year-old boy presented to Casualty after
a fall.

- What is the diagnosis?

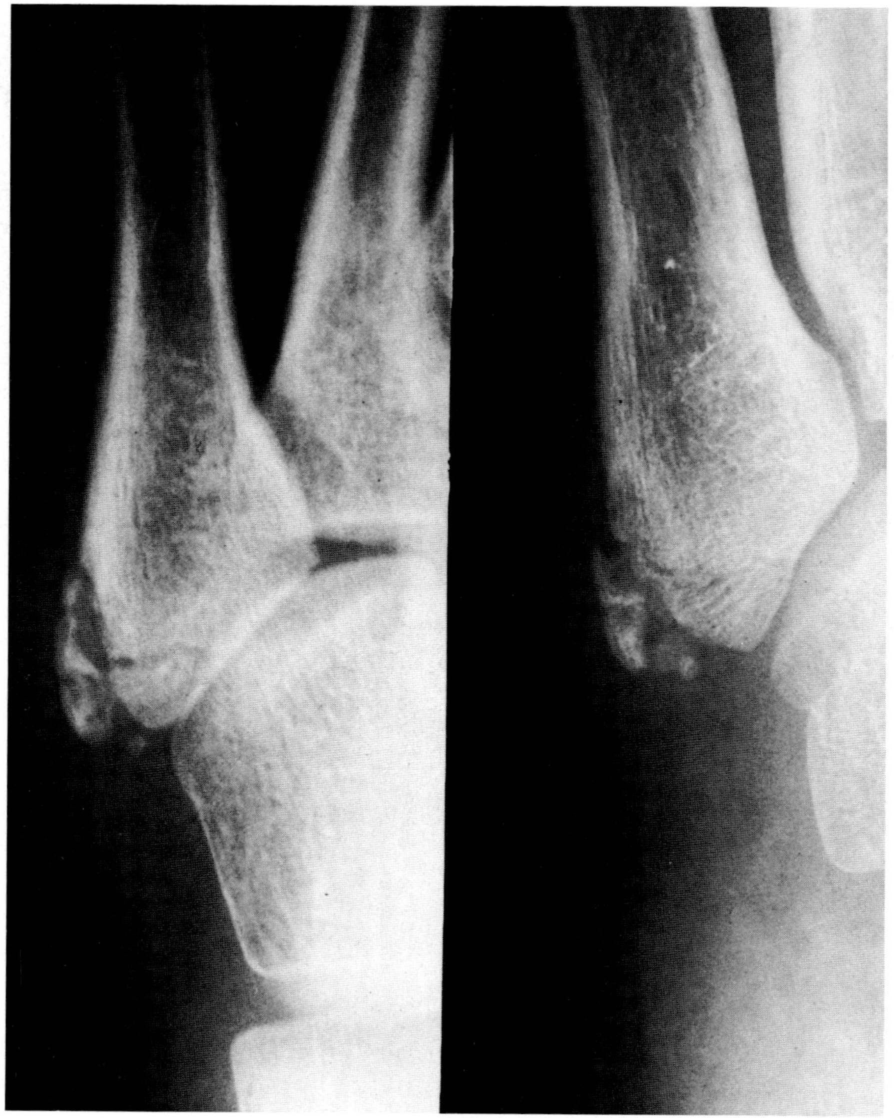

The transverse fracture through the base of the fifth metatarsal is often called a Robert Jones fracture. This common foot injury is due to avulsion of the insertion of the peroneus brevis tendon at the base of the metatarsal during plantar flexion and inversion of the foot. The injury described in 1902 by Robert Jones was of a different nature with a more distal fracture of the metatarsal shaft.

The secondary ossification centre at the lateral margin of the base of the fifth metatarsal should not be mistaken for a fracture. The orientation of the ossification centre is longitudinal whereas the fracture is transverse.

Reference

Rogers, L. F. and Campbell, R. E. (1978) Fractures and dislocations of the foot. *Semin. in Roentgenol.*, **13**, 157-166.

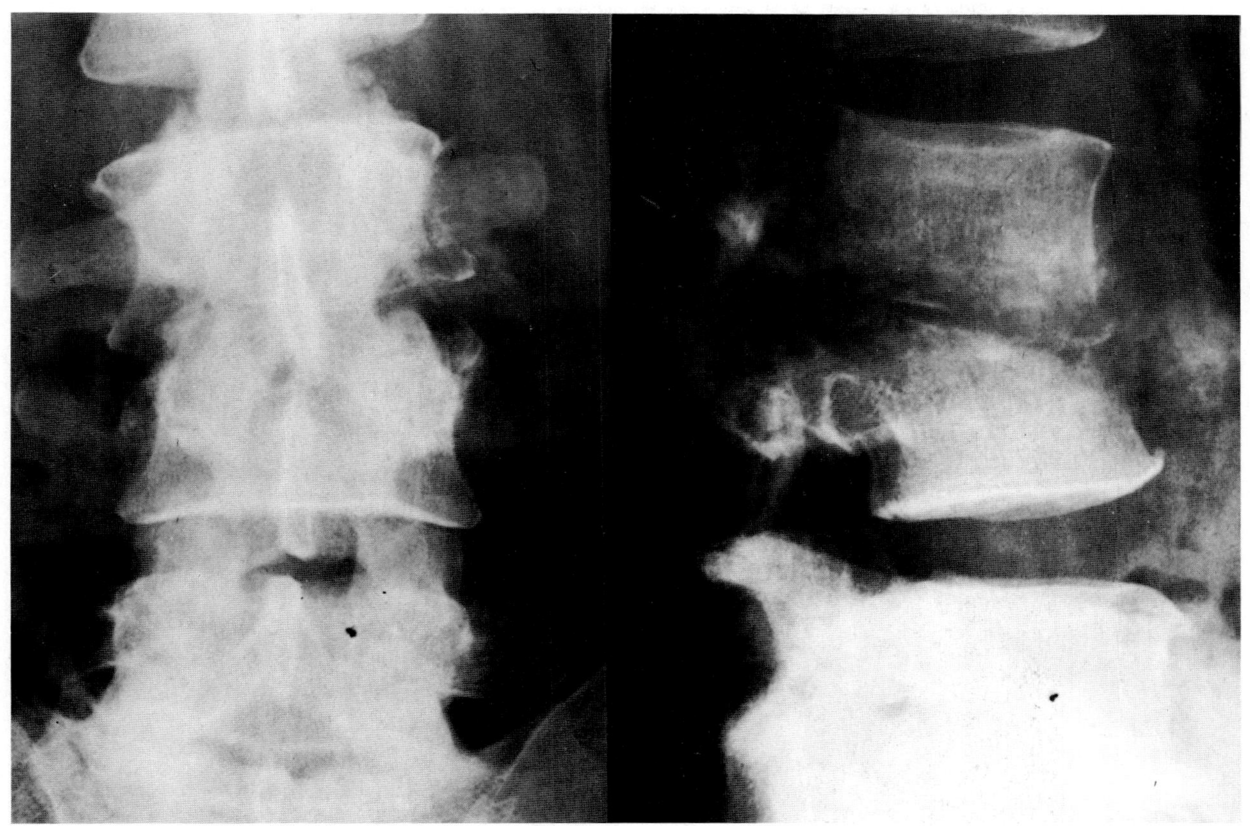

Two months following cystectomy, this 57-year-old white man was admitted with increasing weakness of both lower limbs.

- Describe the appearances.

- What is the most likely aetiology?

A7

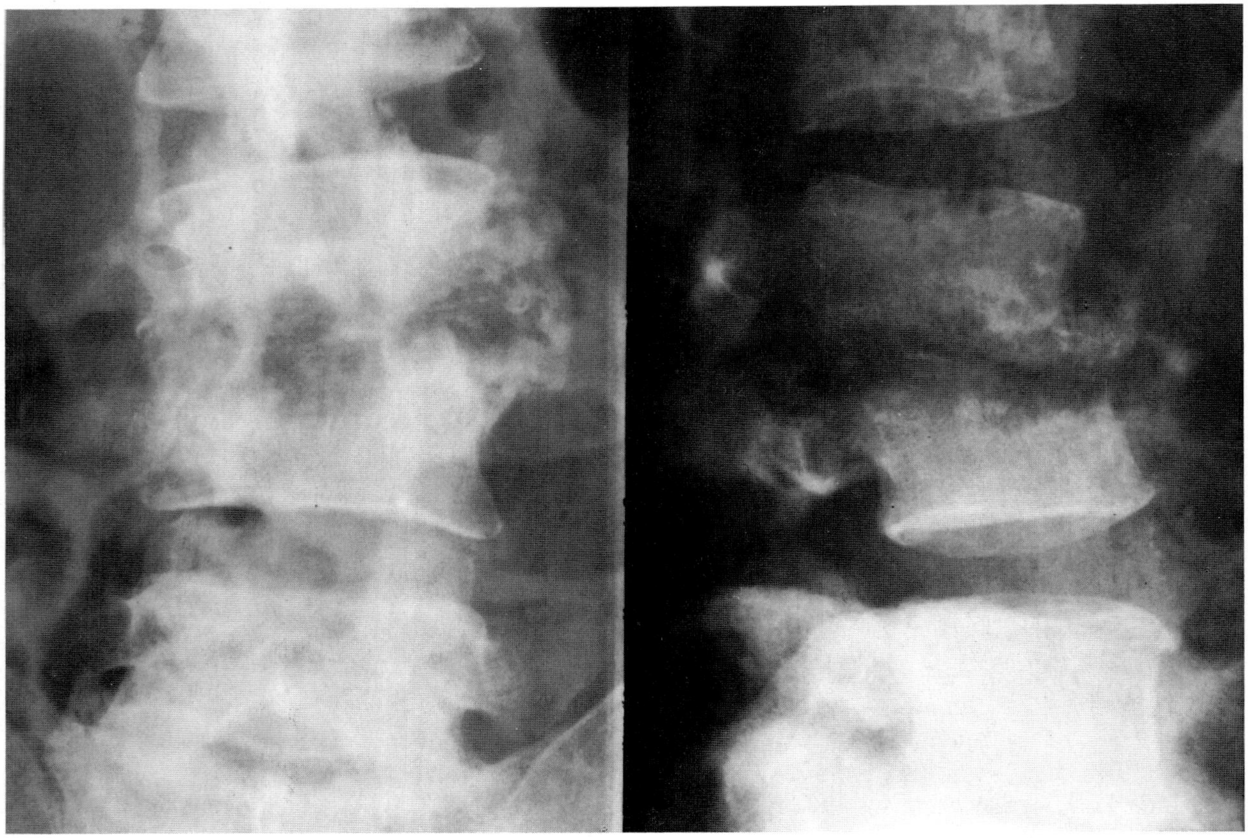

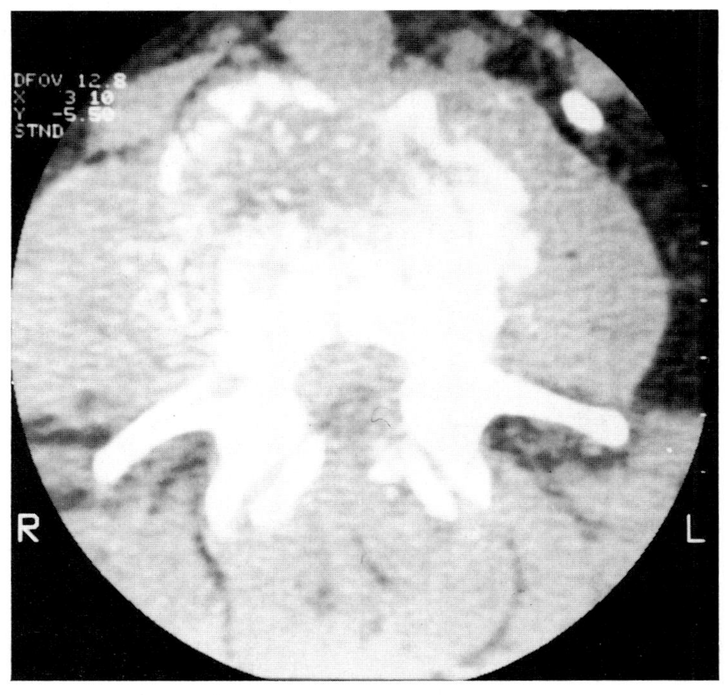

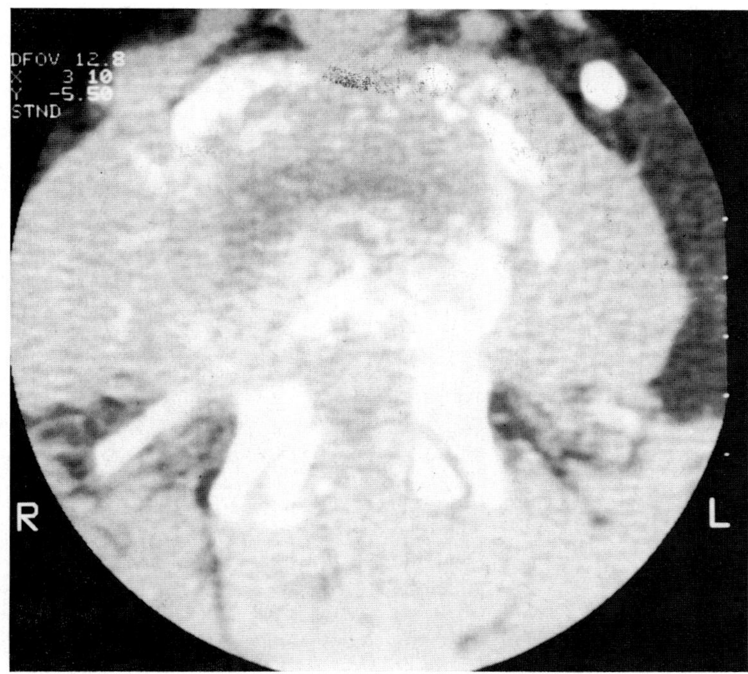

Initial views of the lumbar spine (see page 17) show marked narrowing of the L3/4 disc, loss of definition of the adjacent end-plates, destruction of the anterior thirds of the L3 and L4 vertebral bodies and the formation of new bone anterolaterally. No paravertebral swelling can be identified.

These appearances are consistent with infection. The history, narrowed disc space, new bone formation and absence of a paravertebral abscess tend to favour a pyogenic origin, although in patients of Asian or African origin tuberculous infection can cause similar changes.

Ninety per cent of pyogenic infections are due to *Staphylococcus aureus*, as in this case. Needle or open biopsy is often required to identify the organism and establish its antibiotic sensitivities. Infection is commonly due to spread to the vertebral body bone marrow from a septic focus in the pelvis and is a recognised complication of surgery of the genitourinary tract. Such spread is facilitated by the presence of the valveless prevertebral venous plexus of Batson.

One month following spinal decompression (note laminectomy) and removal of 10 ml of pus, although further bone destruction has occurred, the presence of florid new bone indicates that healing is in progress (see page 18). Ultimately, bony fusion will occur.

The paraplegia in this patient is unusual. It occurs in only one per cent of patients with pyogenic spondylodiscitis, but is reported in up to 35 per cent of TB cases worldwide. The two CT scans demonstrate the extent of vertebral destruction and indicate the epidural encroachment by the infective process.

Q8

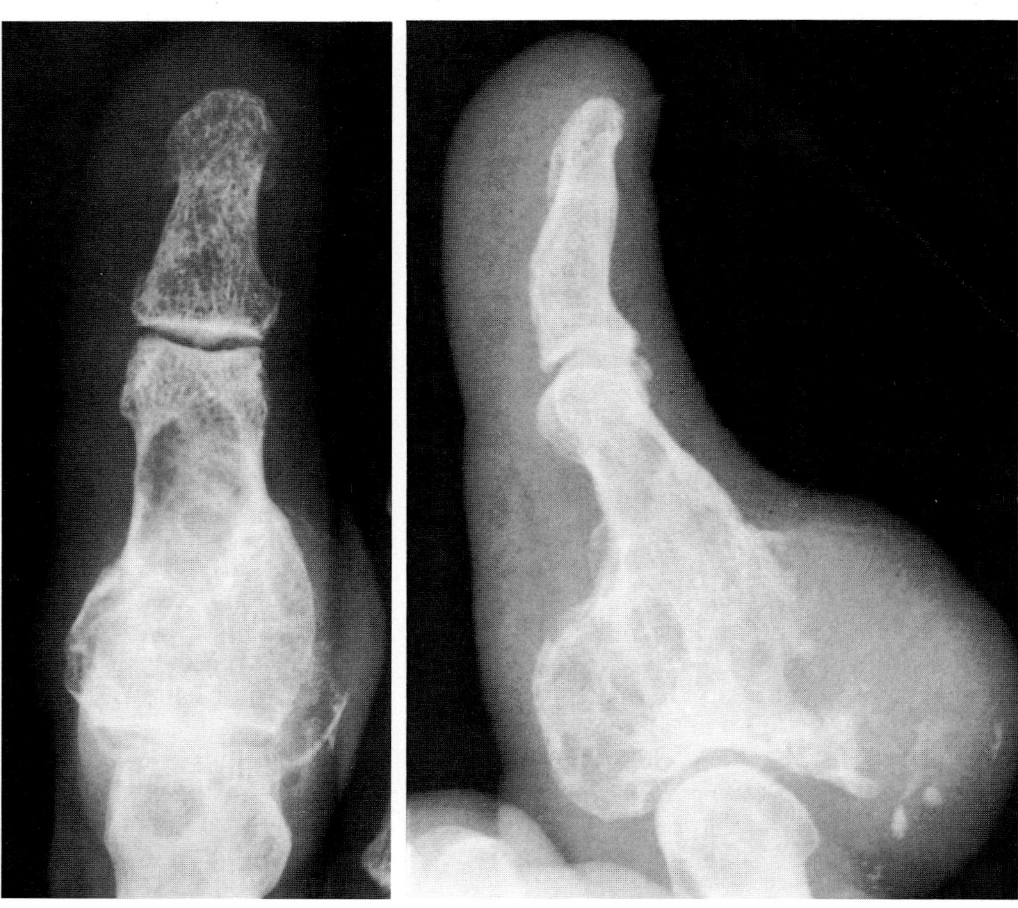

This 35-year-old woman presented initially with a small painless swelling of her middle finger. One year later the swelling was larger but still painless.

- Describe the features.
- Might the lesion be malignant?

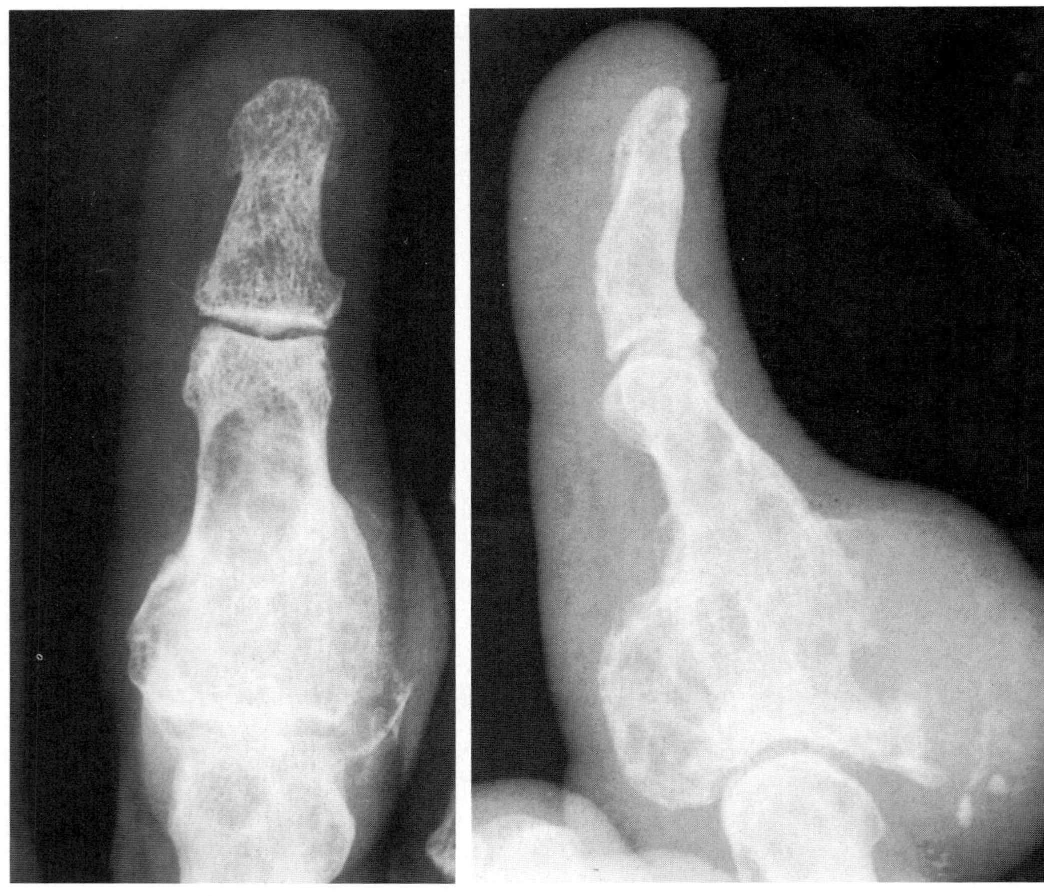

The film shows an expanded, eccentric radiolucent lesion in the middle phalanx which has thinned the overlying cortex, breaching it in places. The narrow zone of transition and sclerosis of the endosteal margin suggest a benign aetiology and the appearances are consistent with an **enchondroma**.

Calcification, which tends to occur in all chondral tumours, is present peripherally. Similar changes are visible in the proximal phalanx. Despite the history of increase in size, the enchondroma still appears benign radiologically with no features suggesting chondrosarcomatous change. The soft tissues seem to be displaced around the lesion but are not swollen and the zone of transition remains narrow.

Although the incidence of chondrosarcomatous transformation is 10-15 per cent in isolated enchondromas of the long bones, it is rare in the hands. Malignant change is usually accompanied by pain and rapid increase in size. In the presence of such clinical indications, reliance should not be placed on radiological evidence of benignity and biopsy must be performed. This was undertaken here and sarcomatous change was excluded.

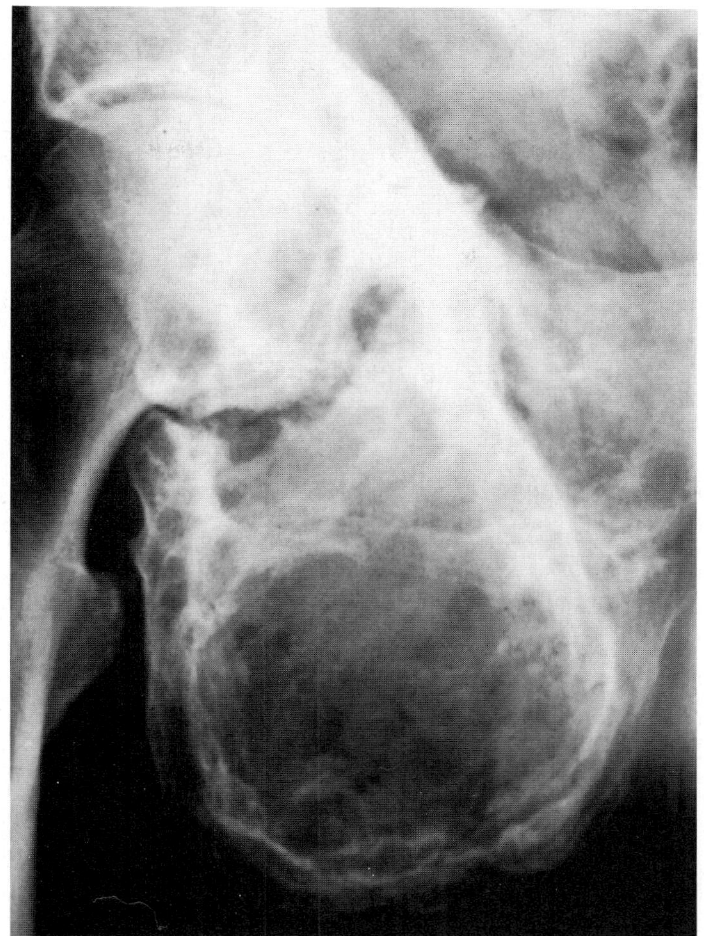

This man complained of discomfort when sitting, of long duration. On examination a non-tender mass was present in the region of the ischial tuberosity.

- What is the diagnosis?

- Would you consider any other causes?

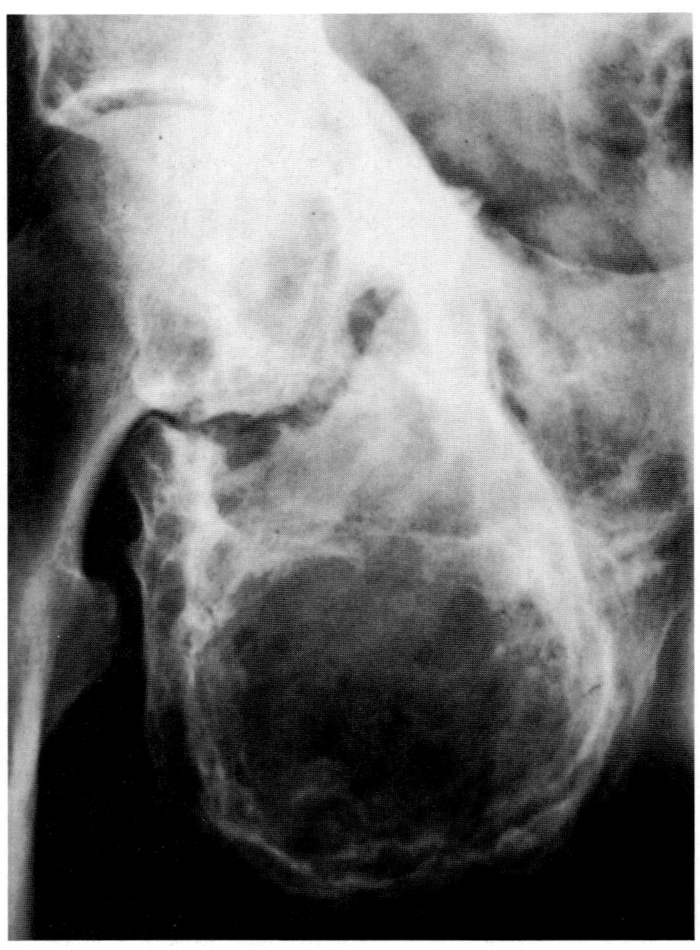

The AP view of the right hip shows a large bony mass below the ischium. The mass is partly fused to the ischium but medially, a fine lucent line of separation is evident. The bony mass has the same general shape as the ischial tuberosity; this is the typical appearance of an old avulsion injury of the non-united ossification centre or apophysis of the ischial tuberosity. Apart from the typical location, such a lesion may suggest a slowly-growing benign tumour of bone.

Avulsion of the apophysis is caused by a strong contraction of the hamstring muscles. This man remembered suffering severe pain in the right hip during a race at school; this was diagnosed at the time as a pulled hamstring. The avulsed apophysis may continue to produce bone and within months of the injury a large bony mass may have appeared. At this stage the appearances are diagnostic and should not be mistaken for myositis ossificans or a calcified haematoma.

Reference

Ellis, R. et al. (1966) Ischial apophyseolysis. *Radiology*, **87**, 646-648.

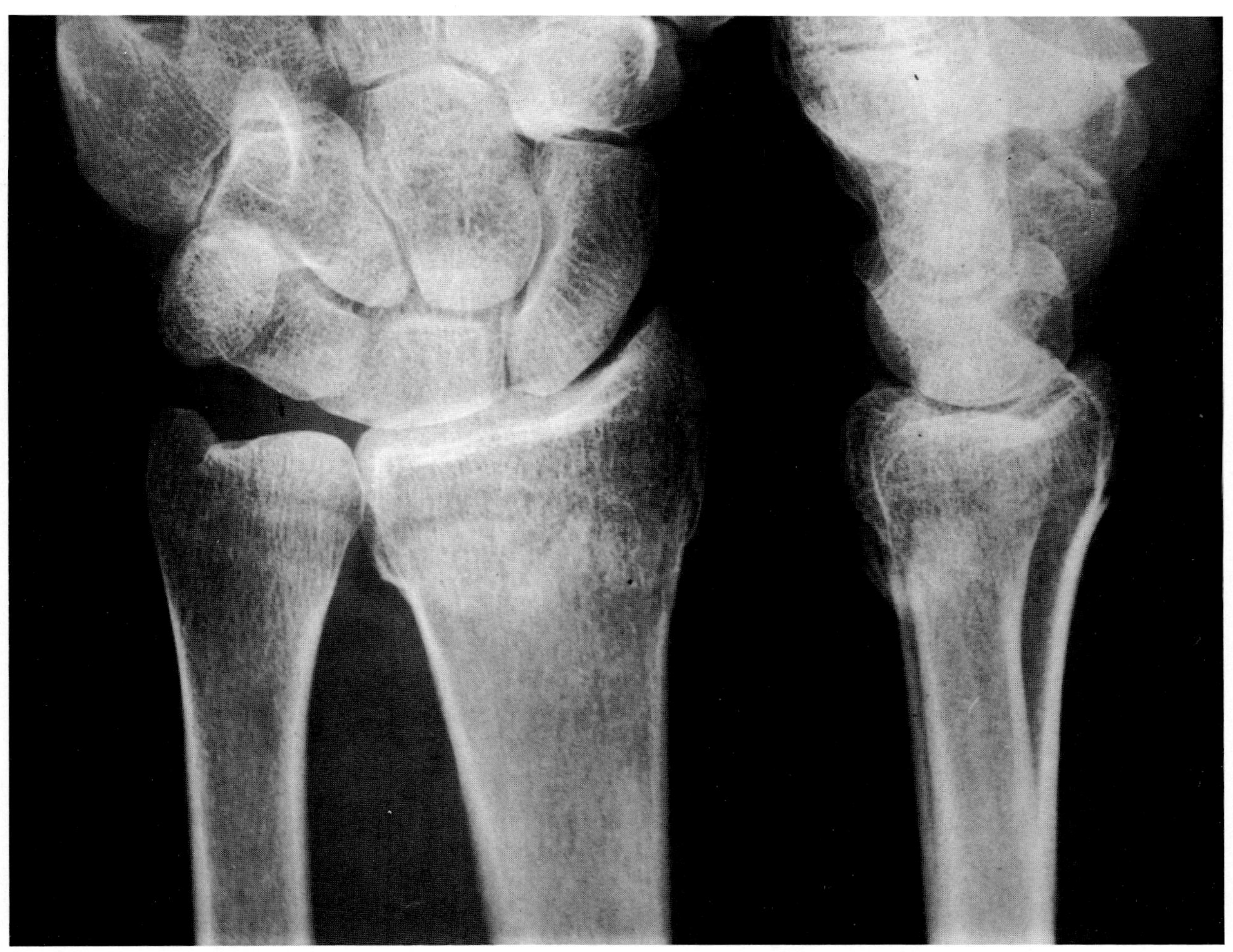

This woman fell while ice-skating.

- Describe the appearance shown on the radiographs.

- What other injuries are commonly associated with this type of fracture?

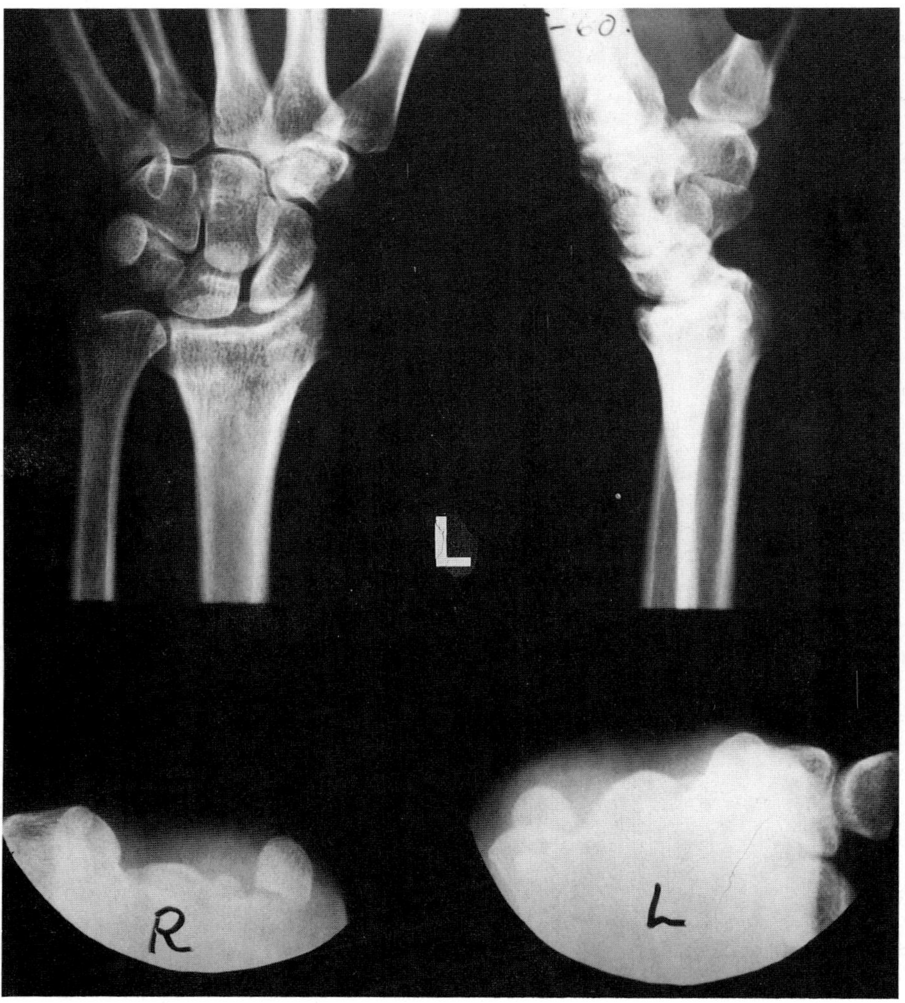

Views of the wrist show a transverse fracture through the distal end of the radius with impaction and dorsal angulation of the distal fragment. This is a Colles' fracture, caused by a fall on to the outstretched hand. Pressure on the thenar eminence impacts the radial fragment and rotates it into a position of supination. This forced supination will result in avulsion of the ulnar styloid in 60 per cent of cases and, less frequently, in a fracture of the distal ulna or dislocation at the radio-ulnar joint.

The example above shows two of the complications which may follow malunion of a Colles' fracture. Persistent dorsal angulation of the radiocarpal joint results in limited flexion of the hand; also the carpal tunnel view shows that the distal radius is encroaching on the carpal tunnel, increasing the likelihood of a carpal tunnel syndrome. The scapholunate distance is abnormally wide in this patient (Terry Thomas sign) suggesting that rupture of the scapholunate ligament with rotatory subluxation of the scaphoid also may have occurred at the time of injury.

Abraham Colles (1773-1843), a Dublin surgeon, and President of the Irish College of Surgeons at the age of 29 years, described the fracture in 1814.

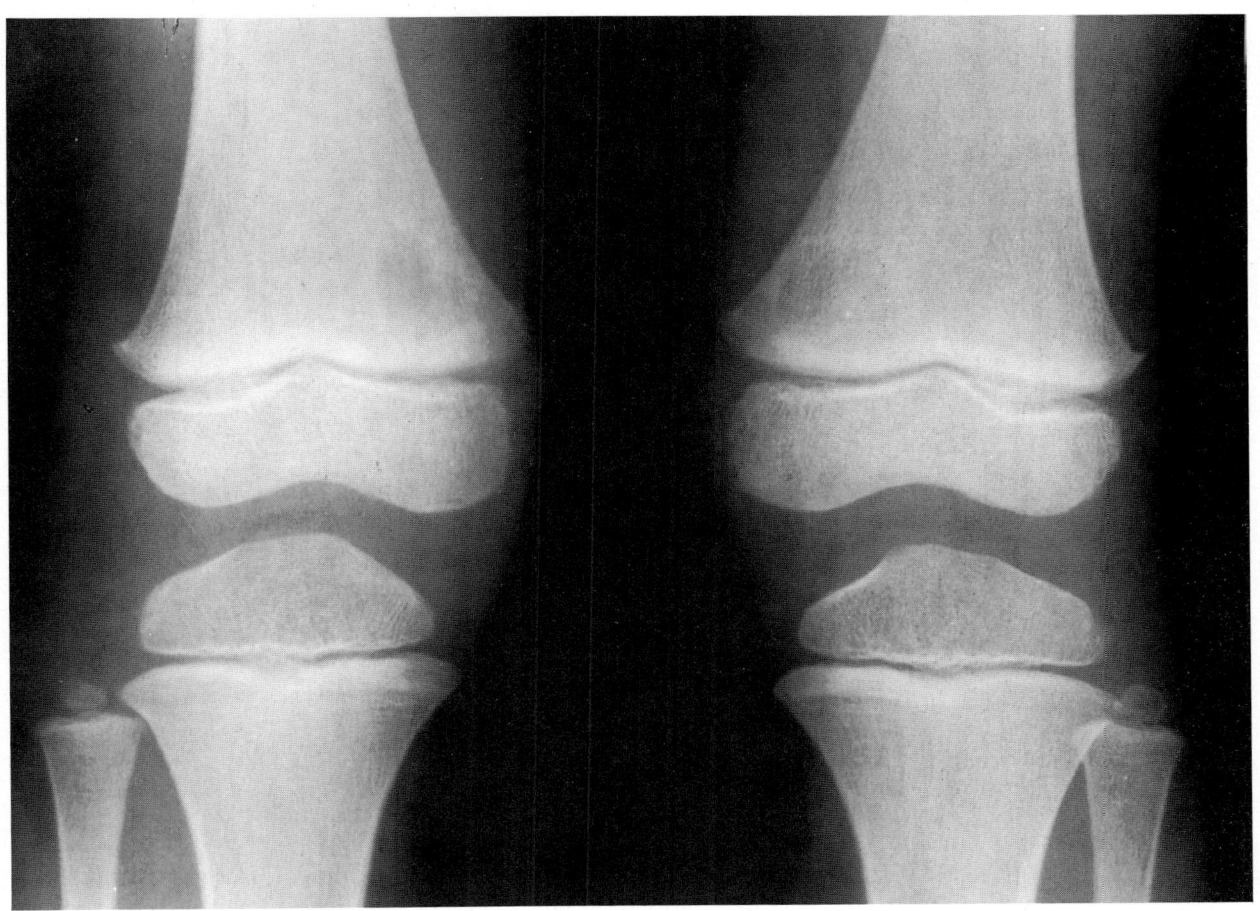

This film was obtained during follow-up of a testicular malignancy in a boy aged 4 years.

- Comment on the radiograph.

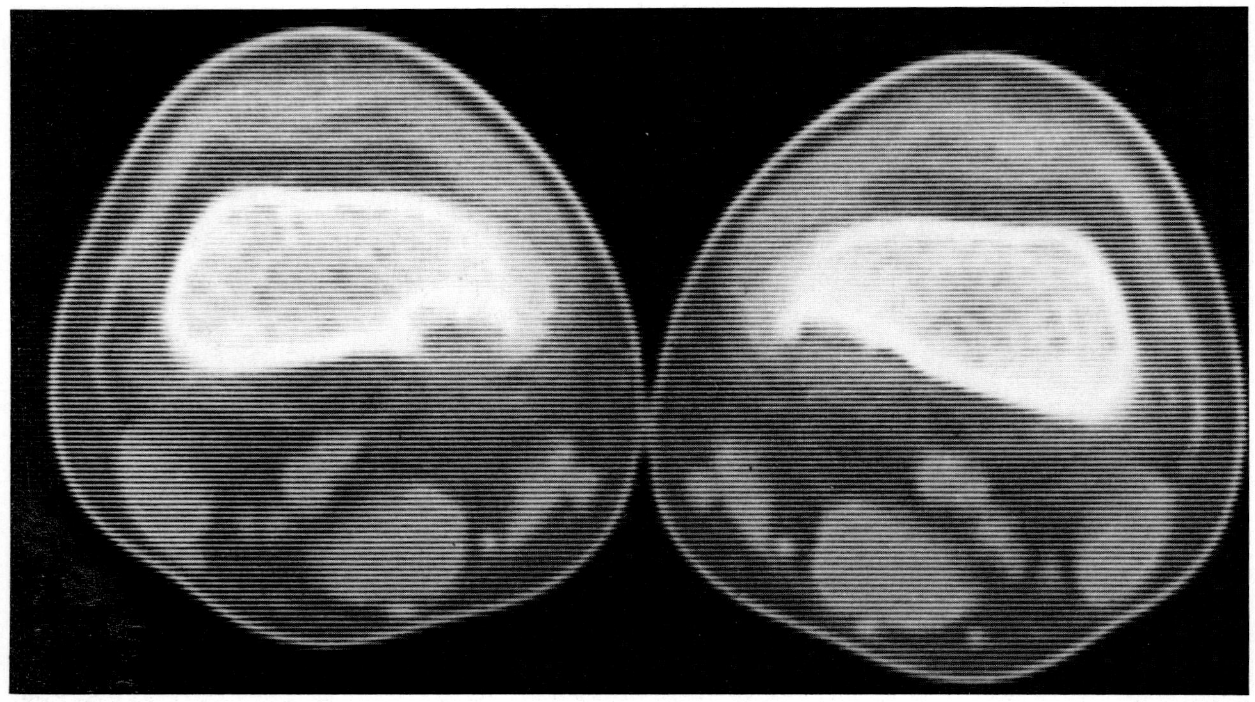

Symmetrical, eccentric, well-defined lucencies with sclerotic rims are present close to the medial margins of both femoral metaphyses. These are consistent with benign cortical defects (non-ossifying fibromas).

Despite the typical radiographic changes, the clinician was suspicious of metastatic spread and requested the CT scan which clearly demonstrates the cortical location of the defects. Undoubtedly lateral radiographs would have confirmed the diagnosis more quickly and at less expense. Unconvinced by radiological assurances, biopsy was undertaken to confirm the pathology.

The distal femoral metaphysis is a common site for both cortical defects and metastases, but the eccentric position and sclerotic margins of these lesions should exclude the latter.

Benign cortical defects are so common and self-limiting that they are regarded almost as normal variants.

The histological appearance is of a fibroblastic matrix encompassing osteoclast giant cells and macrophages containing lipid; the histology is identical to the larger non-ossifying fibroma.

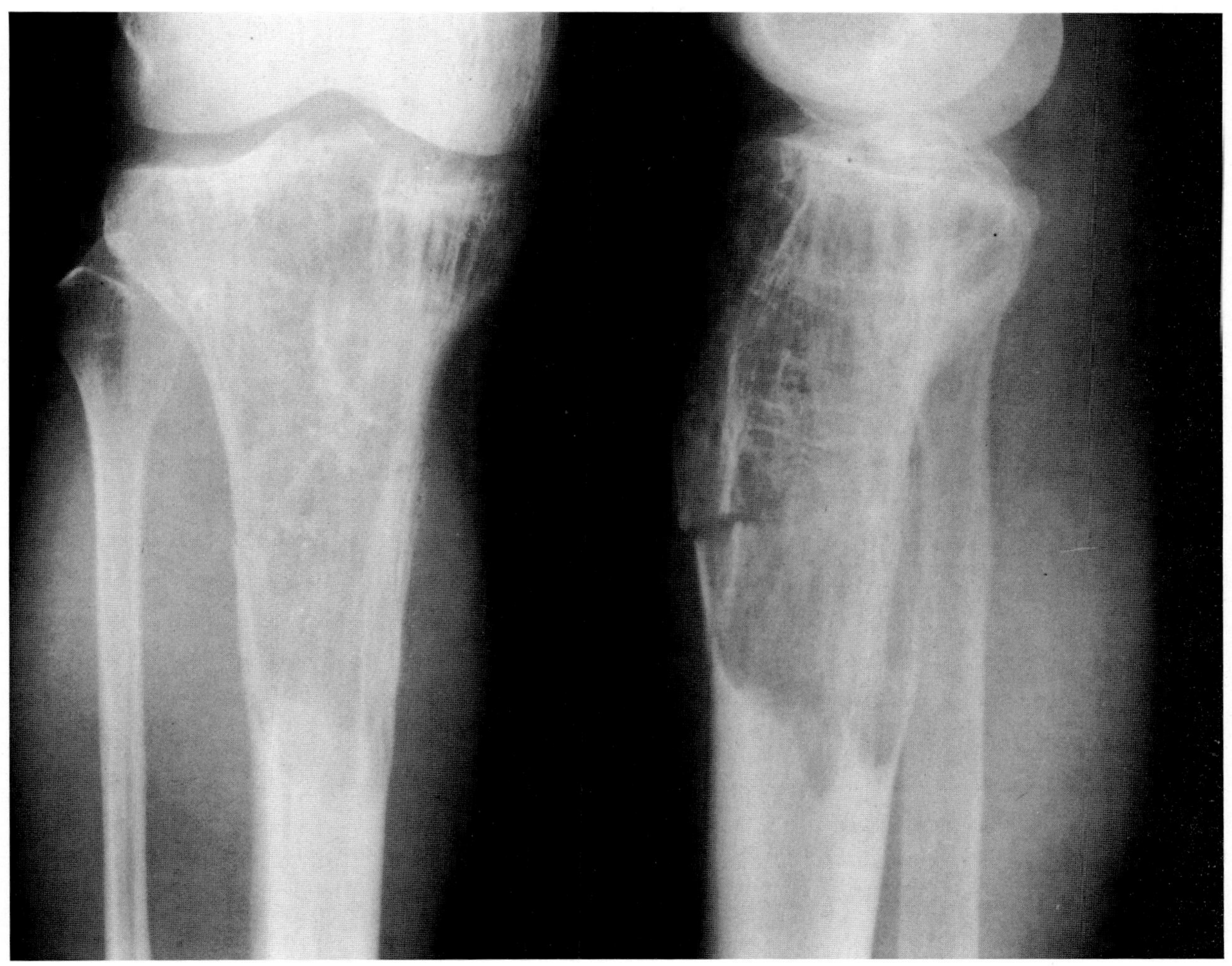

An elderly man presented following a fall.

- Describe the features on the radiograph.

- How could you assess the extent and activity of the underlying disease?

- What other type of fracture characteristically may be found in this condition?

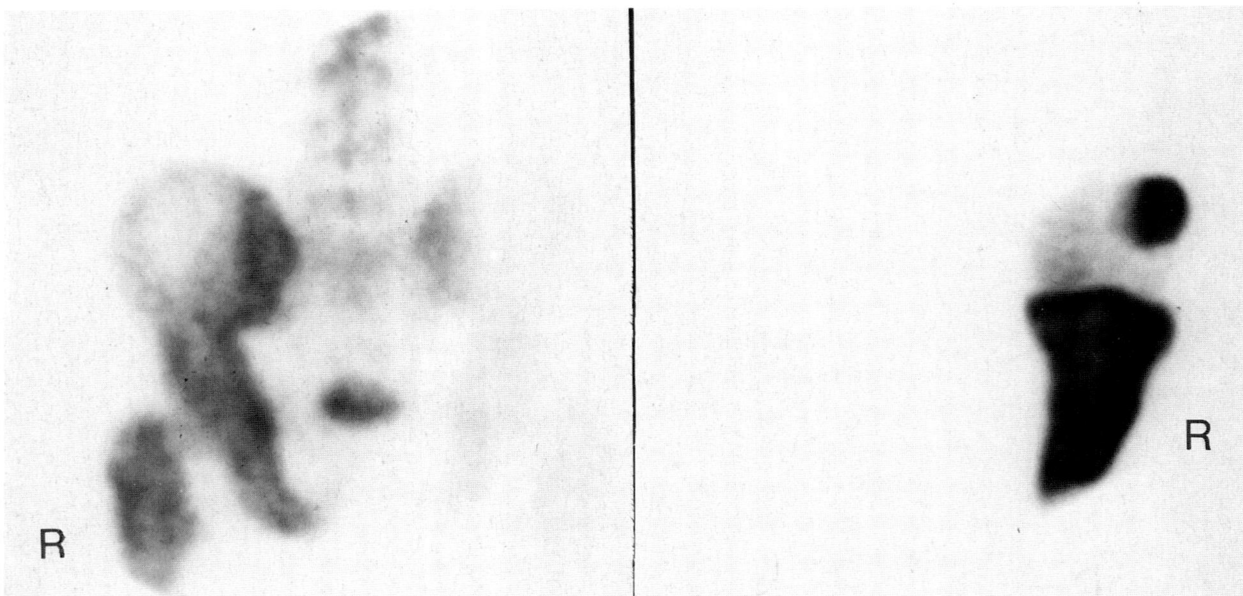

The proximal tibia is expanded by a lesion extending to the subarticular region; it has a V-shaped distal diaphyseal margin. Coarse trabeculation and a pathological fracture are seen. The site and appearances are characteristic of the osteolytic phase of Paget's disease.

Blood flow is high in Pagetoid bone and a ^{99m}Tc diphosphonate bone scan can be used to assess the extent of disease. In this patient the right hemipelvis, femur and patella are also affected.

When polyostotic, Paget's disease commonly involves the spine (75 per cent), skull (65 per cent), pelvis (40 per cent) and proximal long bones (35 per cent). The fibula is often spared.

Pathological fractures in the long bones are frequently horizontal. In Paget's disease, the femur and tibia may become bowed in the course of the disease and stress infractions are common on the bony convexities.

Sir James Paget, F.R.S. (1814-1899) was surgeon to St. Bartholomew's Hospital and Surgeon-Extraordinary to Queen Victoria. Although not the first to observe the disorder, his was the first clearly recorded description.

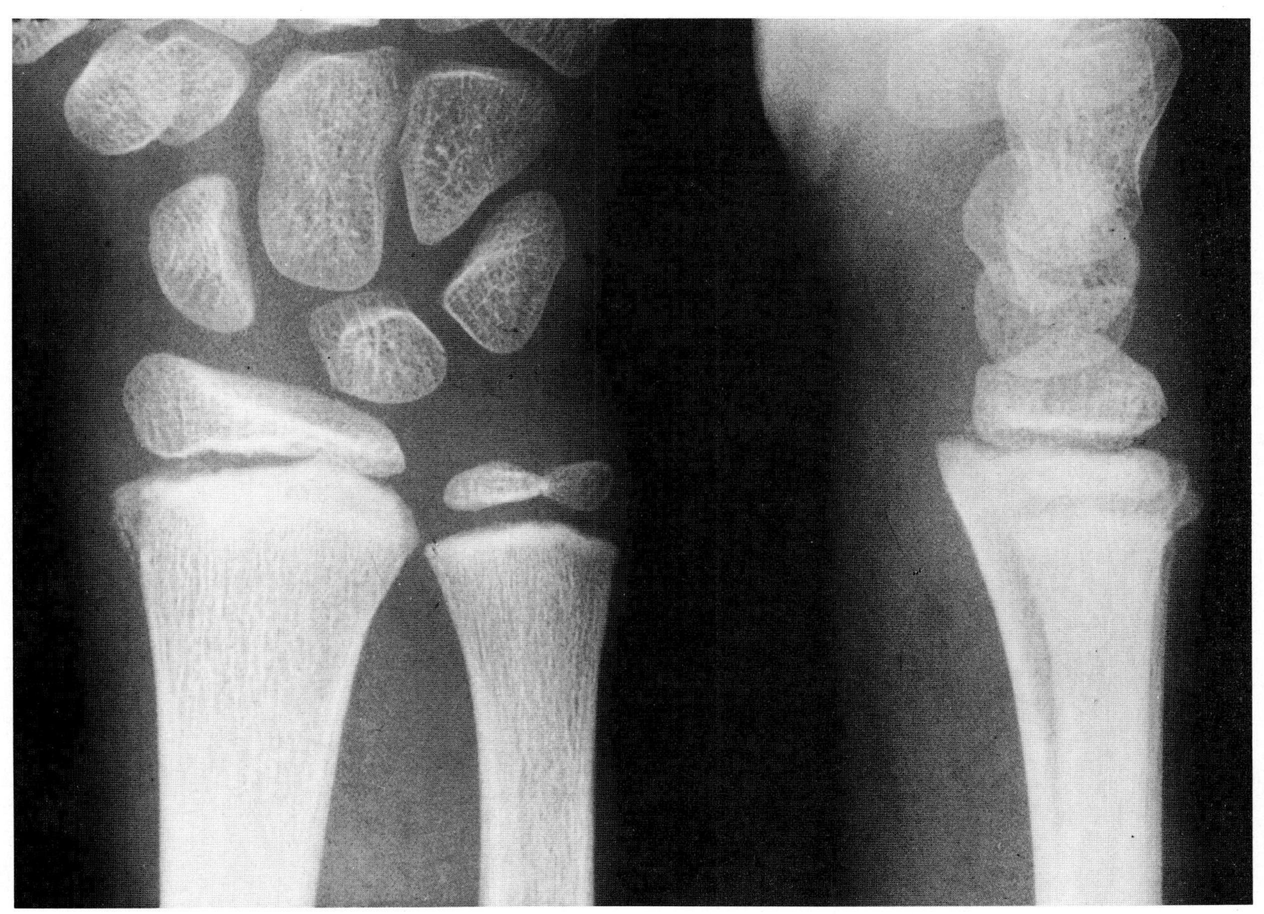

This 12-year-old boy presented to Casualty following a fall.

- How would you classify this injury?

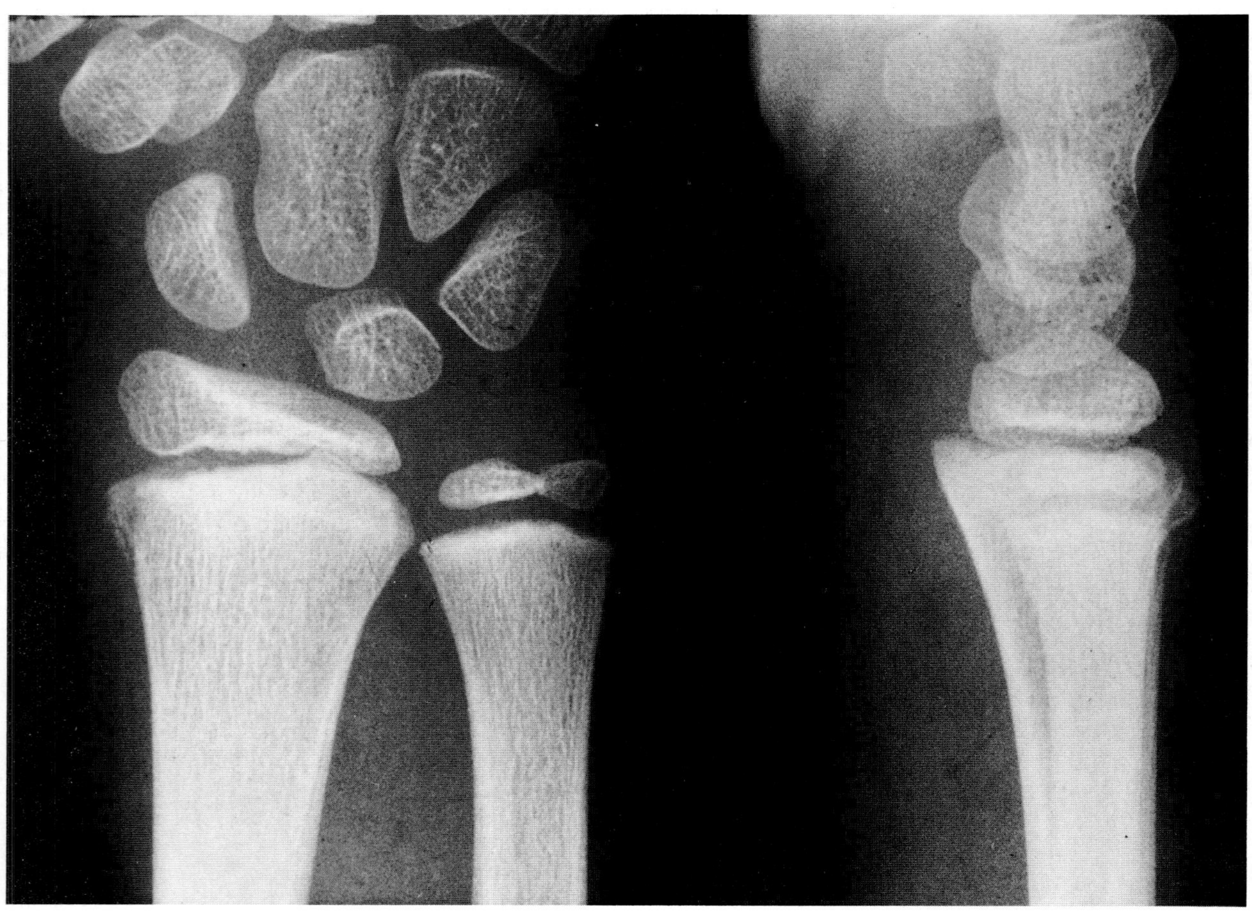

A fracture passes through the lateral margin of the radial metaphysis; asymmetrical widening of the adjacent growth plate is indicative of separation of the radial epiphysis. Epiphyseal injuries are commonly classified by the Salter-Harris system. This case is an example of the commonest form, a Type II injury.

Separations of the distal radial epiphysis are 2-4 times more frequent than epiphyseal separations at other sites. They usually occur in the 10-16 age group and are considered the adolescent counterpart of Colles' fractures, since the epiphysis is often displaced posteriorly to give a 'dinner fork' deformity. This feature however is not evident on the lateral view in this case.

The prognosis following epiphyseal injury depends on the degree of vascular disruption, the final deformity, any subsequent infection and age. Growth retardation or arrest will have a greater effect at an early age, and is more likely to result in significant disability in a weight-bearing limb.

Reference

Rogers, L. F. (1970) The radiography of epiphyseal injuries. *Radiology*, 96, 289-299.

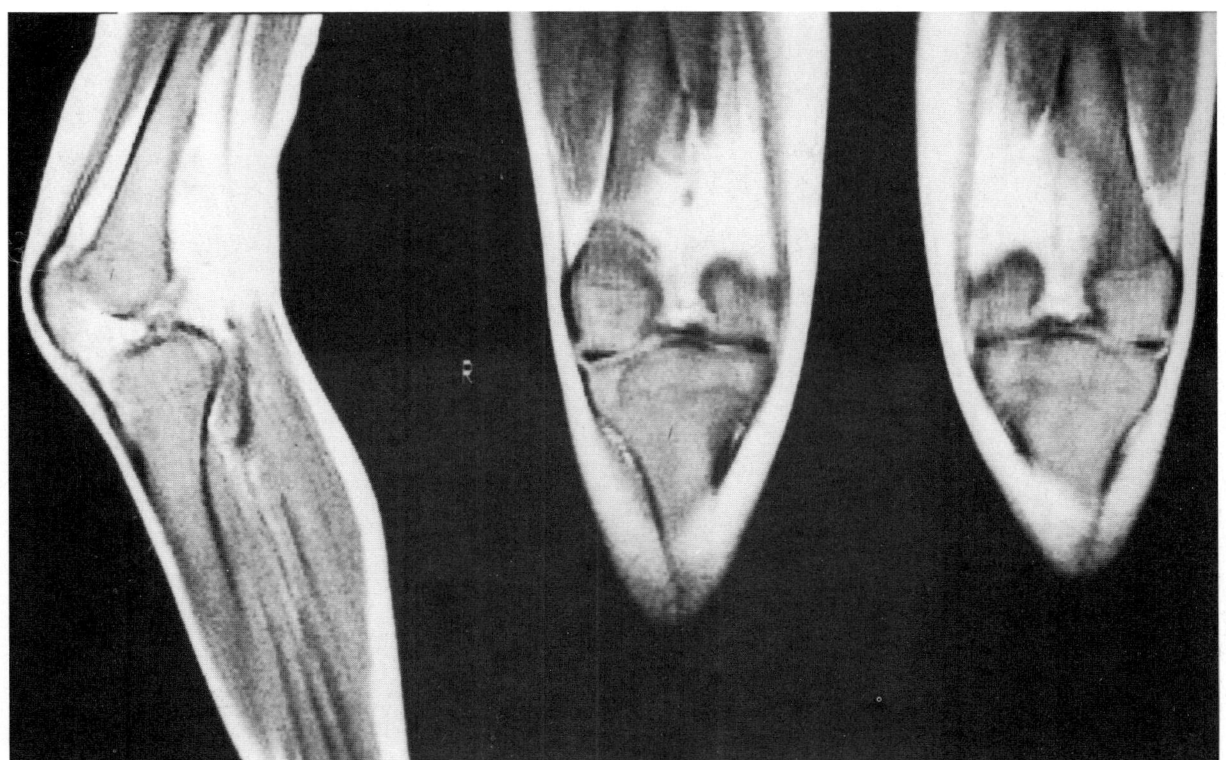

(by courtesy of Dr. med. Klaus Bohndorf, Köln)

This child presented with anaemia and bone pain. A T1-weighted magnetic resonance scan of the knees was obtained.

- What diagnoses would you consider?
- What are the likely plain film appearances?

A14

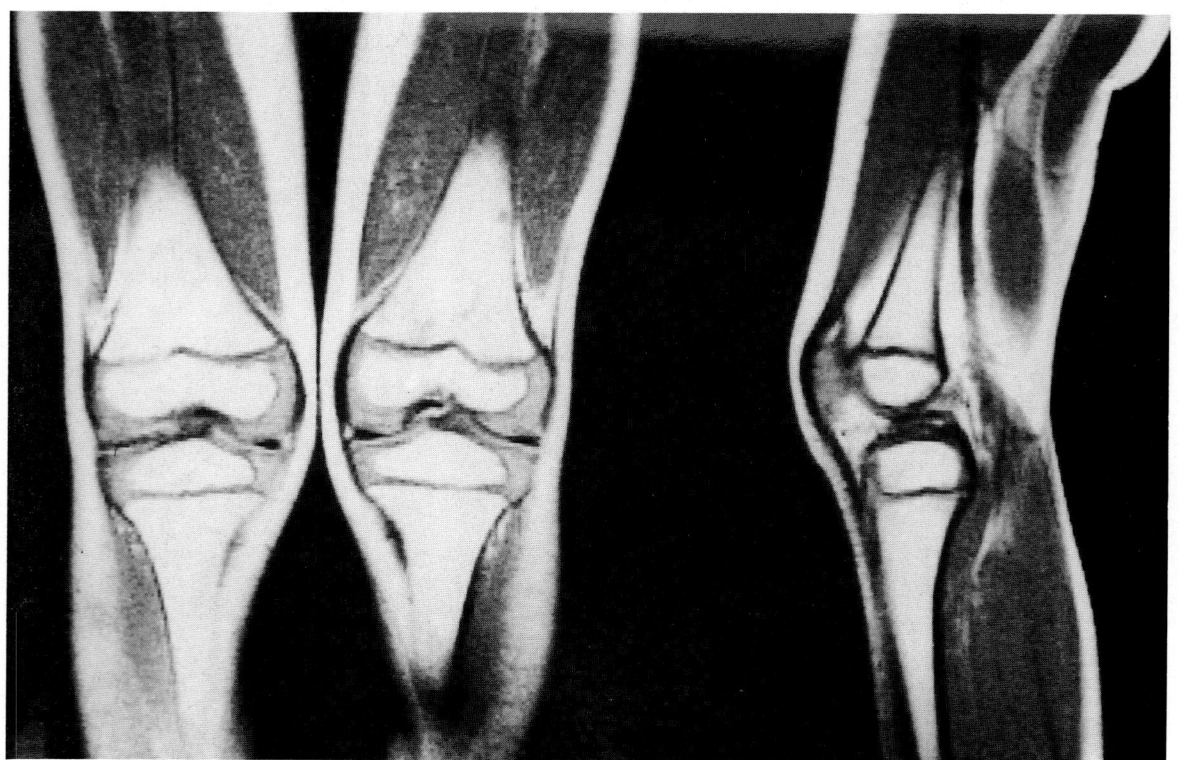

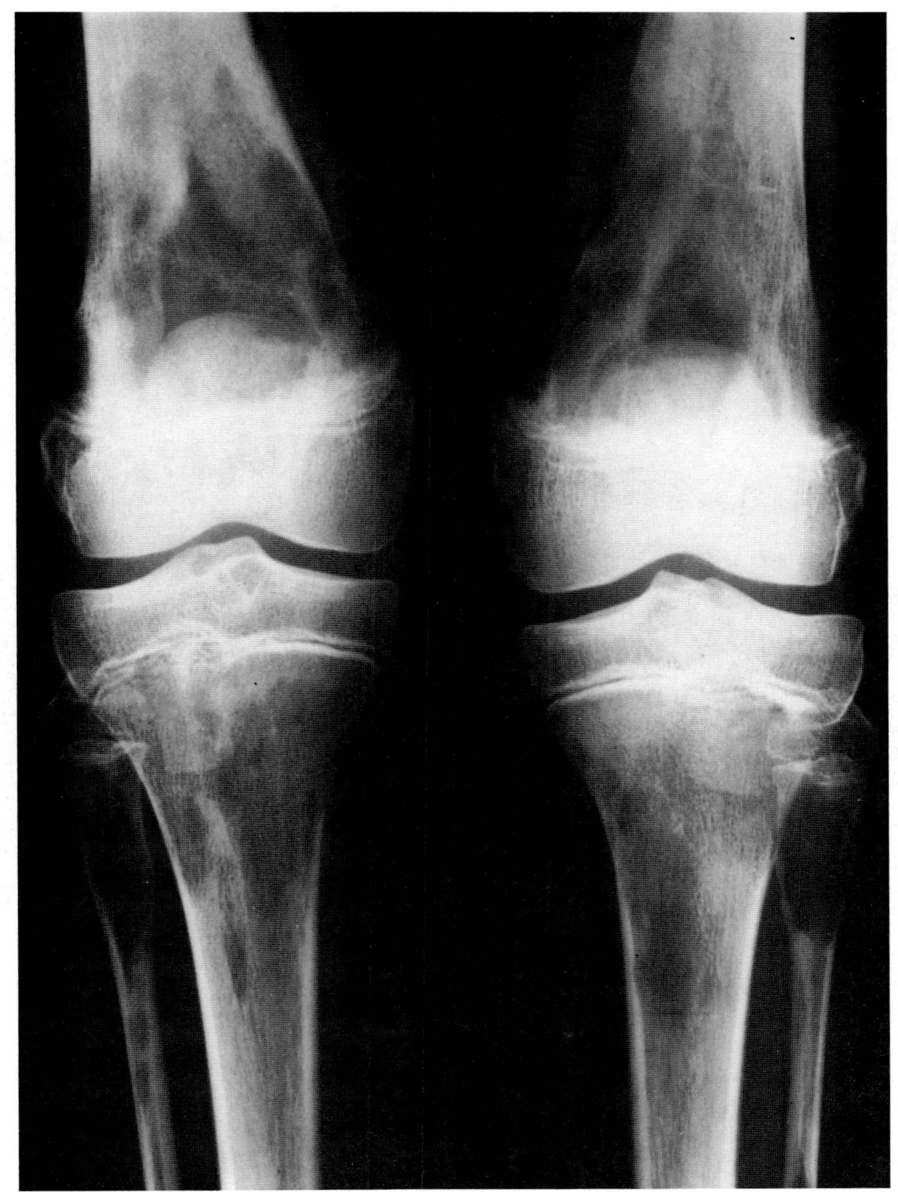

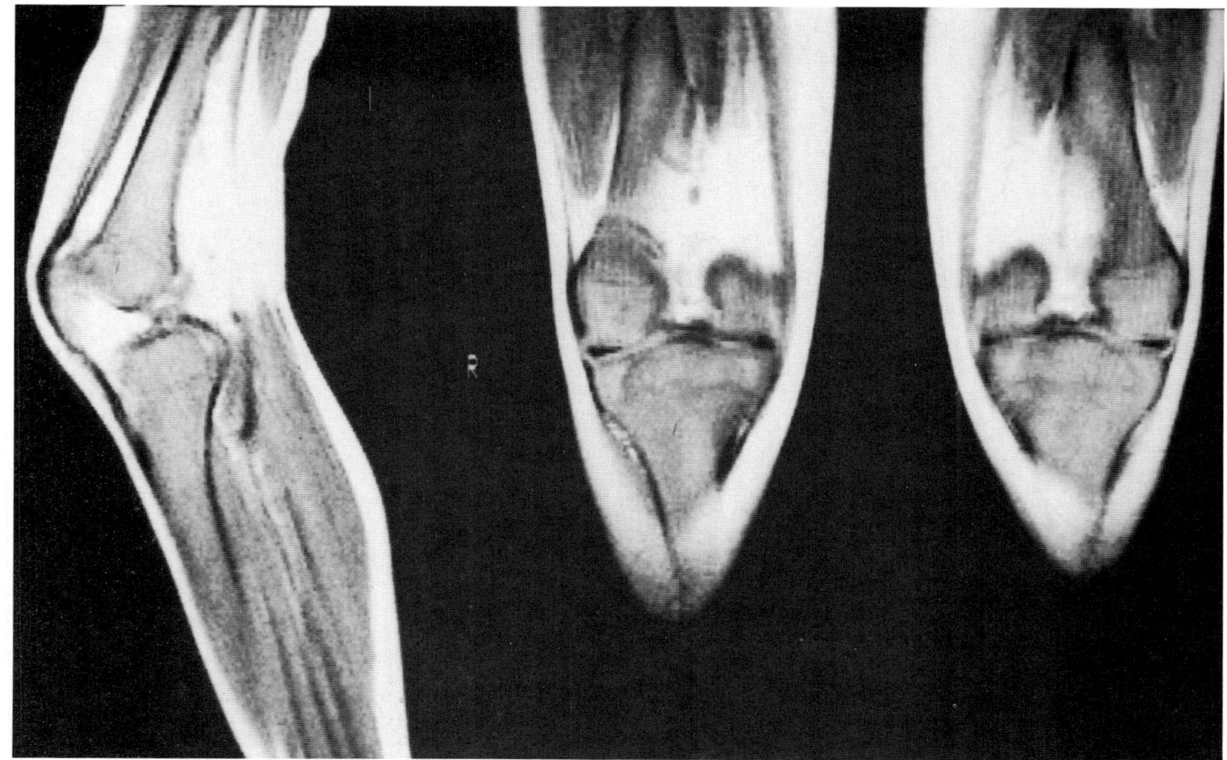

Normal bone marrow contains a large amount of fat and consequently gives a strong signal on magnetic resonance imaging, almost equal in intensity to that of subcutaneous fat, which here appears very white. Any disease process causing infiltration of the marrow, such as leukaemia and neuroblastoma, will reduce the intensity of the signal. Conversely, the signal will be increased in aplastic anaemia and following radiotherapy as the acquired changes are associated with an increase in fat content of the marrow.

In this patient the diffuse reduction in signal in the bone marrow around both knees, compared to the subcutaneous fat, was due to leukaemic infiltration. In MRI the bony cortex gives no signal and appears as a black rim around the marrow. The muscles appear grey. A second MRI scan following successful therapy shows restoration of the marrow signal as a result of replacement of tumour by marrow fat.

The plain film appearances in another child with leukaemia are shown on page 35. Widespread metaphyseal destruction of bone has involved both knees, probably secondary to haematogenous infiltration of bone by leukaemic cells. Other common patterns of involvement in childhood leukaemia are submetaphyseal lucent bands (40 per cent) and osteopenia, which affects the spine in up to 60 per cent of patients. Bone pain is present at presentation in 20-25 per cent of patients.

References

Cohen, M. D. et al. (1984) Magnetic resonance imaging of bone marrow disease in children. *Radiology*, **151**, 715-718.
Parker, B. R., Marglin, S. and Castellino, R. A. (1980) Skeletal manifestations of leukaemia, Hodgkin's disease and non-Hodgkin's lymphoma. *Seminars in Roentgenol.*, **15** (4), 302-315.

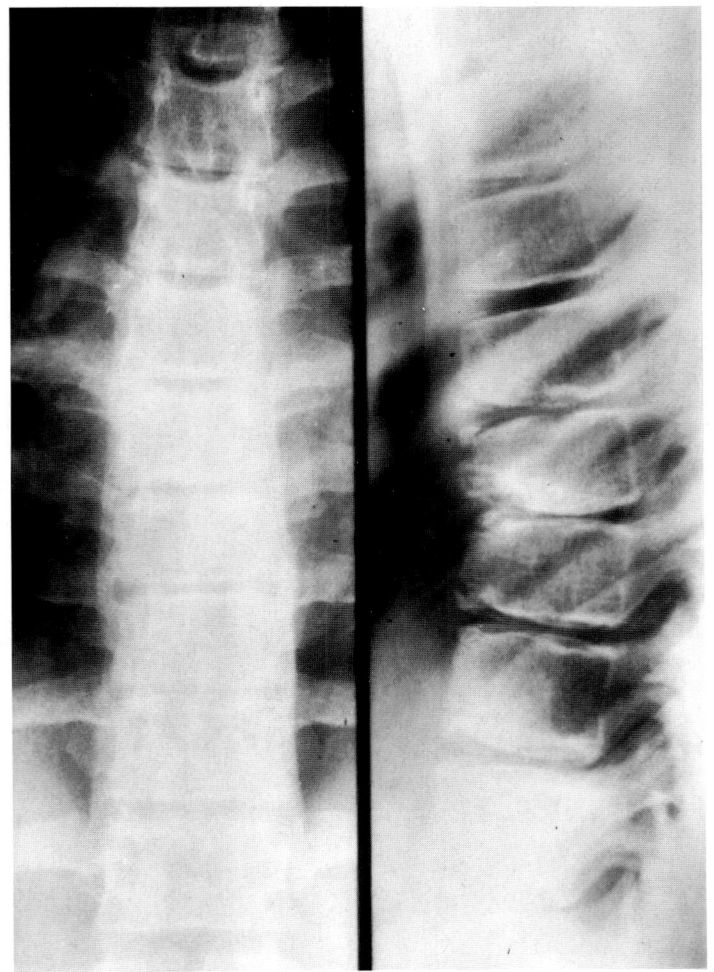

This 13-year-old female gymnast complained of backache.

- What is the cause of these appearances?

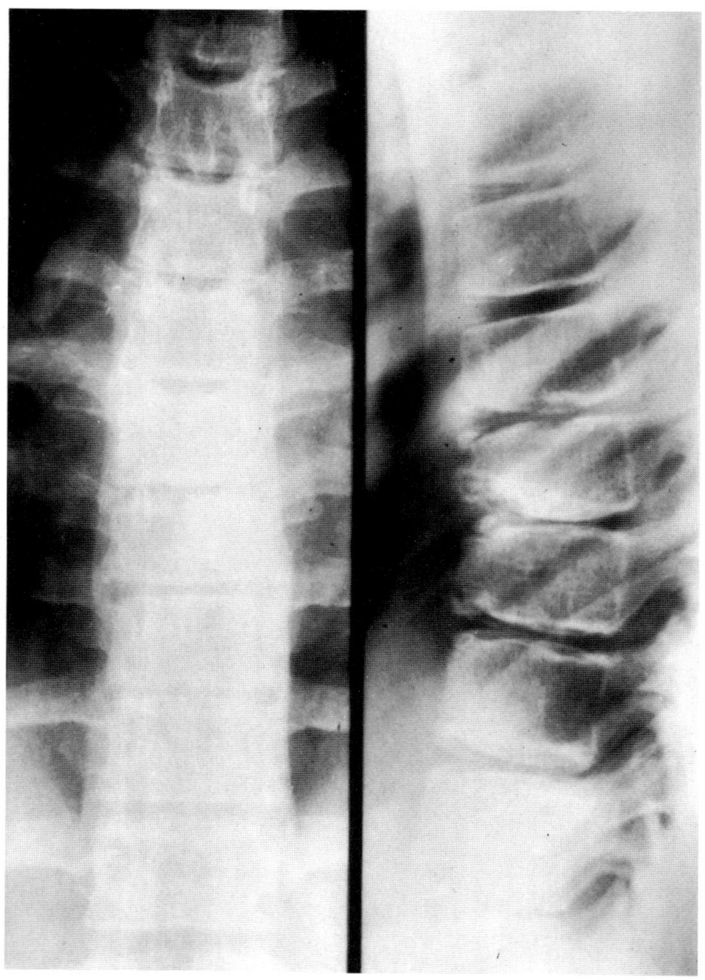

The disc spaces on either side of T7 are narrowed. The irregular deformity of the antero-inferior corner of the body of T7 and reactive sclerosis are typical of the appearances of an early limbus vertebra.

A limbus vertebra results from trauma to the developing spine in adolescence. It is caused by protrusion of disc material through the periphery of the vertebral body end-plate, often anteriorly, separating the ring apophysis from the rest of the vertebral body. A Schmorl's node, in contrast, results from disc herniation through the central portion of the end-plate. This type of trauma is occurring more frequently as sports such as gymnastics and trampolining become more popular with children and adolescents.

It is easier to make the diagnosis in adulthood when a well-defined fragment of bone has developed from the separated ring apophysis. The nature of the lesion may be demonstrated by discography, when contrast medium injected into the nucleus pulposus passes between the vertebral body and the ring apophysis.

Reference

Ghelman, B. and Freiberger, R. H. (1976) The limbus vertebra: an anterior disc herniation demonstrated by discography. *Amer. J. Roentgenol.*, **127**, 854-855.

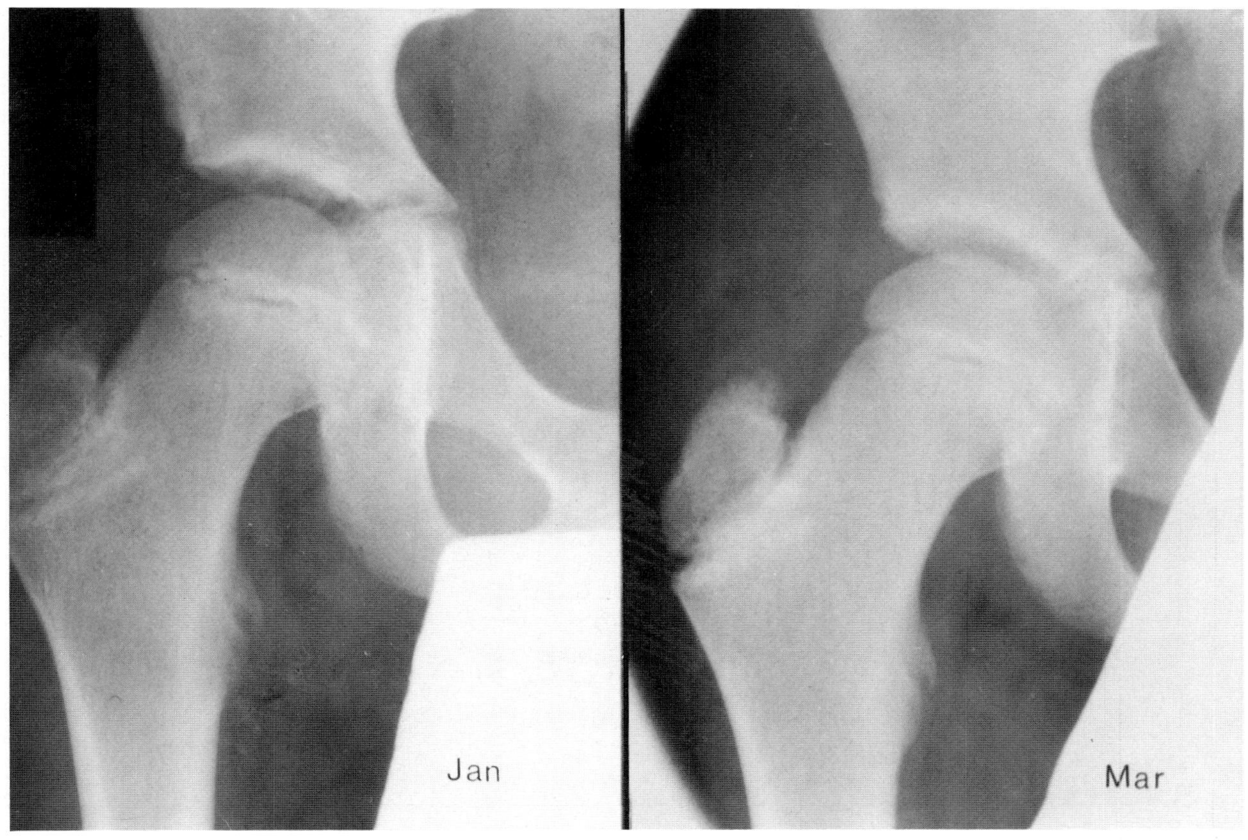

A young boy presented in January with subacute pain and limitation of motion in his right hip.

- What observation was made?

- Is the later film normal? (He was now symptom-free).

- What diagnosis would you give?

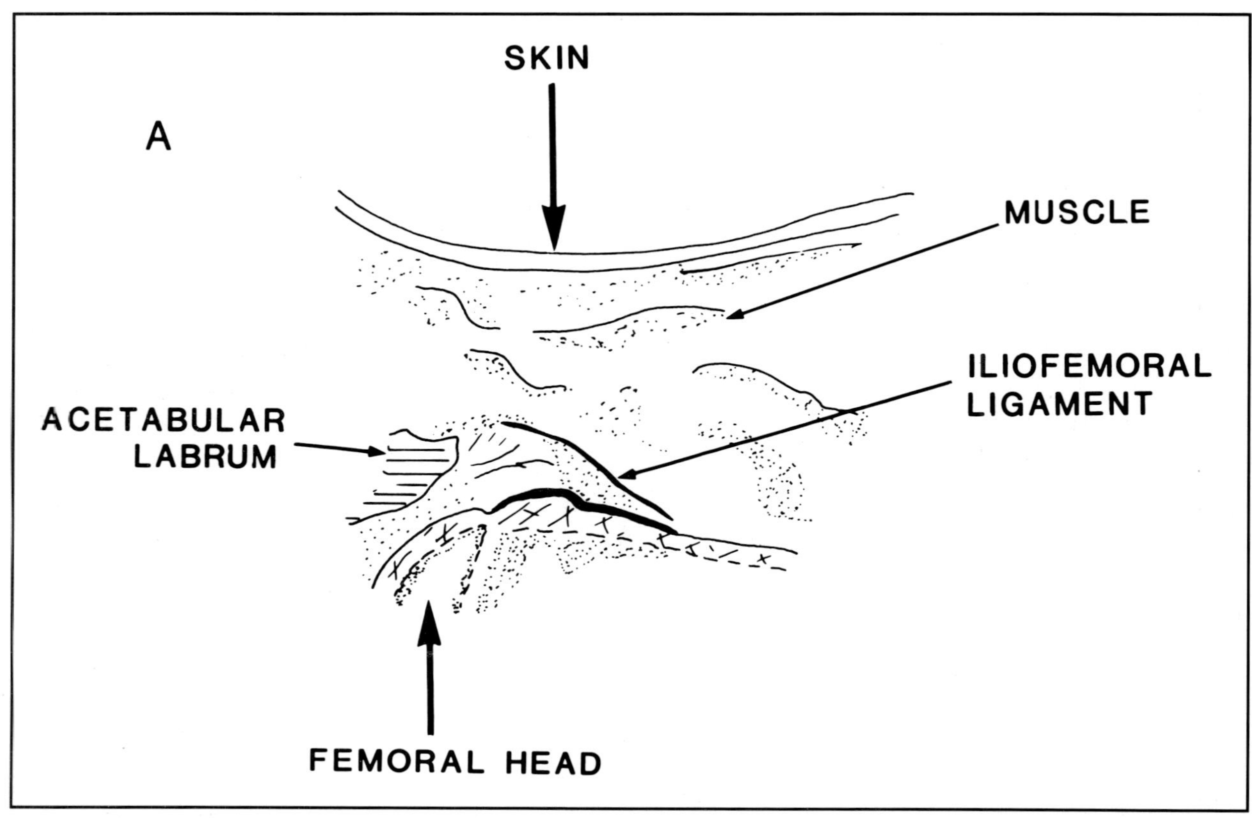

The medial joint space is wide in comparison with the later film. When associated with a painful hip at this age, a joint effusion can often be confirmed. If a pyogenic effusion can be excluded, then non-specific synovitis (irritable hip) is the likely cause. The reason for the widening of the space is not wholly clear. It is unlikely to be caused by an effusion itself and may be the consequence of oedema of the ligamentum teres. When an irritable hip is suspected, the diagnosis can be confirmed by the demonstration of a trans-sonic layer on ultrasonography (see diagrams: A = normal, B = synovial effusion).

Radionuclide scanning often provides a means of discrimination between transient synovitis and Perthes' disease.

References

Carty, H., Maxted, M., Fielding, J. A., Gulliford, P. and Owen, R. (1984) Isotope scanning in the 'irritable hip syndrome'. *Skeletal Radiol.*, **11**, 32-37.

Wilson, D. J., Green, D. J. and MacLarnon, J. C. (1984) Arthrosonography of the painful hip. *Clin. Radiol.*, **35**, 17-19.

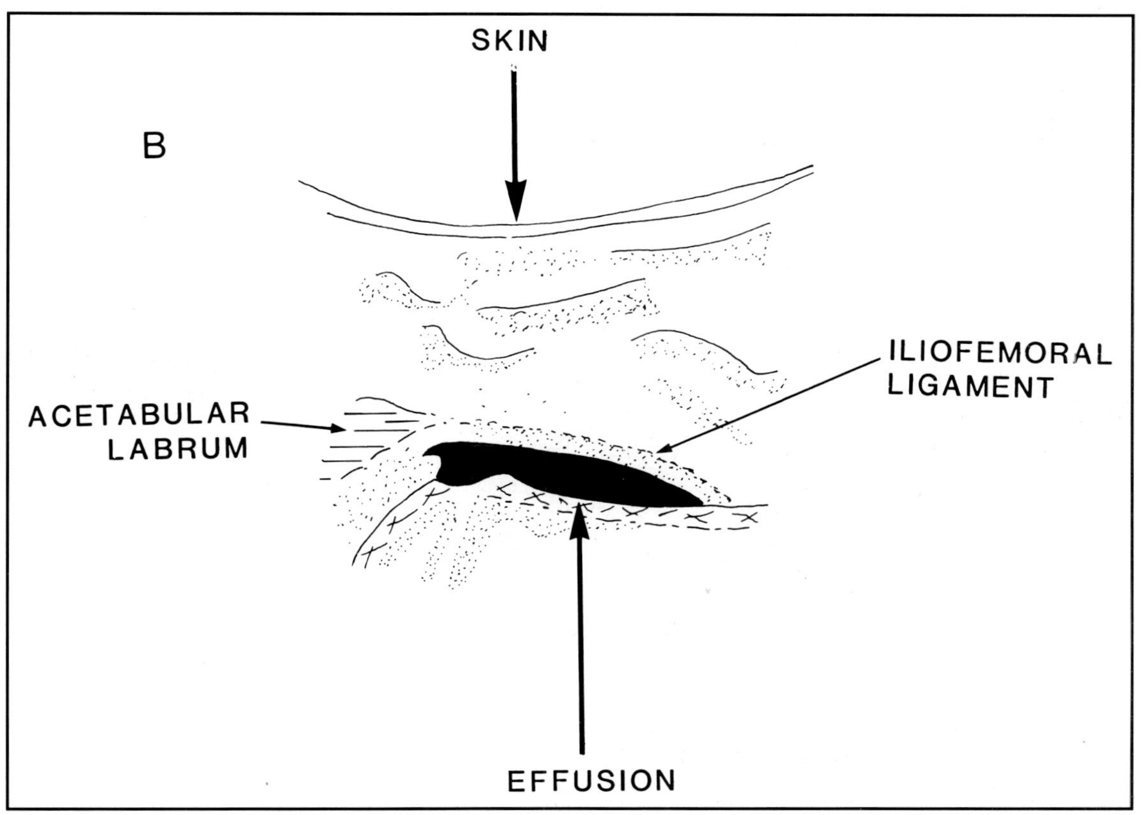

SKIN
B
ILIOFEMORAL
LIGAMENT
ACETABULAR
LABRUM
EFFUSION

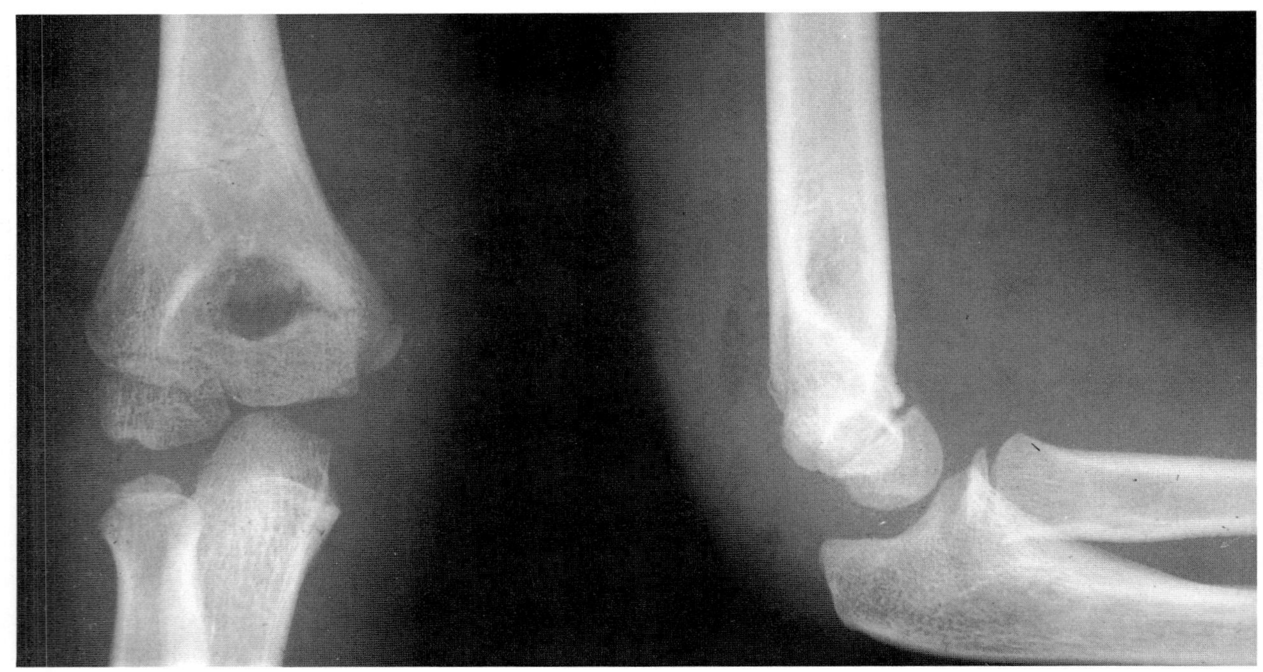

This 8-year-old boy was seen in Casualty following a fall.

- Describe the abnormal features.
- How common is this injury?

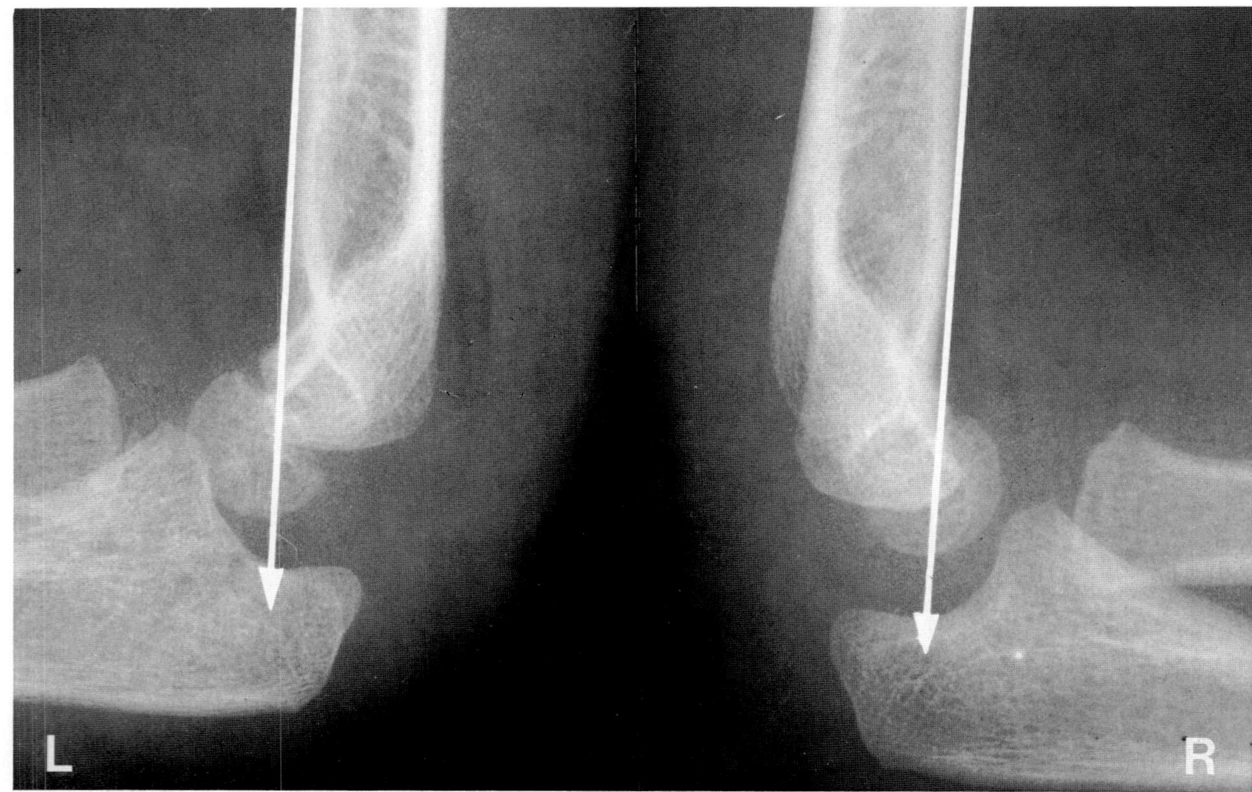

The radiolucent anterior and posterior fat pads which are normally closely applied to the humerus have been displaced outwards. The anterior fat pad is often just visible in the lateral view of the normal elbow, but the posterior fat pad is never seen and its displacement is a reliable sign of an effusion within an intact elbow joint capsule (the fat pad sign).

Ninety per cent of children with a positive fat pad sign have a fracture, which in this case is supracondylar. Supracondylar humeral fractures comprise 60 per cent of elbow fractures in children and should be specifically excluded in all trauma cases. The fracture line is not always visible and the anterior humeral line can be useful in evaluation. This line is drawn along the anterior humeral cortex and passes though the middle third of the capitulum in approximately 95 per cent of normal elbows. It will pass through the anterior third in approximately 95 per cent of supracondylar fractures. It is of no value in this patient as the fracture is undisplaced and the line passes through the middle third of the capitulum, but the fracture is in any case easily visible.

In the example above, the right elbow is normal whilst the left is the site of a supracondylar fracture. Unusually, the majority of the capitulum lies in front of the anterior humeral line.

Reference

Rogers, L. F., Malave, S. Jr., White, H. and Tachdijan, M. O. (1978) Plastic bowing, torus and greenstick fractures of the humerus: radiographic clues to obscure fractures of the elbow in children. *Radiology*, **128**, 145-150.

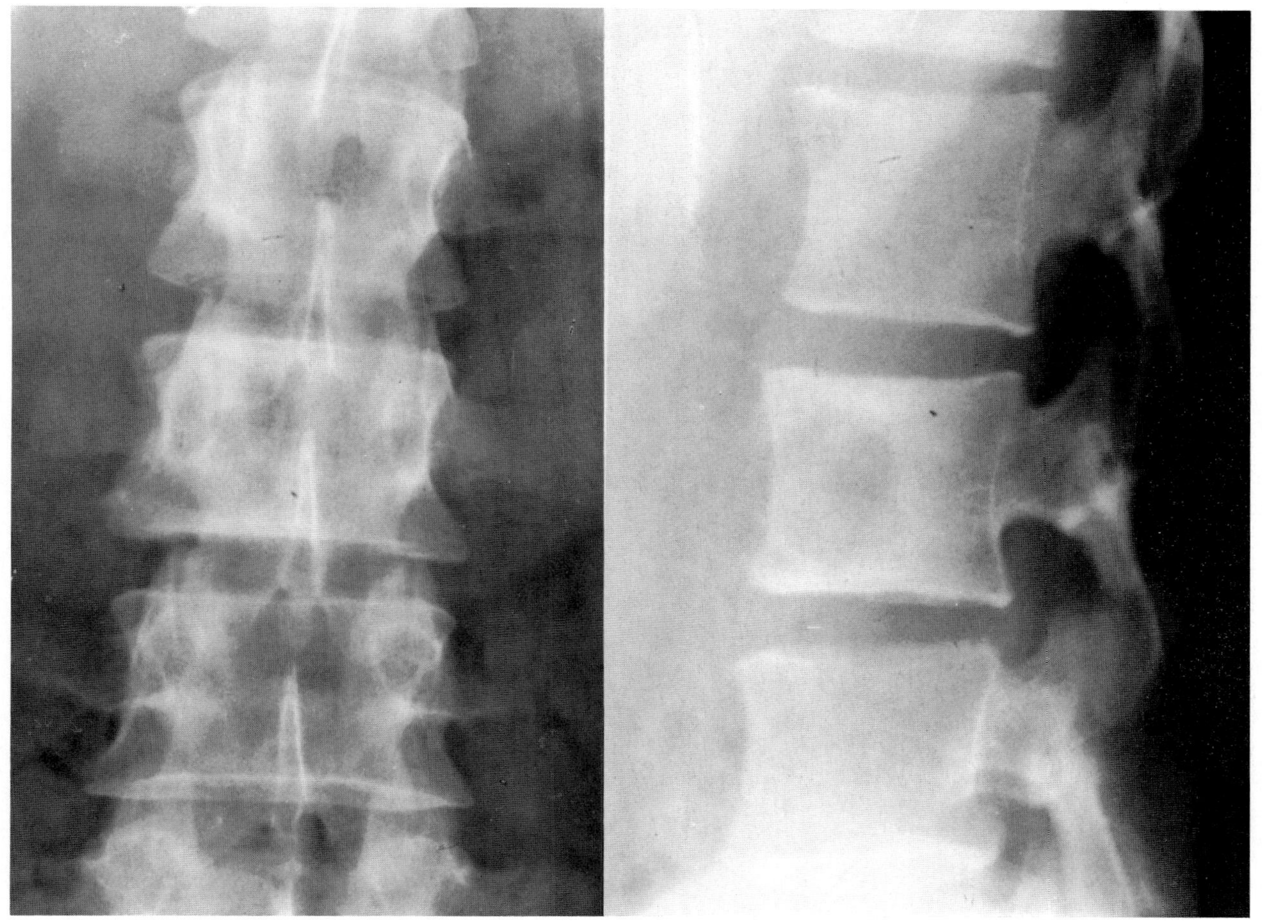

This Tanzanian man had an 18-month history of backache which had started after a period of heavy lifting.

- What is the most likely diagnosis?

- How would the appearances differ in a white patient?

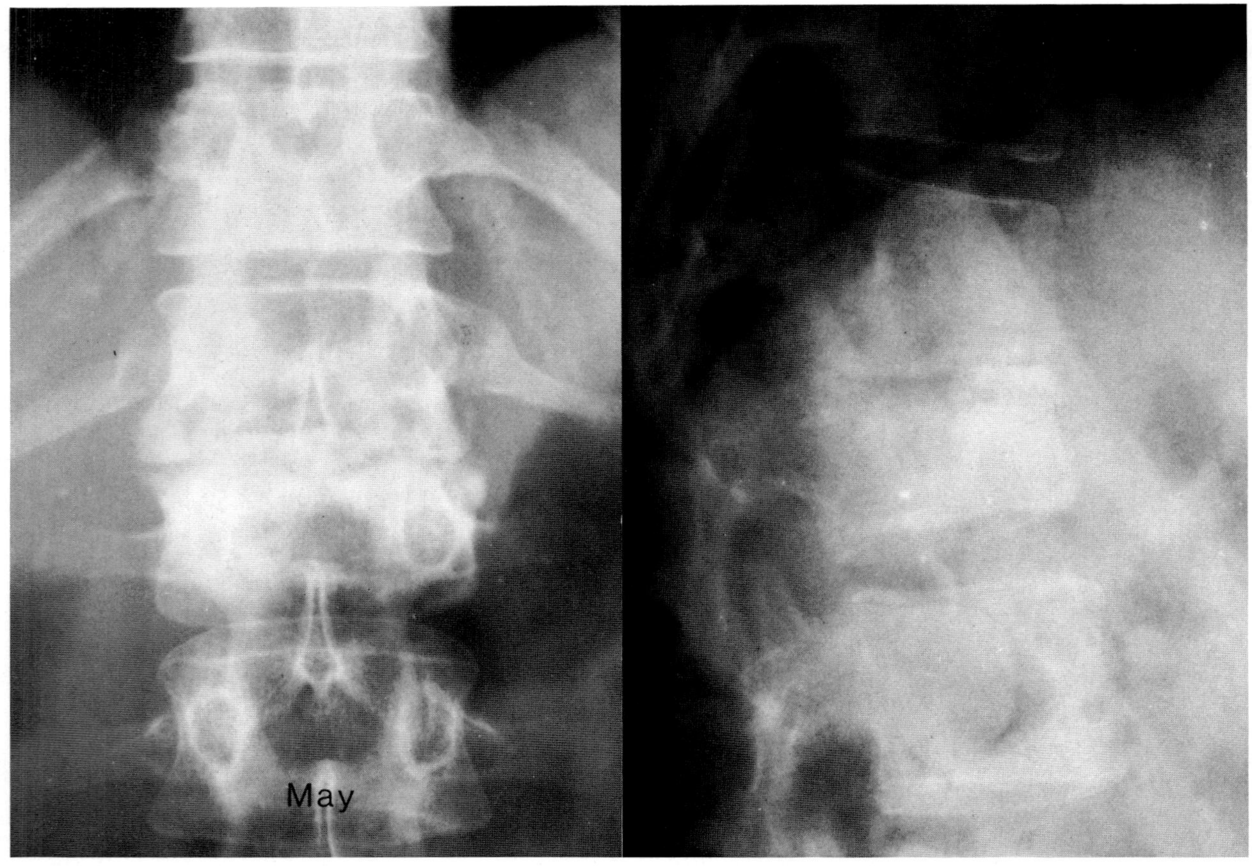

A destructive lesion is present in the anterior part of the body of L3. The adjacent periosteal reaction and surrounding sclerosis suggest an infective aetiology. In a black patient the intact end-plates and lack of involvement of the adjacent disc spaces and vertebral bodies are in keeping with tuberculosis. The diagnosis was confirmed by aspiration of acid-fast bacilli from a soft tissue swelling which had appeared over the iliac crest.

The case above illustrates the typical appearances of tuberculosis in a white patient. Infection starts in the anterior part of the vertebral body and spreads across the end-plate to involve the adjacent disc and vertebral body. The end-plates become ill-defined and the disc space narrowed. Reactive sclerosis and a periosteal reaction are rare. If spinal tuberculosis of this type is left untreated, progressive wedging of the involved vertebral bodies leads to angulation and gibbus formation.

Reference

Chapman, M., Murray, R. O. and Stoker, D. J. (1979) Tuberculosis of the bones and joints. *Seminars in Roentgenol.*, **14**, 266-282.

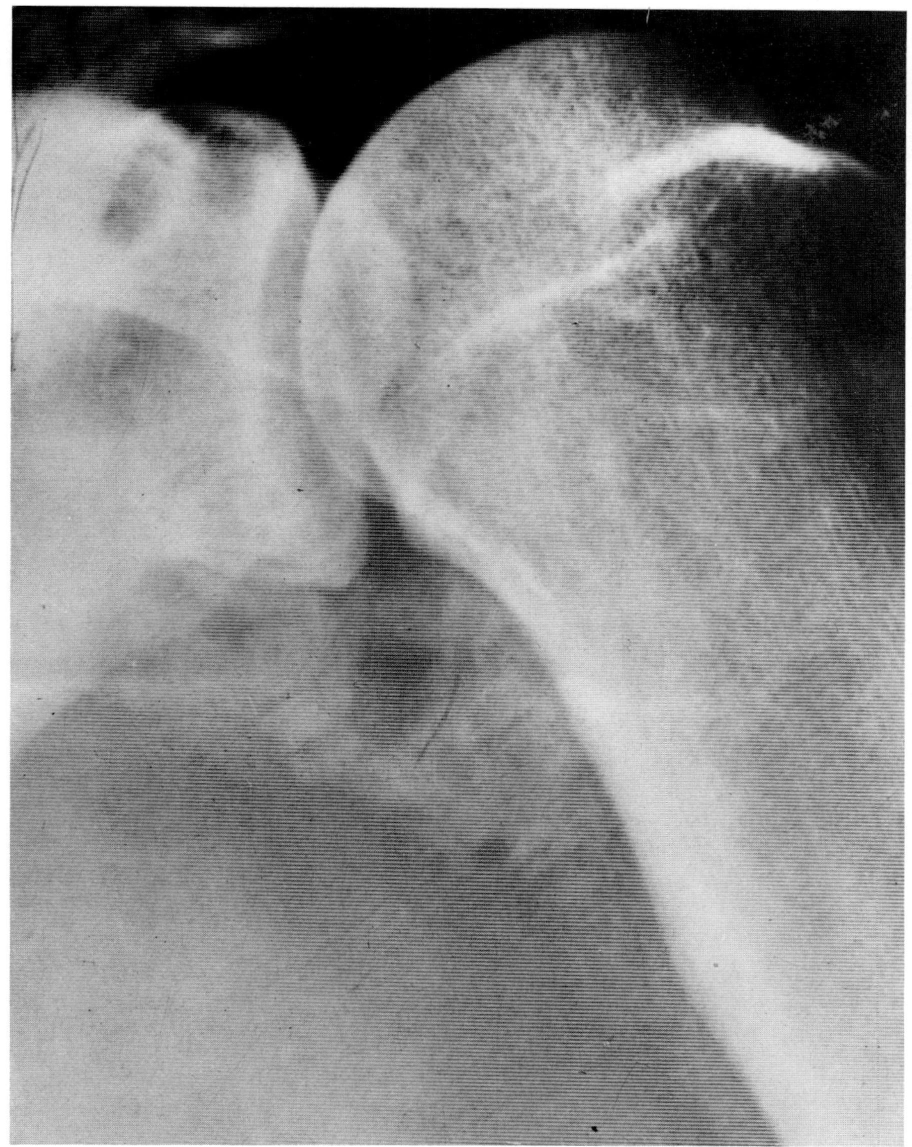

This 52-year-old man had been admitted with a head injury two months earlier.

- What are the appearances due to?

- In what other condition is this appearance commonly found?

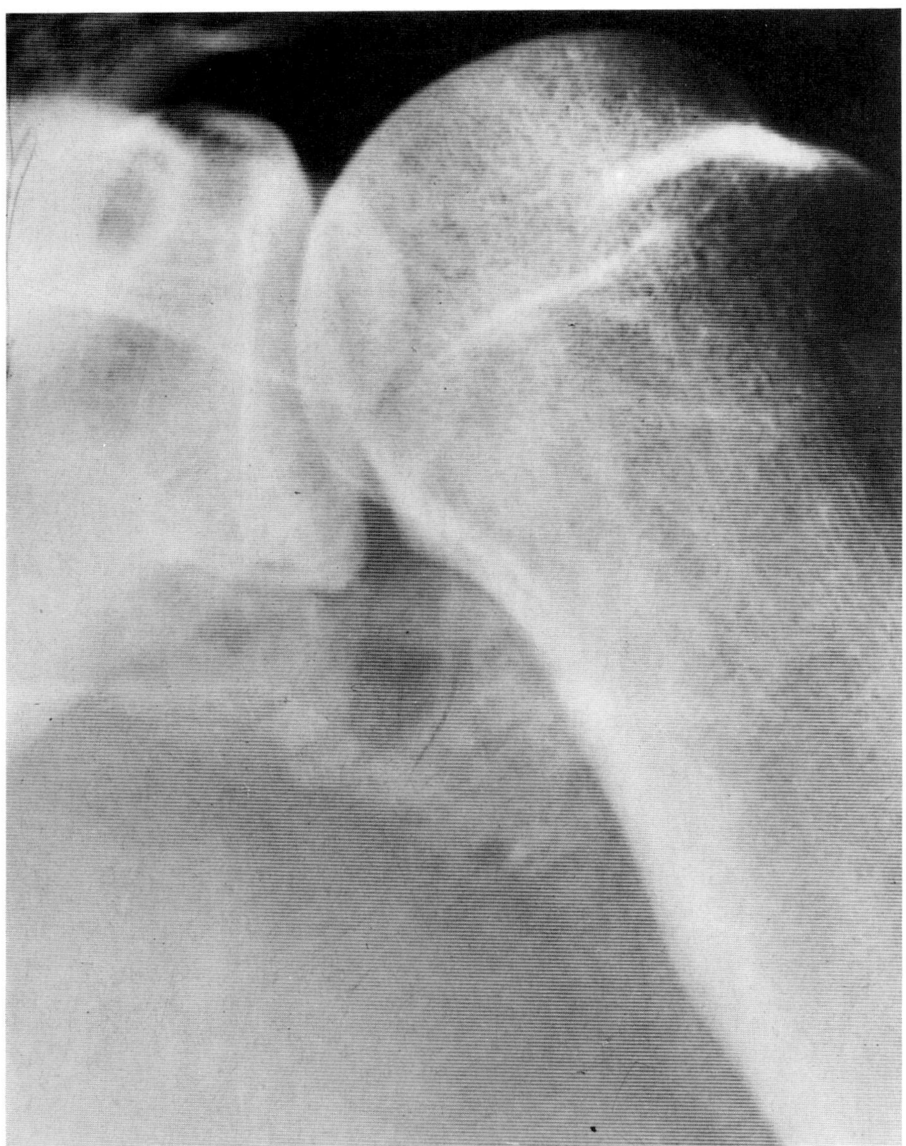

Soft tissue ossification is present below the left shoulder joint. Periarticular new bone formation is a well-known complication of paraplegia but may also occur following head injury, as in this case. The patient had sustained a fracture of the left temporal bone and developed an extradural haematoma. He remained unconscious for five weeks following evacuation of the haematoma.

The heterotopic new bone usually appears 2-6 months after injury and may be the result of passive manipulation of the limbs in an unconscious patient. It is most frequent around the hip, knee and shoulder joints and tends to be more extensive in young men. Patients may be asymptomatic or complain of pain and restricted joint movement.

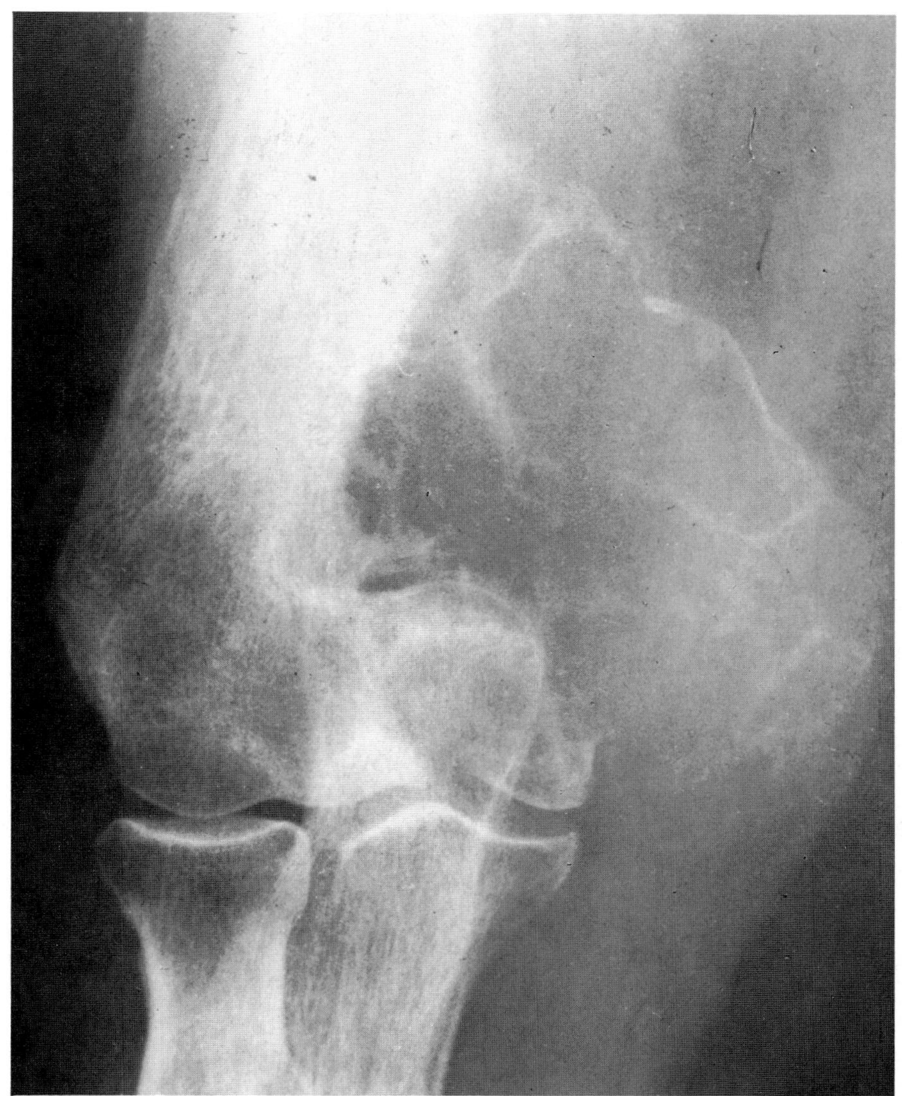

This 75-year-old woman complained of pain in her elbow.

- What is the most likely diagnosis?

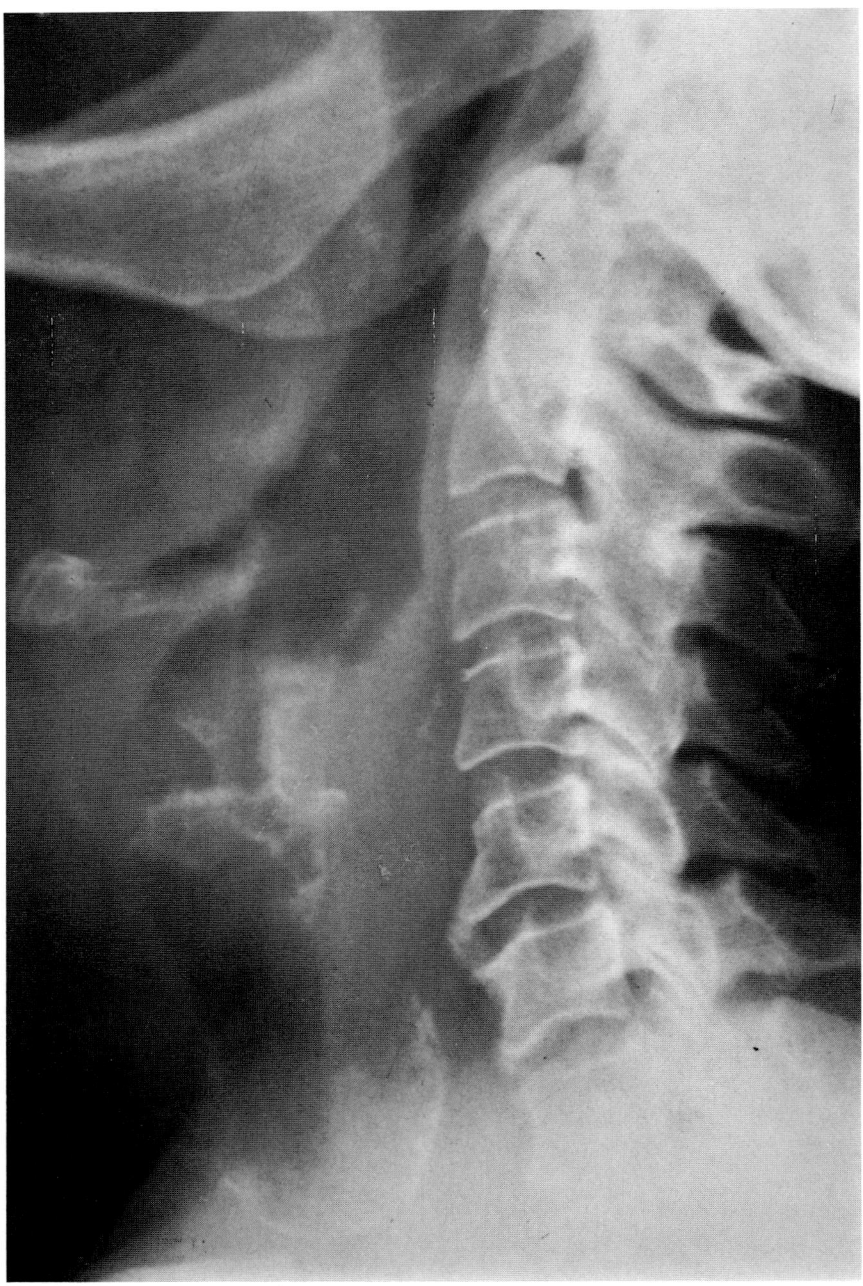

An expanded lytic lesion is present in the medial aspect of the distal end of the humerus. The lesion has thinned the overlying cortex, breaching it in places, and involves the articular surface.

In an elderly patient, the most likely diagnosis is a metastasis. Metastases of such an expansile and lytic nature are usually secondary to carcinoma of thyroid or kidney. In a young adult, a giant-cell tumour would be more likely. This patient had a thyroid carcinoma and a lateral projection of the neck (above) shows the calcification within it.

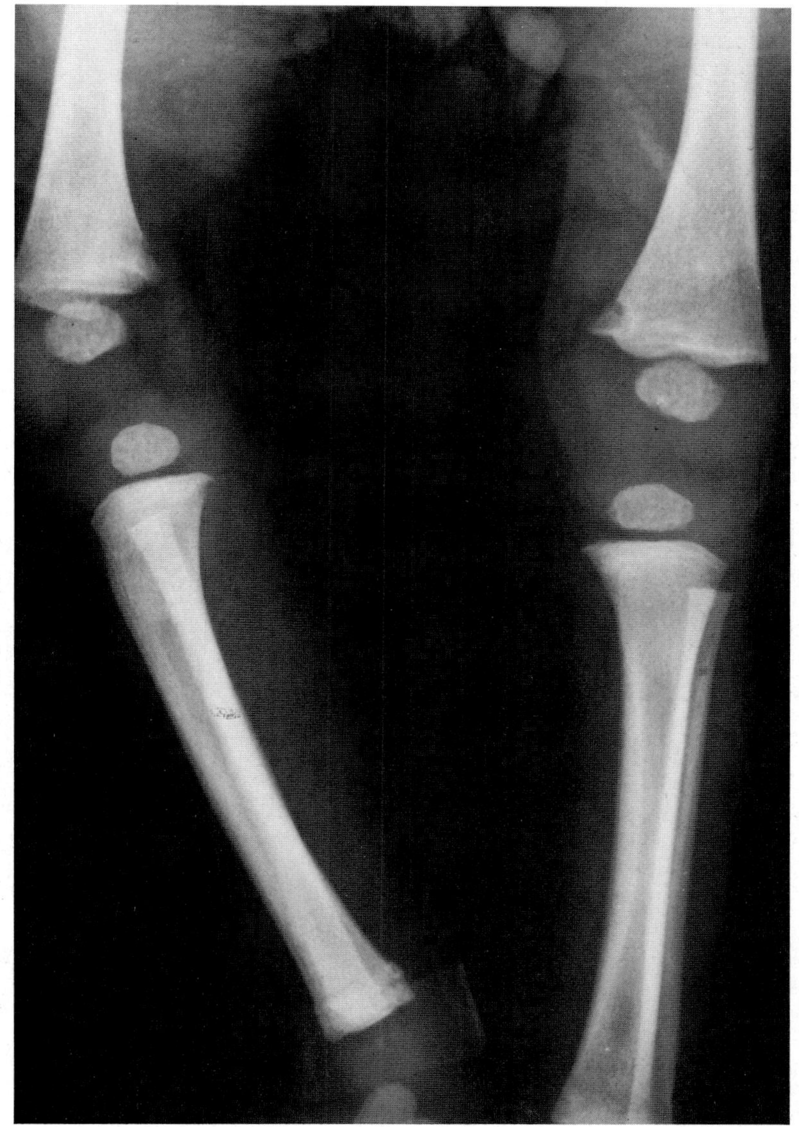

This 18-month-old child was referred for investigation.

- What would you do next?
- Are the appearances typical?

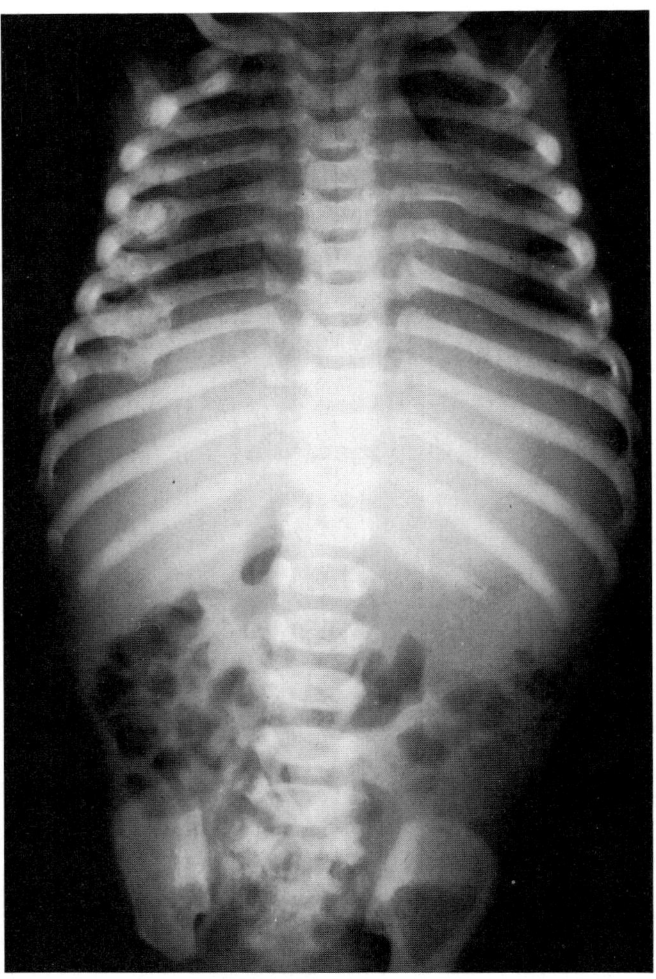

Healing fractures are seen at the metaphyseal margins of both distal femurs and in the right tibial distal metaphysis. Epiphyseal-metaphyseal fractures of long bones in small children are classically associated with non-accidental injury. A skeletal survey in this child revealed multiple anterior and posterior rib fractures in different stages of healing (chest film above) and multiple skull fractures. Metaphyseal marginal fractures may be the result of severe twisting injuries and can be accompanied by considerable periosteal reaction.

This pattern of injury is well-described, but not universal, in non-accidental injury. The majority of fractures in the long bones are transverse or spiral, and multiple fractures are found in only a quarter of cases. Even in the presence of a single, but unexplained fracture, the suspicion of a non-accidental aetiology must be maintained until it can be excluded.

Reference

Kogutt, M. S., Swischuk, L. E. and Fagan, C. J. (1974) Patterns of injury and significance of uncommon fractures in the battered child syndrome. *Amer. J. Roentgenol.*, **121**, 143-149.

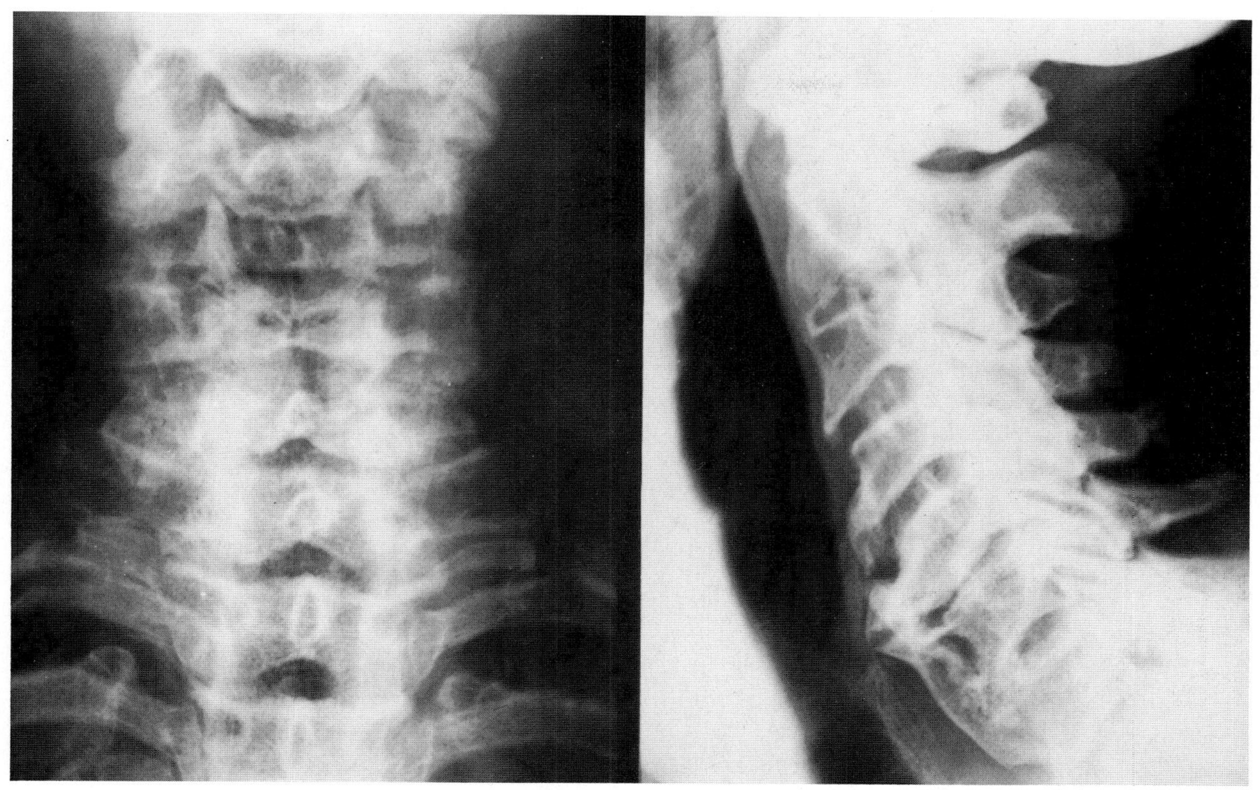

This 70-year-old man complained of neck stiffness.

- How does this condition differ from ankylosing spondylitis?

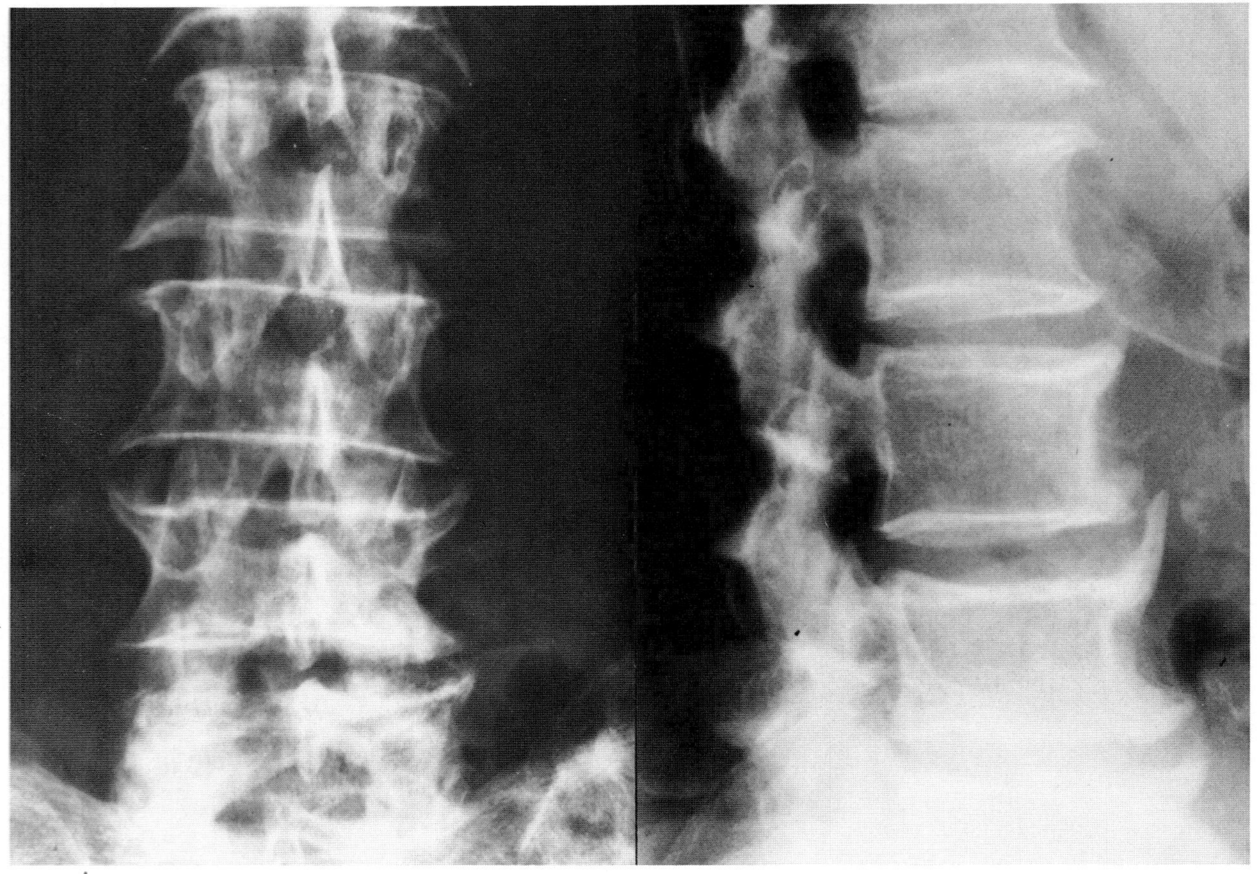

Extensive ossification of the anterior longitudinal ligament and anterolateral paravertebral tissues is present between C4 and C7. Bony excrescences protrude at the discovertebral junctions in the remainder of the cervical spine. Apart from degenerative narrowing of the C5/6 disc, the disc spaces are preserved and the apophyseal joints are unaffected. The bony density is normal.

The appearances fulfil the criteria for the diagnosis of diffuse idiopathic skeletal hyperostosis (DISH), a condition affecting the middle-aged and elderly where flowing ossification is generally present along the anterolateral aspects of at least four contiguous vertebral bodies. Although commonest in the thoracic region, any part of the spine may be involved. In this case, the lumbar spine was also affected (see above). Involvement of the cervical spine may cause dysphagia.

Ankylosing spondylitis is differentiated by its more delicate syndesmophytes, ankylosis of the apophyseal and sacro-iliac joints and sometimes by the difference in age incidence.

Reference

Resnick, D. and Niwayama, G. (1976) Radiographic and pathological features of spinal involvement in DISH. *Radiology*, 119, 559-568.

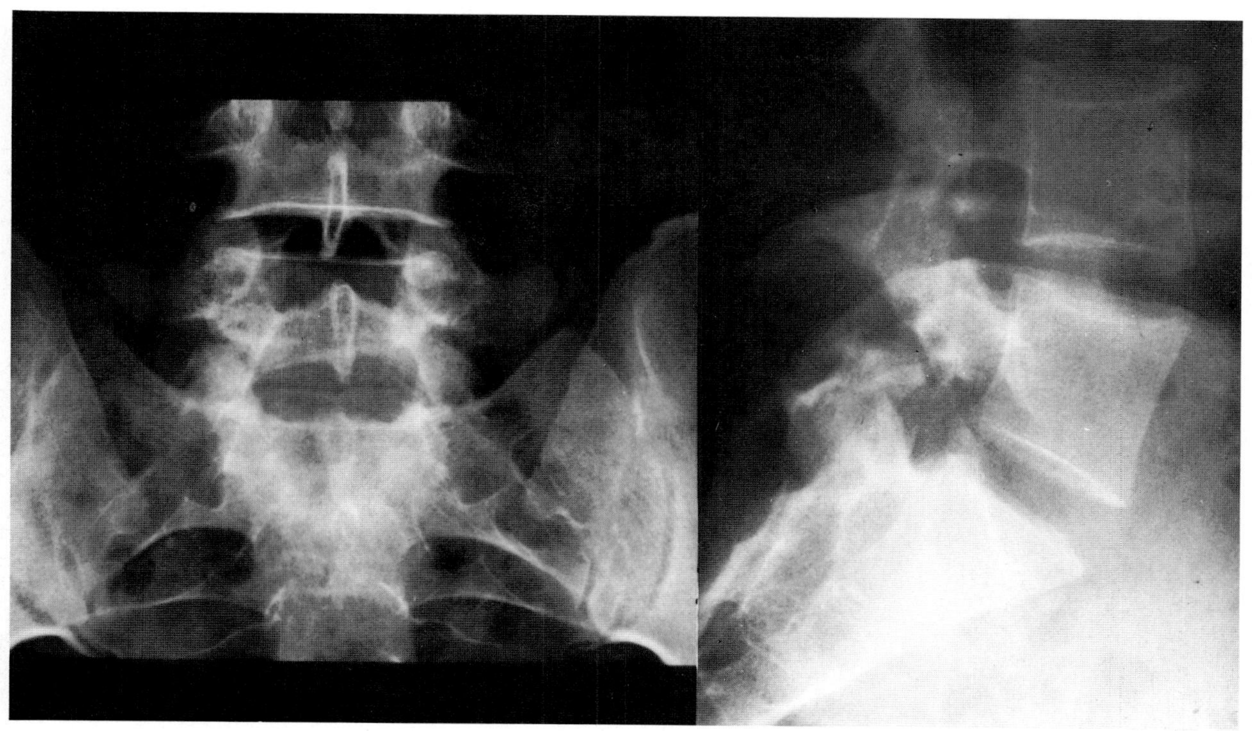

This 38-year-old woman had developed low back pain following an RTA one year earlier.

- What do the radiographs show?

- What further projection would be useful?

- Are the appearances likely to be related to the RTA?

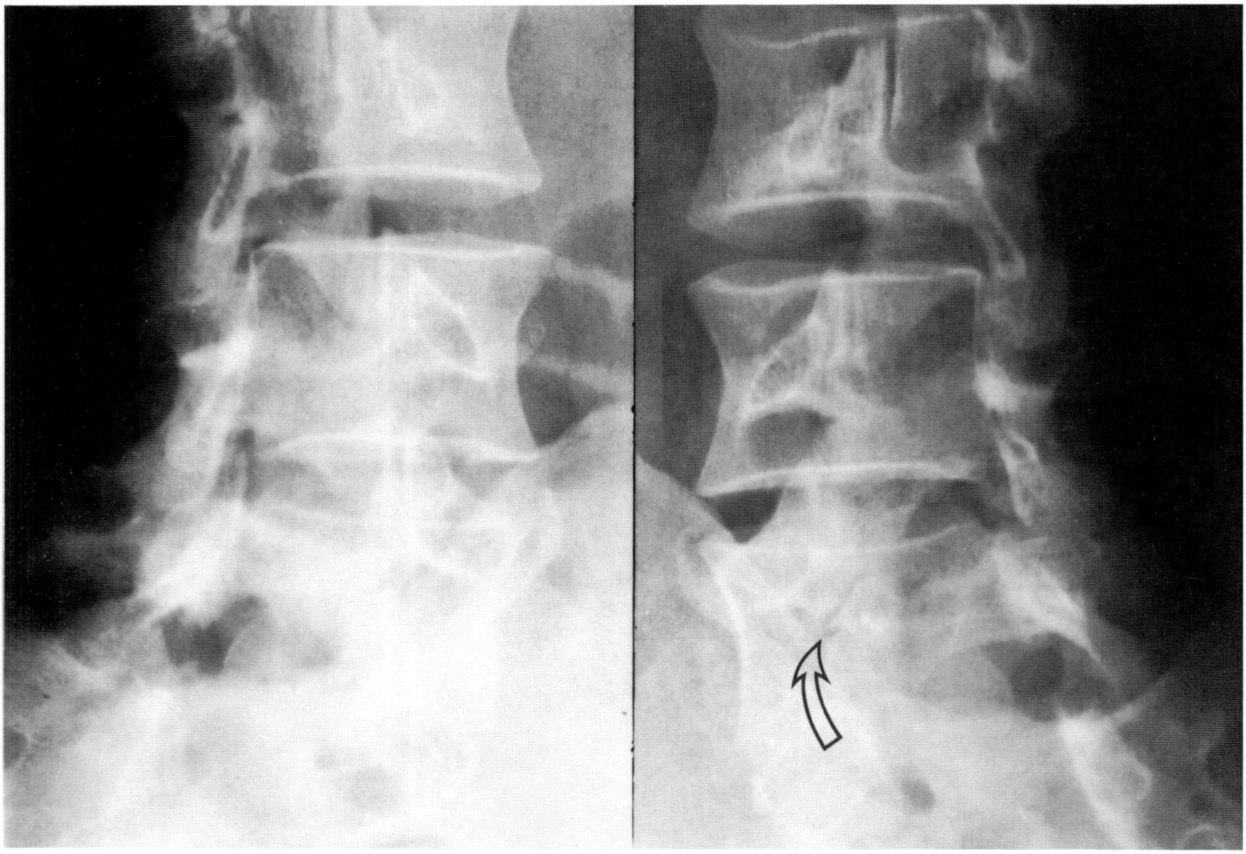

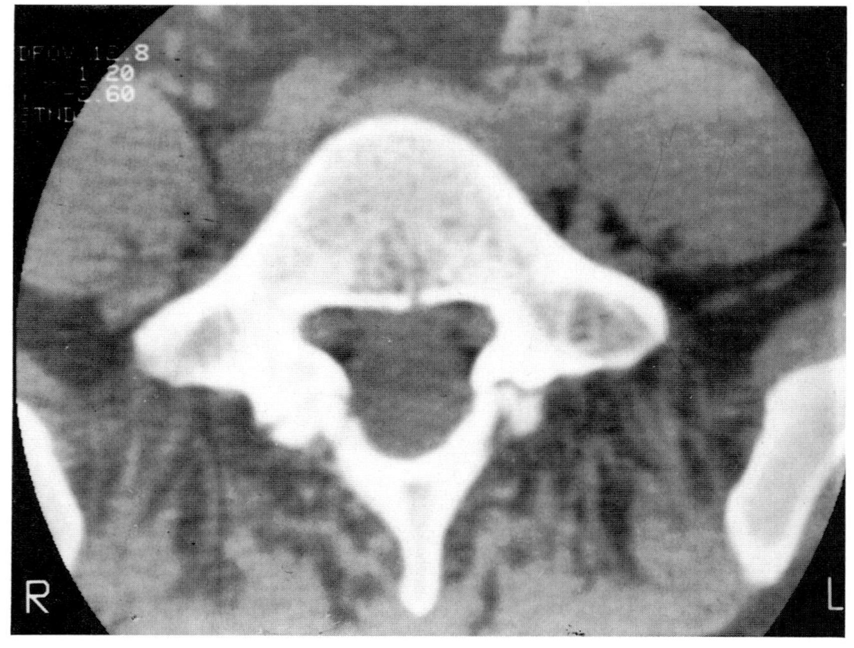

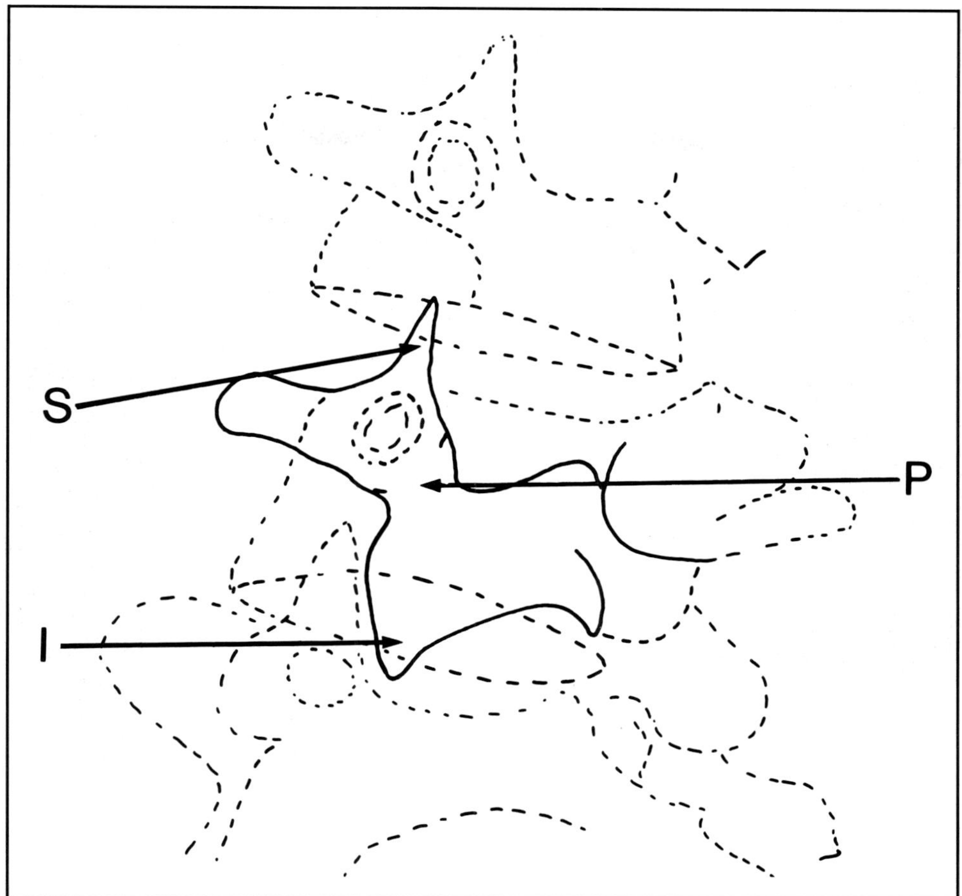

A defect of the pars interarticularis is shown at L5 on the lateral view. The AP view confirms a break in the right pars but the appearances on the left are inconclusive. Oblique views in this case confirmed the bilateral defects (arrow, page 56).

It is useful to know whether the defect is bilateral, since vertebral stability is dependent on intact neural arches. A bilateral pars defect will allow forward movement of the vertebral body and may result in secondary disc derangement.

The pars interarticularis is best demonstrated with an oblique view in which it forms the neck of the 'Scottie dog', as shown in the diagram above. The ear of the dog is the superior articular process (S), its front leg is the inferior articular process (I) and the pars interarticularis of L4 (P) is the dog's neck.

As there is no movement of the vertebral body the patient has a spondylolysis. When movement has occurred, the condition is termed a spondylolisthesis; it is usual to assess the degree of forward slippage of the upper vertebral body as a percentage of its AP diameter.

Pars defects may be caused by an identifiable injury but most are stress fractures commonly occurring in the lower lumbar spine. Such defects are essentially ununited fractures, as shown on the CT scan.

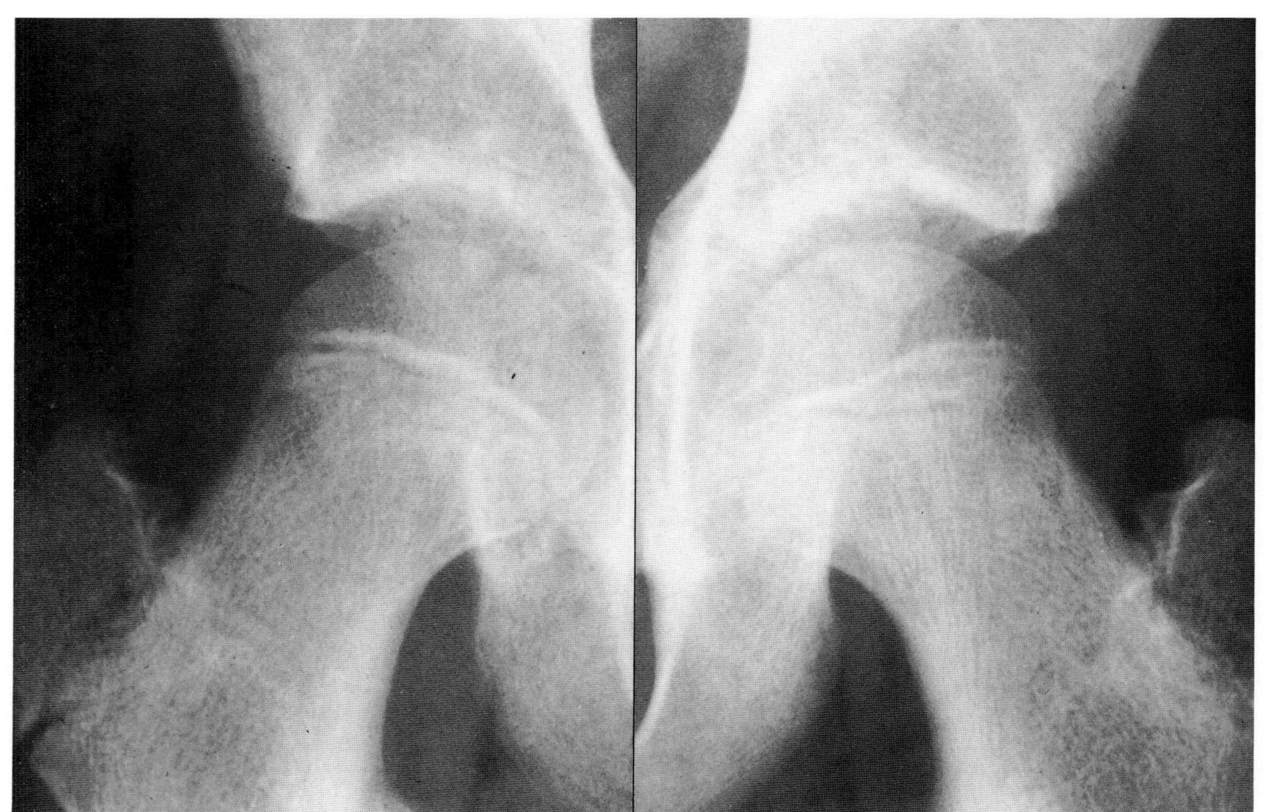

This 13-year-old girl presented with a painful hip.

- Describe the abnormalities.
- What is the diagnosis?
- What other radiograph should be obtained?

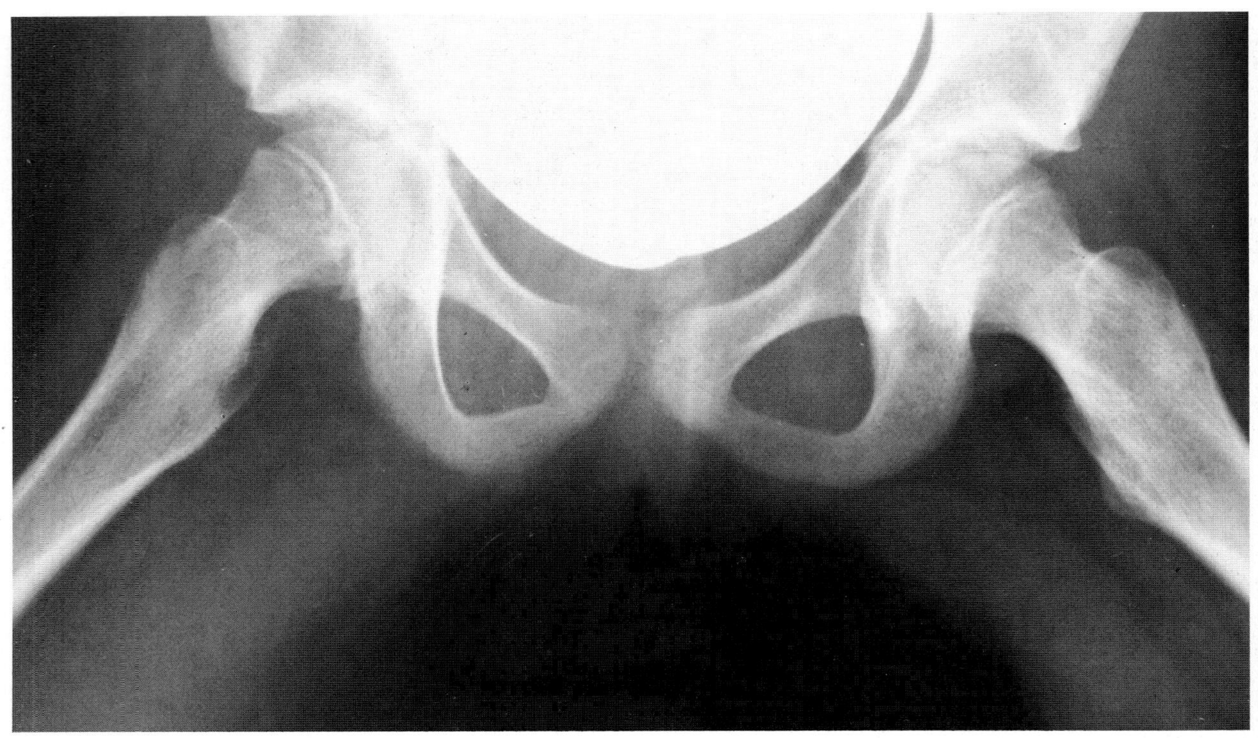

The appearances on the anteroposterior views of both hips are those of a slipped right femoral epiphysis. The radiological signs are mild osteopenia of the femoral epiphysis and neck, reduction in height of the epiphysis and widening of the lateral part of the growth plate. A line drawn along the lateral margin of the femoral neck barely passes through the epiphysis.

The manifestations of a slipped epiphysis may be subtle on the AP view. When the condition is suspected, it is essential to obtain either a frog lateral or a Billing projection to confirm the epiphyseal displacement, which is usually in a posterior direction. This deformity is demonstrated above in the frog lateral view of the same patient. Both hips should be examined on every occasion as the condition is bilateral in 20-25 per cent of cases.

References

Billing, L. and Eklof, O. (1984) Slip of the capital femoral epiphysis: revival of a method of assessment. *Pediatr. Radiol.*, **14**, 413-418.

Bloomberg, T. J., Nuttall, J. and Stoker, D. J. (1978) Radiology in early slipped femoral capital epiphysis. *Clin. Radiol.*, **29**, 657-667.

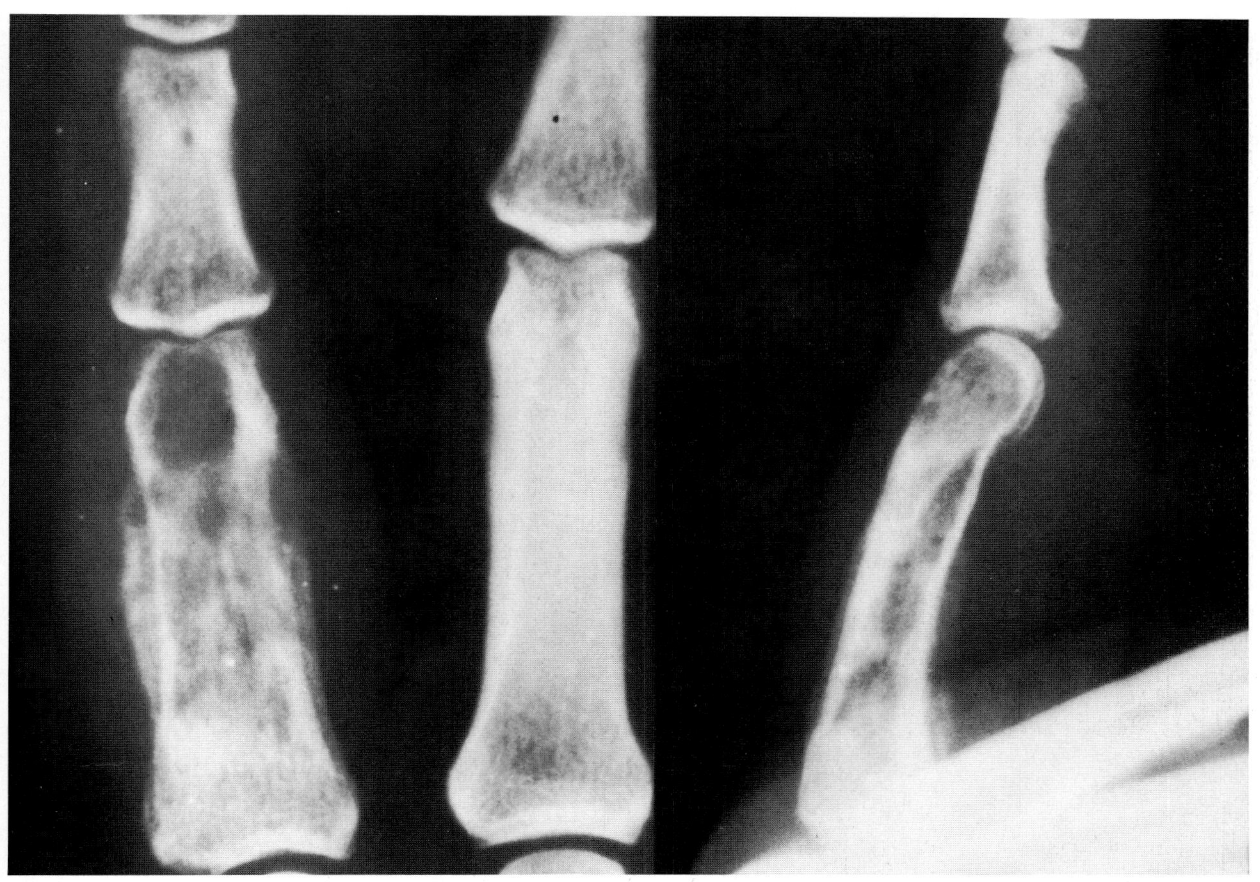

This black woman presented with soft tissue swelling of her index finger.

- What differential diagnosis would you consider?

- How do the appearances in this condition differ in childhood?

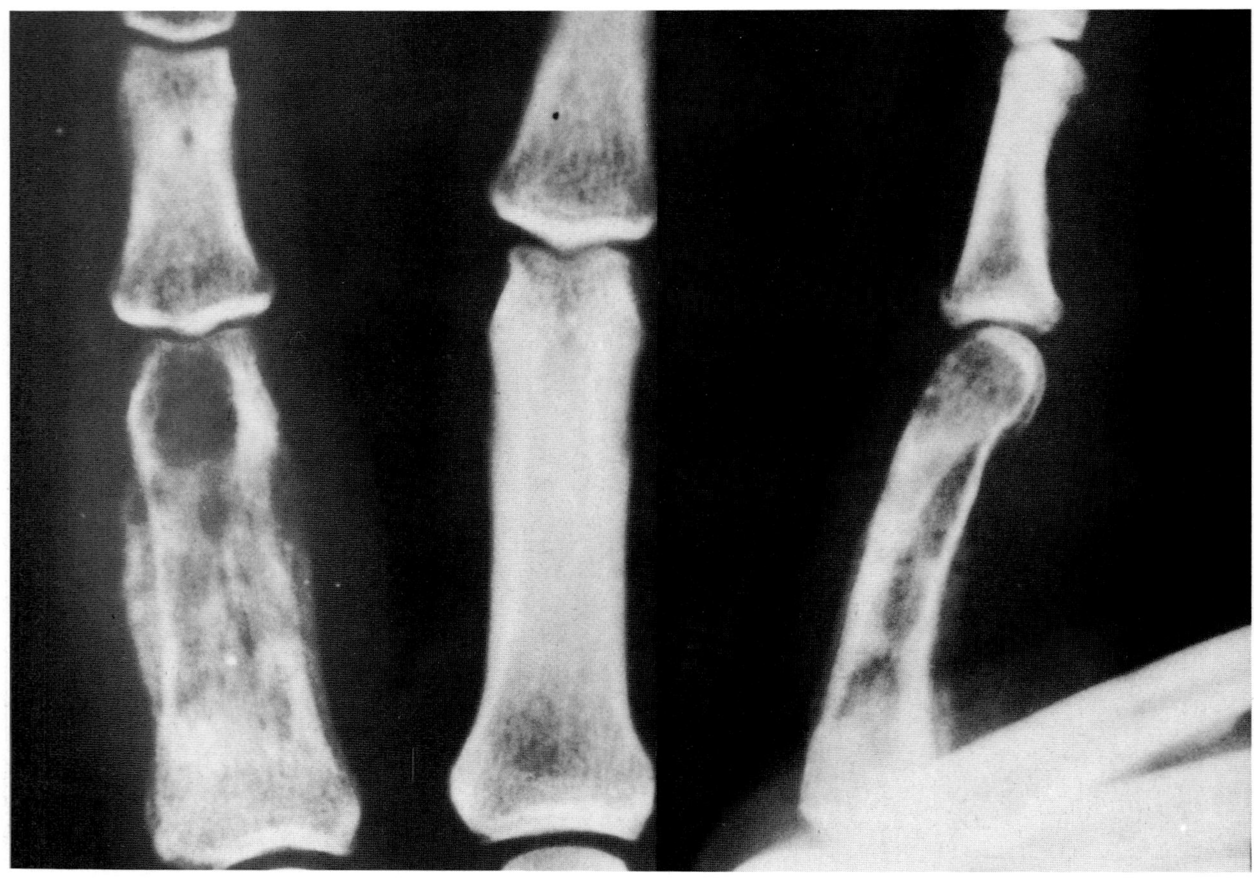

The lytic destruction, exuberant periosteal reaction and the surrounding soft tissue swelling indicate an infective process in the proximal phalanx of the index finger which is probably extending into the base of the middle phalanx.

It is not usually possible to distinguish radiologically between pyogenic and tuberculous osteomyelitis, although tuberculous osteomyelitis has a longer duration and is more likely to cross the adjacent joint. In this case acid-fast bacilli were aspirated from the affected phalanx.

Tuberculous dactylitis of the small bones of the hands and feet occurs most frequently in the under-five age group but can affect adults. The involved bone may sometimes show marked expansion and a cystic appearance, termed spina ventosa (a small bone blown up with air). Spina ventosa and multiple bone involvement are both more common in the younger age group. Sickle cell anaemia and syphilitic dactylitis should be included in the differential diagnosis in a child.

Reference

Chapman, M., Murray, R. O. and Stoker, D. J. (1979) Tuberculosis of the bones and joints. *Seminars in Roentgenol.*, 14, 266-282.

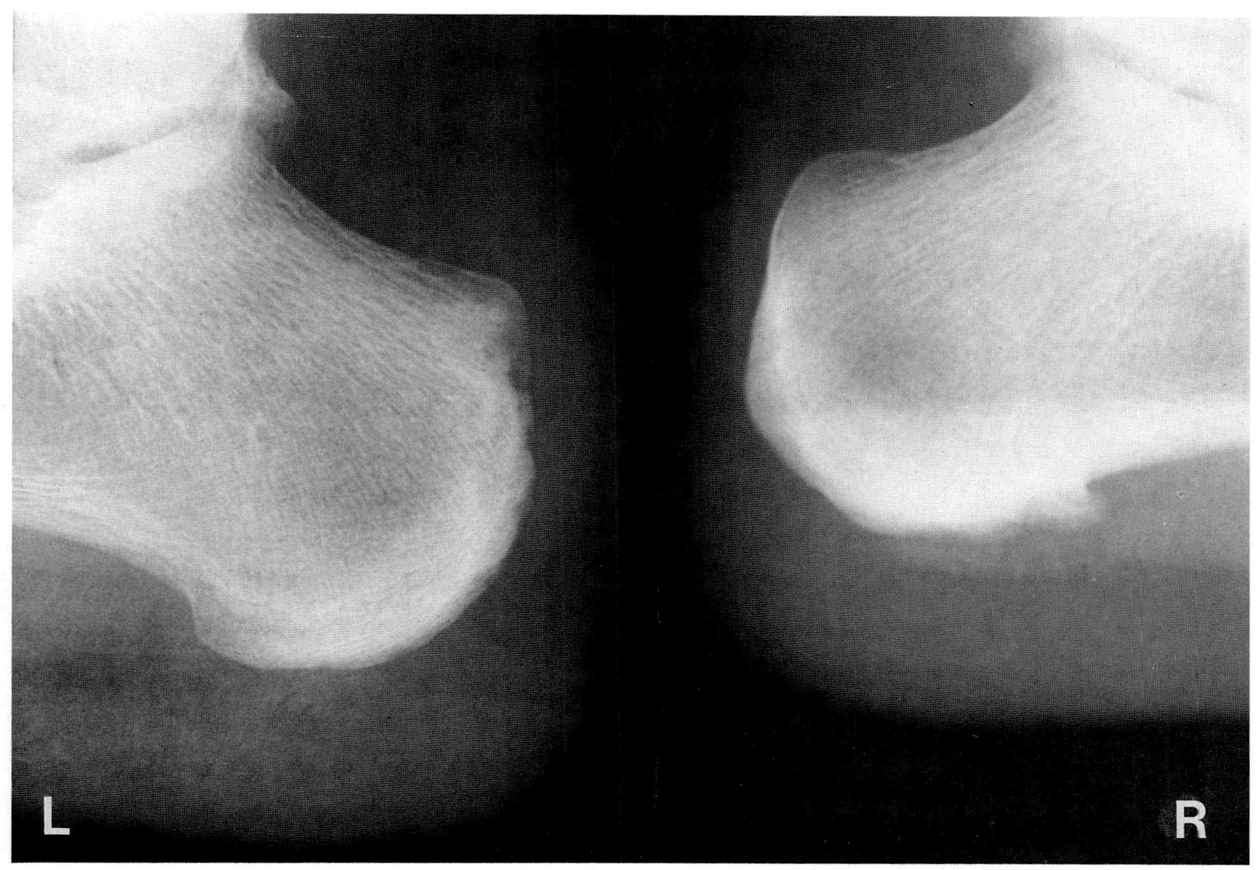

This 25-year-old man complained of painful heels.

- Describe the appearances and give a differential diagnosis.

- What questions would you ask the patient?

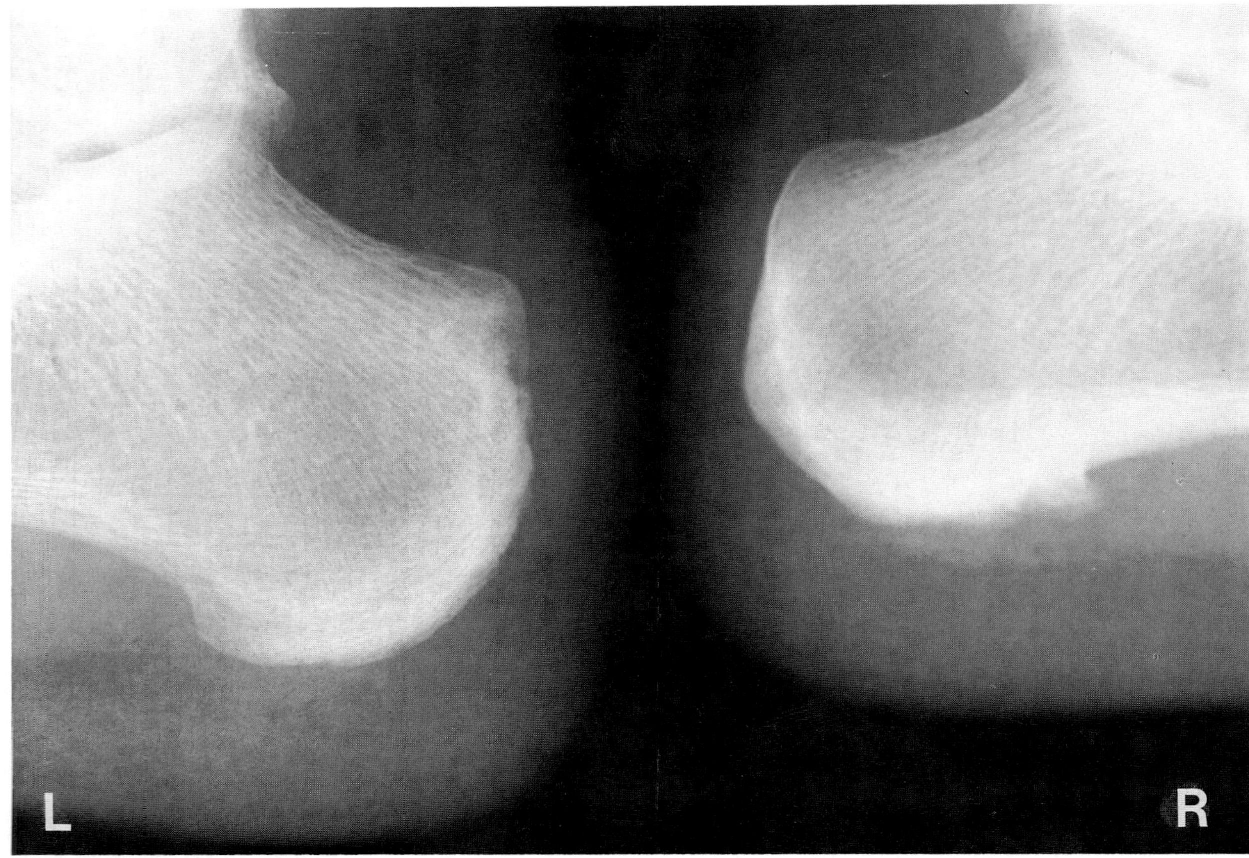

The lateral view of the left heel shows erosions on the posterior aspect of the calcaneus at and above the site of insertion of the Achilles tendon; an opacity in the adjacent soft tissues has obliterated the outline of the tendon and is due to a retrocalcaneal bursitis. On the right, hyperostosis and an ill-defined spur have developed on the plantar surface of the calcaneus.

The findings are consistent with an inflammatory synovial process; rheumatoid arthritis and Reiter's disease are the most likely causes. As the patient was suffering from urethritis and gave a history of recent conjunctivitis and joint pains, a diagnosis of Reiter's disease was made.

Calcaneal involvement affecting the posterior and/or plantar surfaces occurs in 25-50 per cent of patients with Reiter's syndrome and may be the only manifestation of the disease. A retrocalcaneal bursitis often precedes the development of erosions and plantar spurs. Unlike rheumatoid arthritis, posterior spurs are rare. Similar plantar spurs with florid periostitis may be seen in ankylosing spondylitis and psoriasis.

Reference

Resnick, M. D., Feingold, M. L., Curd, J., Niwayama, G. and Goergen, T. G. (1977) Calcaneal abnormalities in articular disorders. *Radiology*, **125**, 355-366.

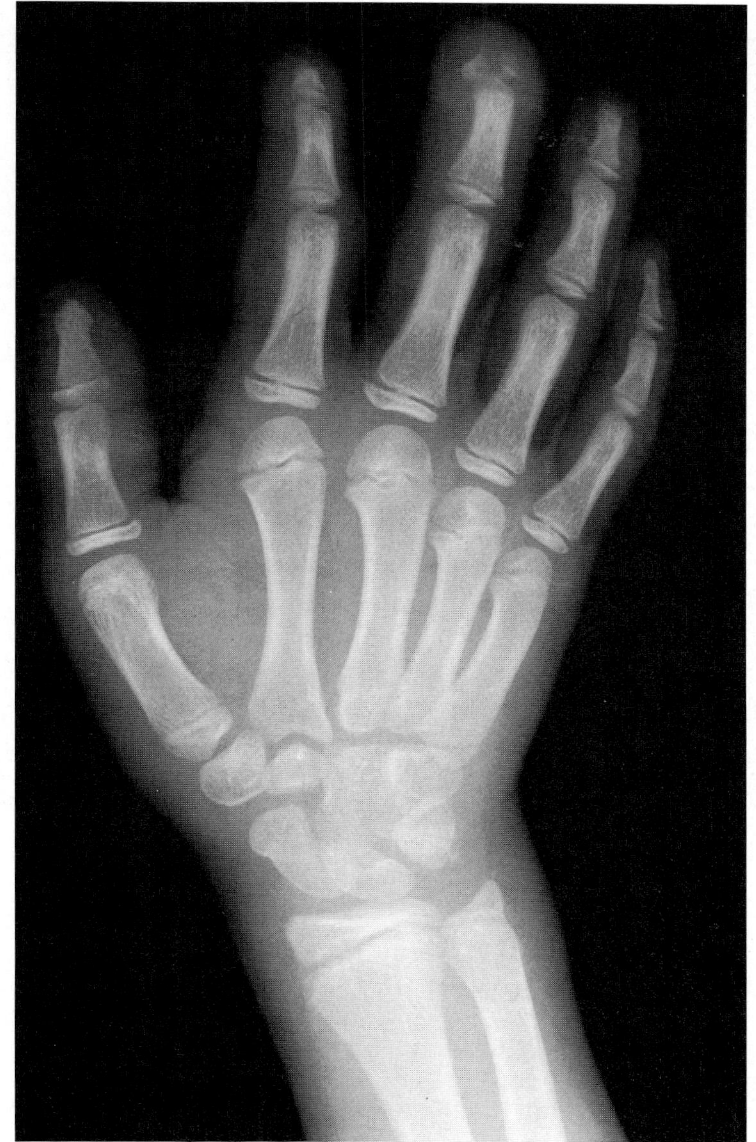

Since the age of 18 months, this 10-year-old girl had developed a progressive foot deformity.

- Describe the appearances in the hand.

- What diagnoses would you consider?

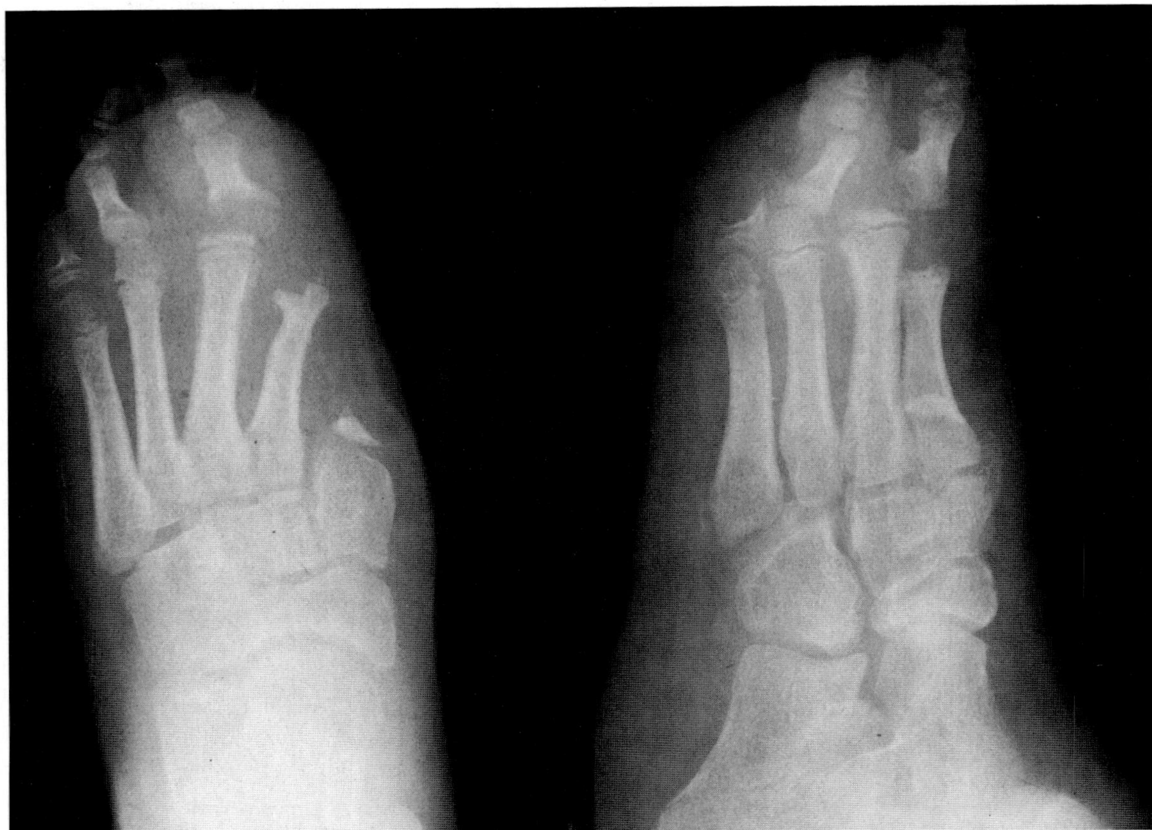

Acro-osteolysis is present in the index, middle and ring fingers. Soft tissue swelling and a fracture of the terminal phalanx is also evident in the middle finger.

Although these appearances could have resulted from trauma or thermal injury, the history of a progressive foot deformity and the normal bone density should suggest a neuropathic aetiology with multifocal involvement. Such changes in syringomyelia are confined to the upper limbs and in myelomeningocele to the lower limbs. The history is inconsistent with leprosy which typically also may affect the interphalangeal joints in the hands.

This child was able to jump from a height without feeling any pain and the diagnosis was one of congenital insensitivity to pain. Pain sensation is reduced in this condition but touch and temperature sensation are usually preserved. The lower extremities are often more severely affected than the upper extremities and the radiograph of this patient's feet (see above) shows widespread phalangeal and metatarsal resorption. The periosteal reaction is due to osteomyelitis secondary to soft tissue ulceration and infection. Fracture, epiphyseal separation and dislocation are frequent in neuropathic conditions. This patient had sustained a fracture through the proximal left humerus and dislocation of the humeral head. The radiograph on page 67 demonstrates the characteristically clear line of demarcation at the site of fracture, suggestive of surgical resection. The non-union and amorphous mineral deposits in the surrounding soft tissues are also typical. Evidence is accumulating that support and protection of a part following injury will avoid or reduce the subsequent deformity.

Reference

Murray, R. O. (1957) Congenital indifference to pain with special reference to skeletal changes. *Brit. J. Radiol.*, 30, 2-6.

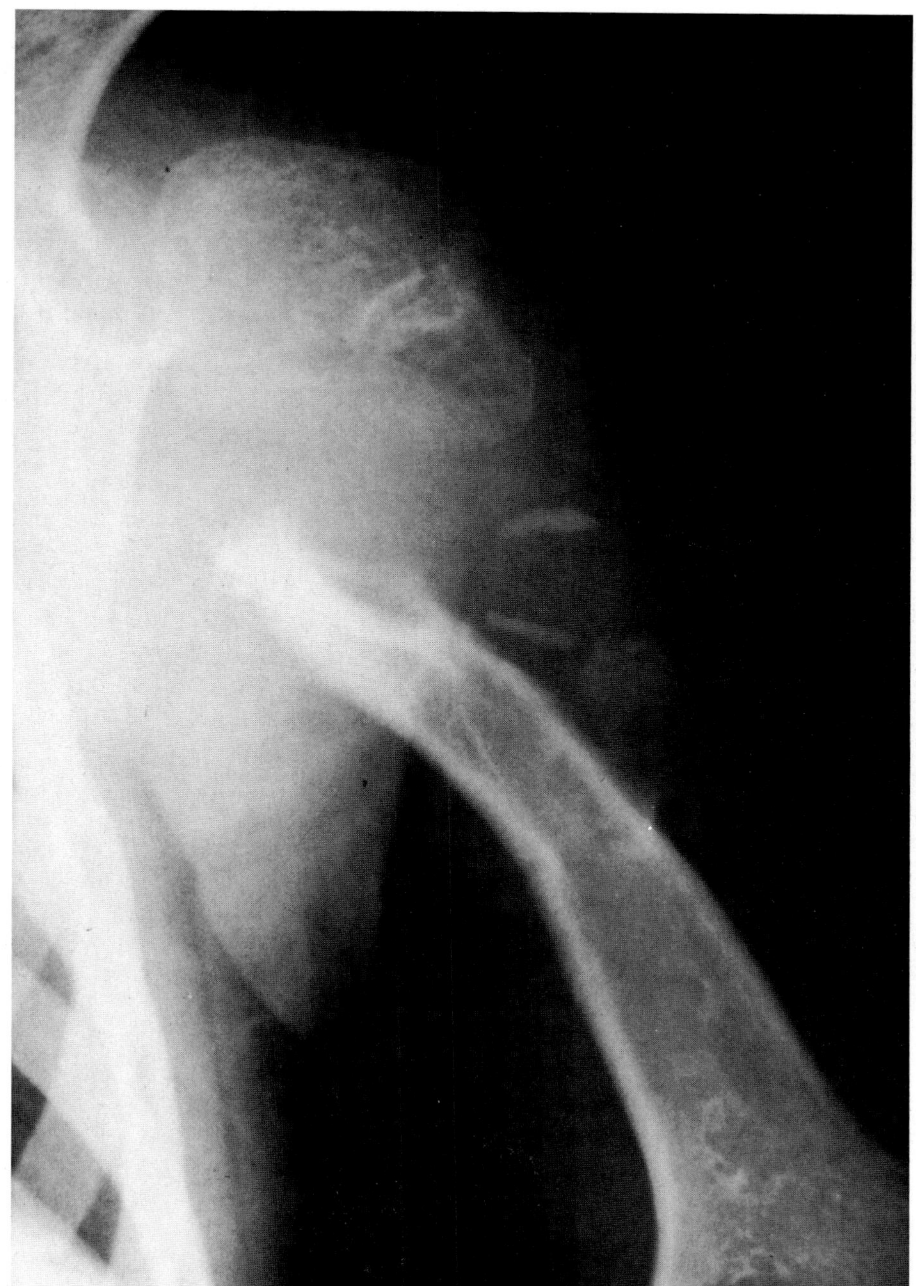

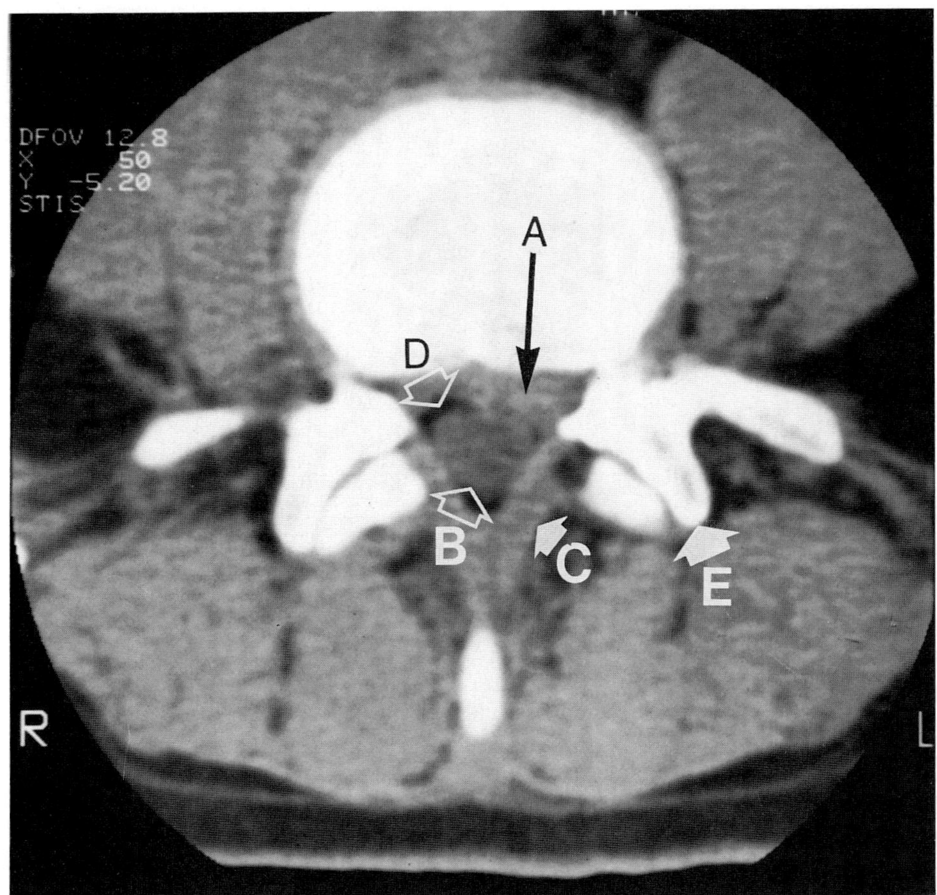

This 39-year-old man developed acute onset low back pain radiating down the left leg. These CT scans have been performed at the level of the L4/5 disc and the L5 vertebral body.

- Identify the structures labelled A-E.

- What is the cause of his pain?

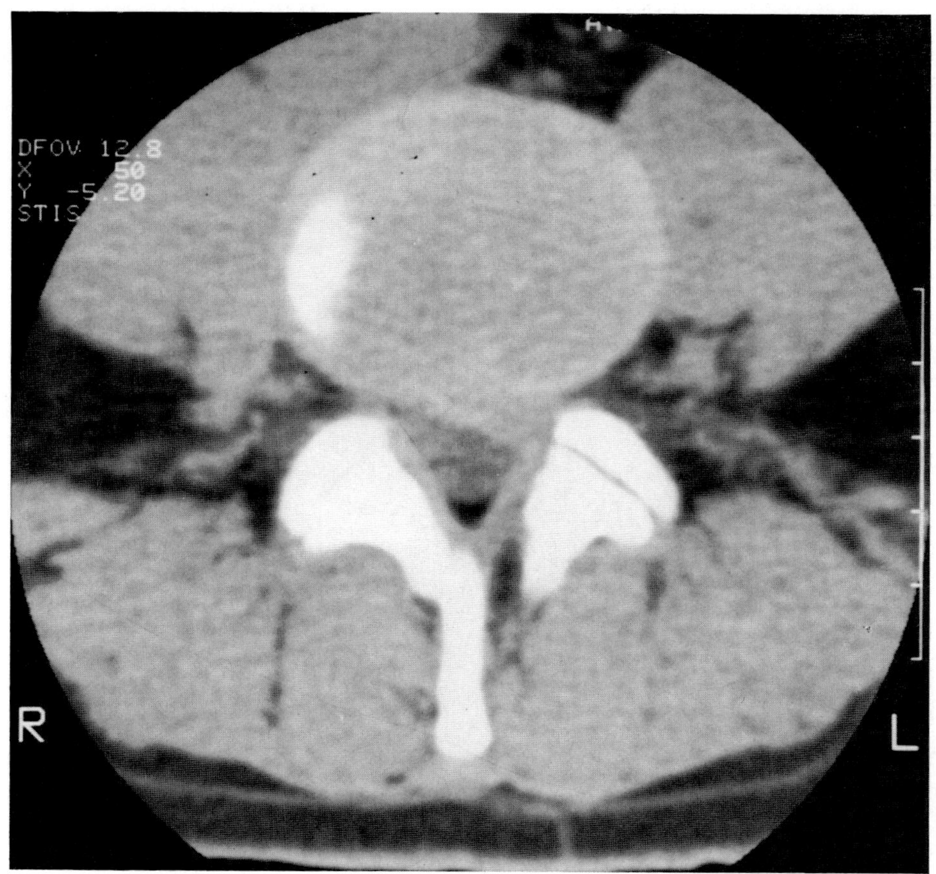
DFOV 12.8
X 50
Y -5.20
STIS
R
L

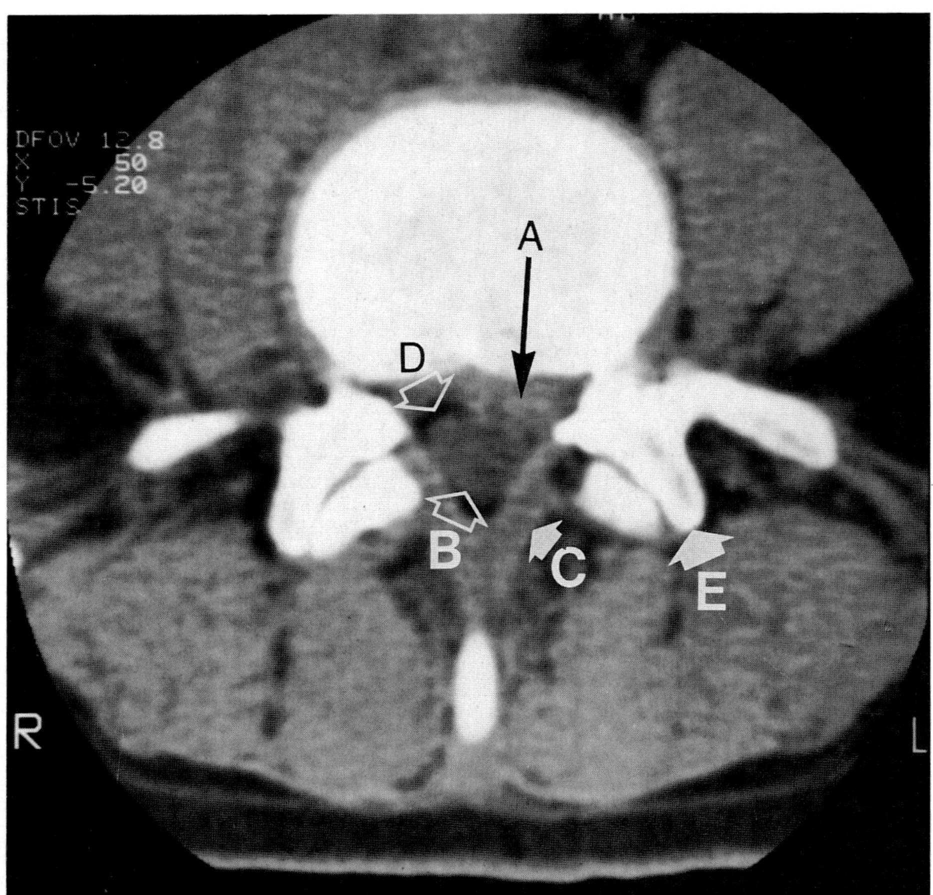

A   Intervertebral disc

B   Theca containing cauda equina

C   Ligamentum flavum

D   Epidural fat

E   Inferior articular facet

Posterolateral herniation of the L4/5 disc has resulted in compression of the left L5 nerve root, and of the epidural fat and thecal sac. Note is made of the incidental narrowing of the L4/5 intervertebral foramina and the right lateral recess at L5 by degenerative hypertrophy of the apophyseal joints.

CT can provide a good demonstration of lumbar disc pathology because the abundant epidural fat allows differentiation of the soft tissues within the vertebral canal.

The posterior margin of the normal lumbar disc has a mid-line concavity. If the nucleus pulposus herniates through the anulus fibrosus, it will cause bulging of the disc margin if confined by the posterior ligament. If material is extruded into the epidural canal, fragments may migrate along the canal.

CT scans may be difficult to interpret when scar tissue replaces epidural fat following laminectomy and discectomy.

Reference

Teplick, J. G. and Haskin, M. E. (1983) CT and lumbar disc herniation. *Radiol. Clin. N. Amer.*, **21**, 259-288.

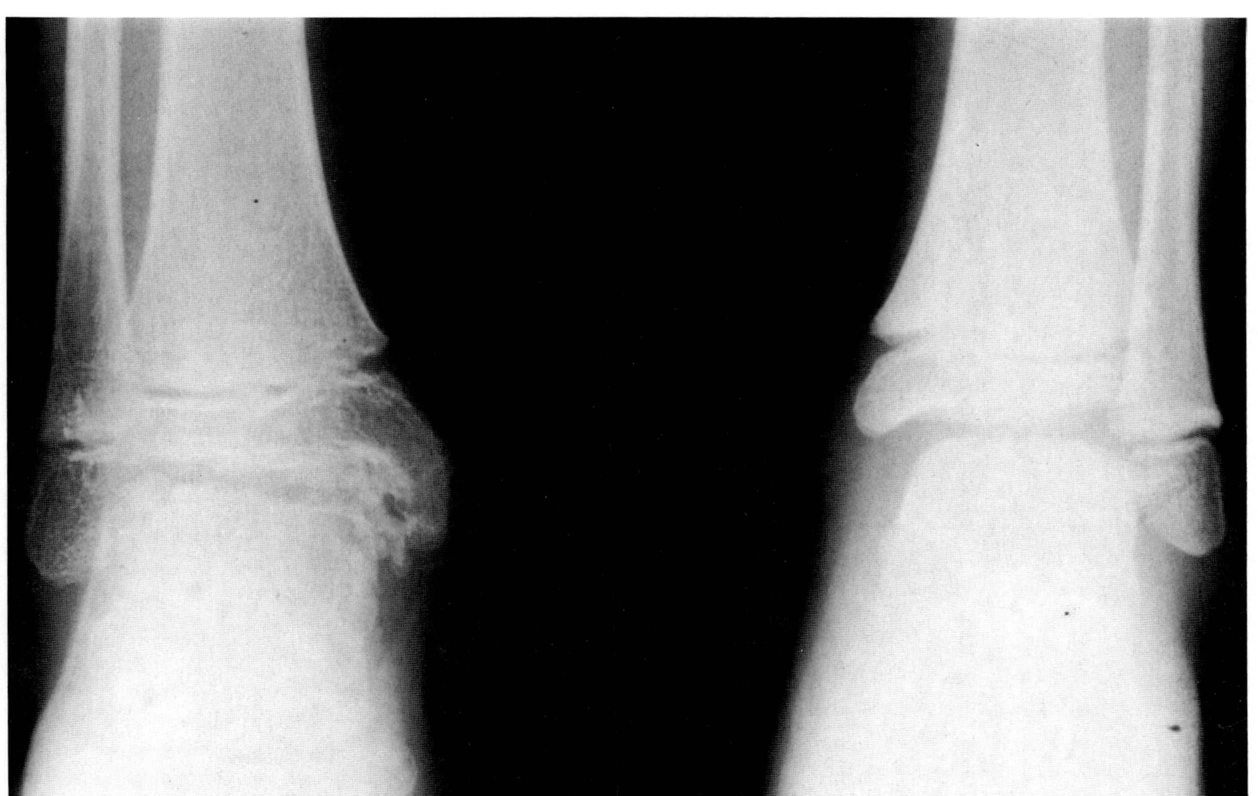

This child complained of a hard painless swelling over his right ankle.

- Describe the abnormalities.

- What might you see on a radiograph of the knees?

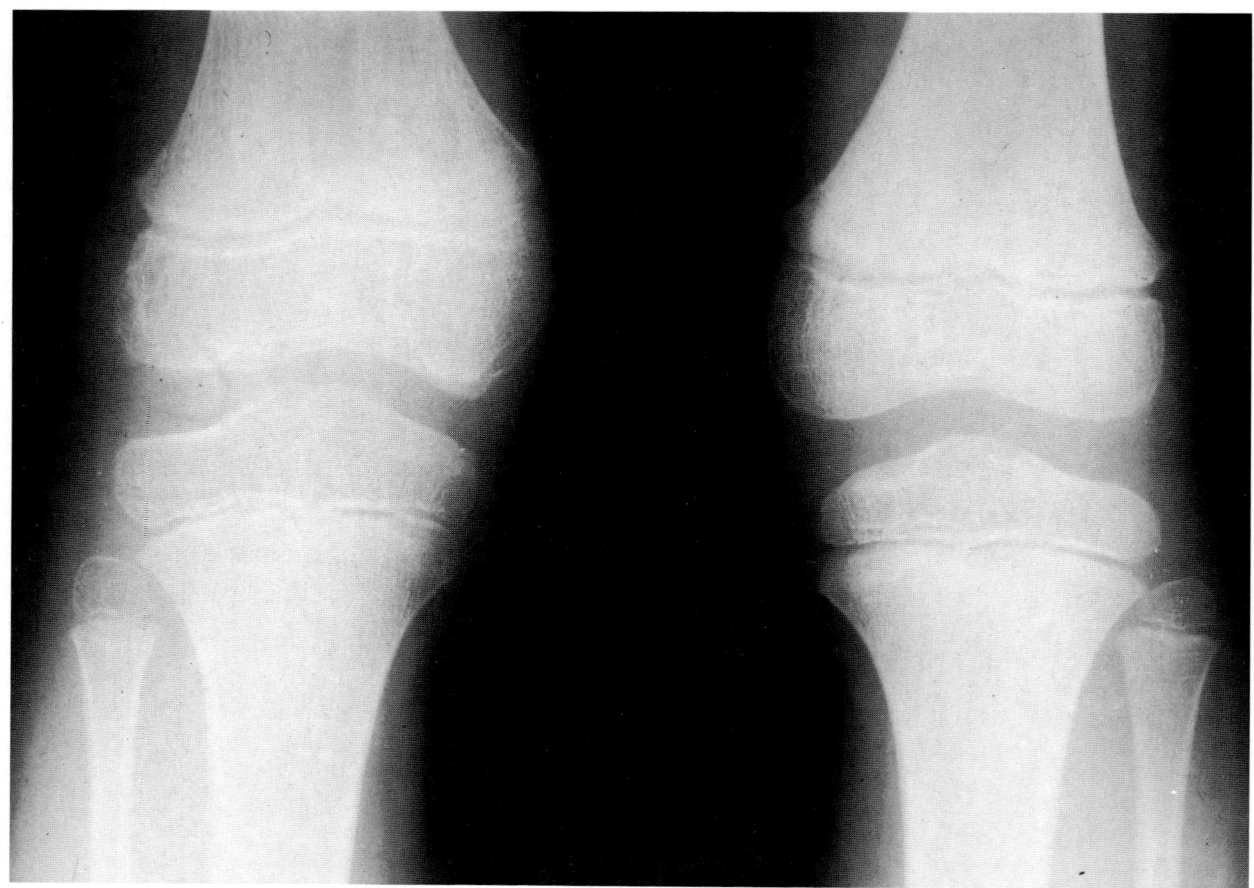

Asymmetrical, irregular enlargement of the medial halves of the right tibial epiphysis and talus is associated with irregularity of the articular surfaces and talar slanting. Localised fusion of the tibial growth plate has occurred.

A radiograph of both knees also shows enlargement of the medial halves of the right distal femoral and proximal tibial epiphyses. The left ankle and knee are normal.

The epiphyseal abnormalities in dysplasia epiphysealis hemimelica (Trevor's disease) are usually confined to one side of the affected limb, more commonly the medial side. The disorder shows a male predominance, and patients present in childhood with painless swelling or deformity of a limb. There is often associated muscle wasting. The changes do not progress after puberty and secondary degenerative change is unusual. It is a rare disease and its aetiology is uncertain, although histologically the lesion resembles an osteochondroma.

David Trevor (1906-1988), a consultant orthopaedic surgeon at the Royal National Orthopaedic Hospital in London, described ten cases involving the ankle in 1950. A report of a single case had been made by Mouchet and Belot in 1926.

Reference

Fairbank, T. J. (1956) Dysplasia epiphysialis hemimelica (tarso-epiphysial aclasis). *J. Bone Joint Surg.*, **38-B**, 237-257.

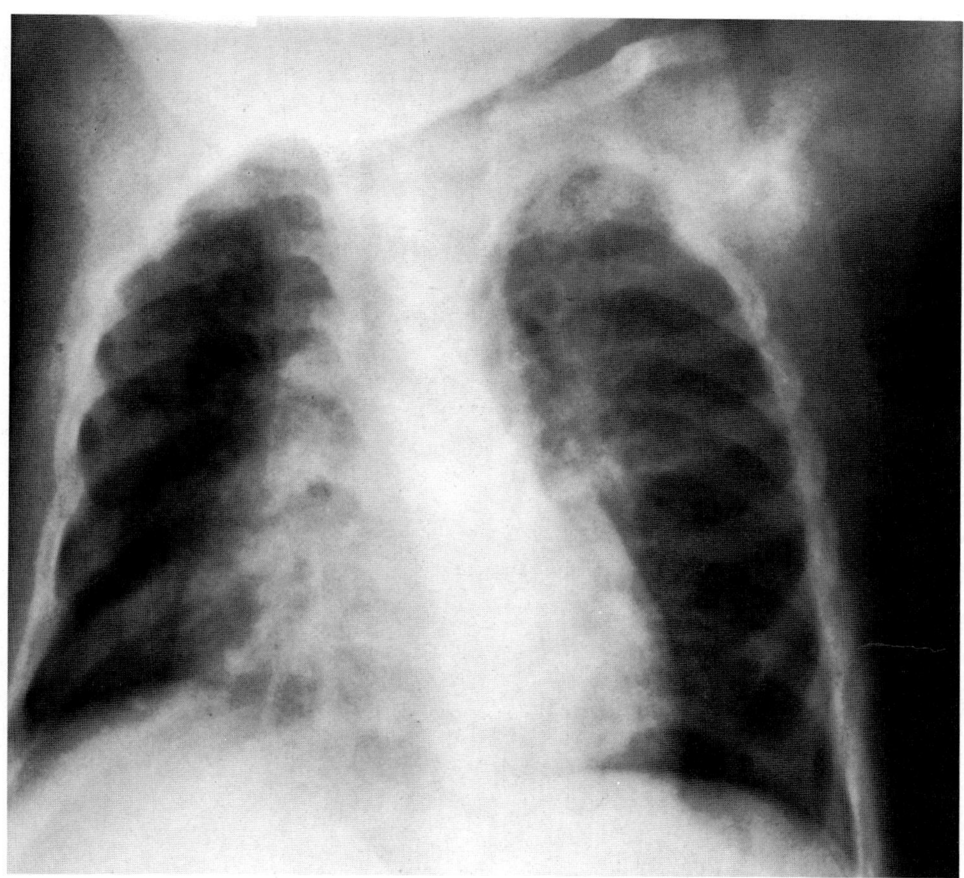

This 18-month-old black child was reluctant to stand and had swollen wrists.

- What abnormalities are shown on the chest radiograph and what is the diagnosis?

- What is the mechanism of the radiographic changes seen in this condition?

- Where else may radiographic changes be seen in this disease?

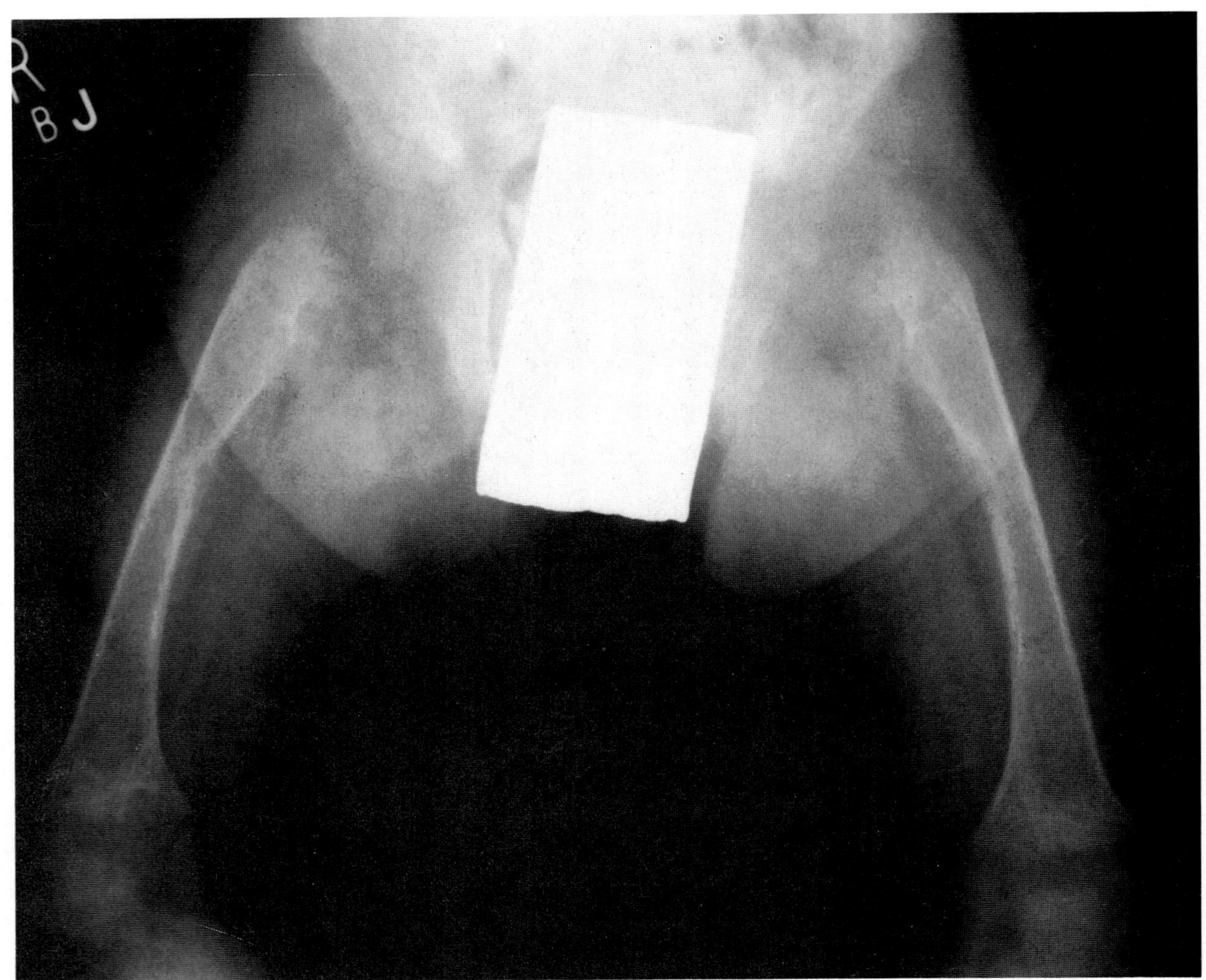

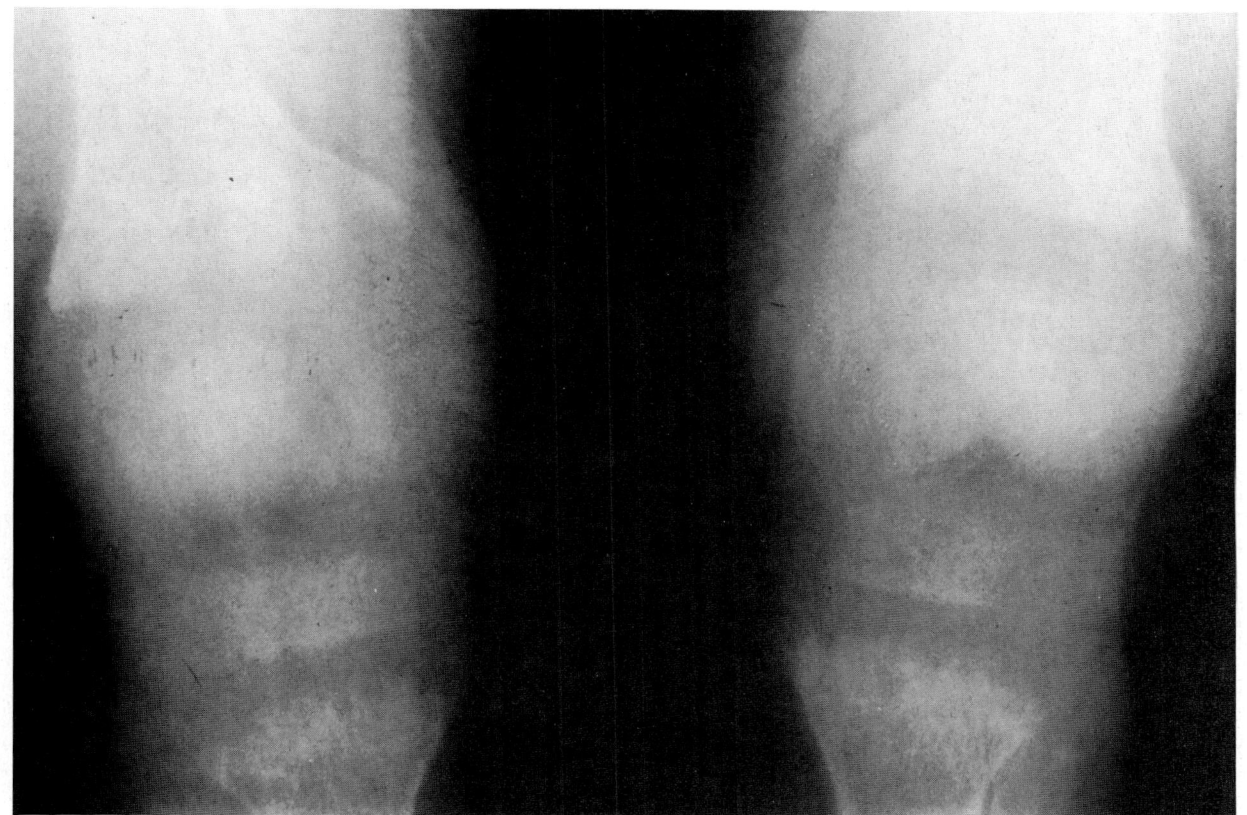

This child has severe rickets. The bones are poorly mineralised and splaying and irregularity are present in the anterior ends of the ribs (the radiological counterpart of the rachitic rosary) and the left proximal humeral metaphysis.

Rickets results from inadequate mineralisation of osteoid in developing bone and is due to a deficiency of vitamin D as a result of inadequate intake, defective absorption or disturbed metabolism.

The effects of rickets are most apparent in areas of rapid growth, such as the distal femur, both ends of the tibia, the distal forearm bones, proximal humerus and costochondral junctions. The sites of maximum radiological change depend on the age of the child. This patient had a serum calcium level of 1.8 mmol/l (normal = 2.15-2.70 mmol/l) and a vitamin D level of 5 nmol/l (normal = 20-100 nmol/l in winter, 25-150 nmol/l in summer). Dietary assessment revealed an inadequate intake of both vitamin D and calories. The disease is prevented by adequate exposure to sunlight, not available in the northern hemisphere.

Radiographic manifestations include marked irregularity of the zone of provisional calcification (on the metaphyseal side of the growth plate) and apparent widening of the growth plate. In weight-bearing regions (classically wrists when crawling, knees when walking) stress causes metaphyseal splaying, and bowing of the long bones. Skeletal maturation is retarded and bone density reduced.

Looser's zones (pseudo-fractures) are less common in rickets than in osteomalacia but are present in both femora in this case.

Reference

Steinbach, H. L. and Noetzli, M. (1964) Roentgen appearance of the skeleton in osteomalacia and rickets. *Amer. J. Roentgenol.*, **91**, 955-972.

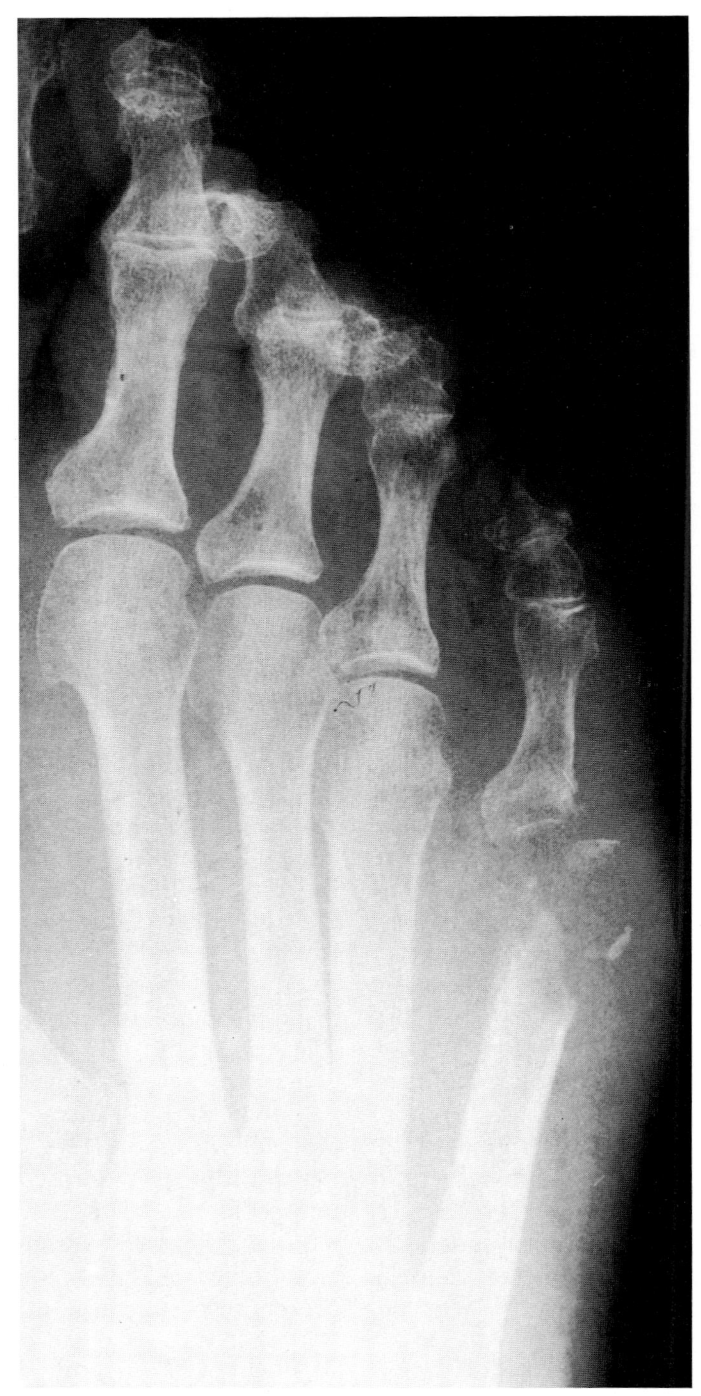

This elderly patient was suffering from a chronic disorder. He had developed an ulcer on the sole of his foot.

- What is the cause of these appearances?
- What changes would you expect following treatment?

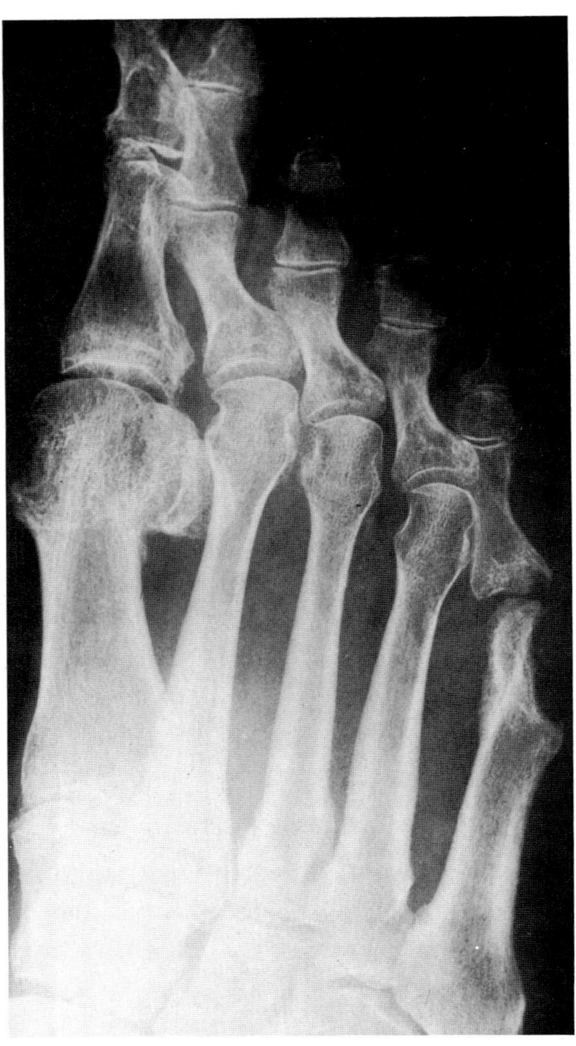

The initial film shows bony resorption and soft tissue swelling around the fifth metatarsophalangeal joint. Fragments of bone lie in the soft tissues and a periosteal reaction is present. The preservation of bony density is typical of a neuropathic disorder; the tapering of the metatarsal supports a diabetic aetiology. Some of the bone destruction may be due to secondary infection. Changes at the first metatarsophalangeal joint may be caused by associated gouty arthritis.

The patient was an insulin-dependent diabetic. The film above was obtained three months later and demonstrates the reconstitution of bone which typically follows improved diabetic control.

Atheromatous involvement of the vascular supply to the nerves is considered to be the most important factor in diabetic neuropathy. The tarsal and tarsometatarsal joints are usually affected by a destructive process, whereas tapering resorption is more frequent at the metatarsophalangeal joints. Reconstitution of bone may not be complete, resulting in metatarsal shortening, subluxation of the phalangeal heads and ulceration over the bony prominences subject to pressure.

Reference

Kellett, M. A. (1967) The radiologic features of diabetes mellitus. *Radiol. Clin. N. Amer.*, 5, 239-248.

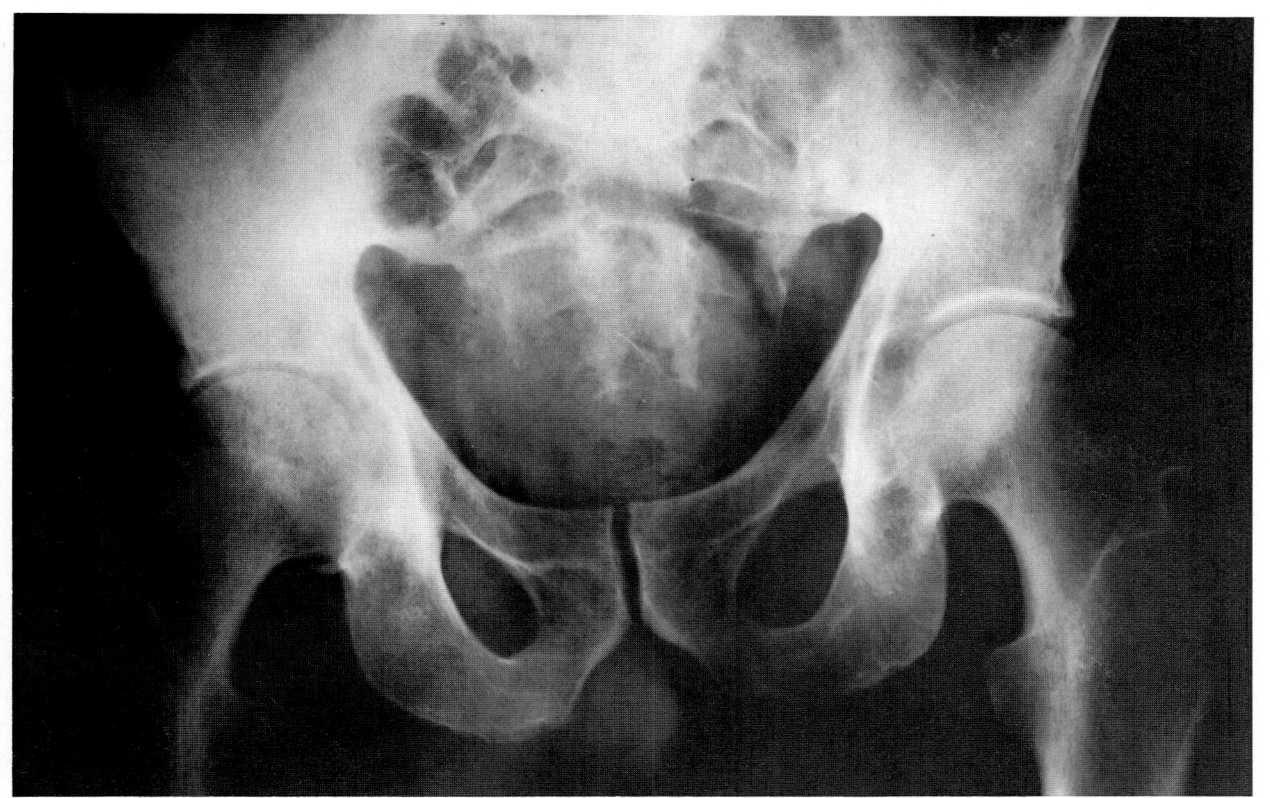

This 60-year-old man complained of right hip pain.

- What is the likely cause of his symptoms?

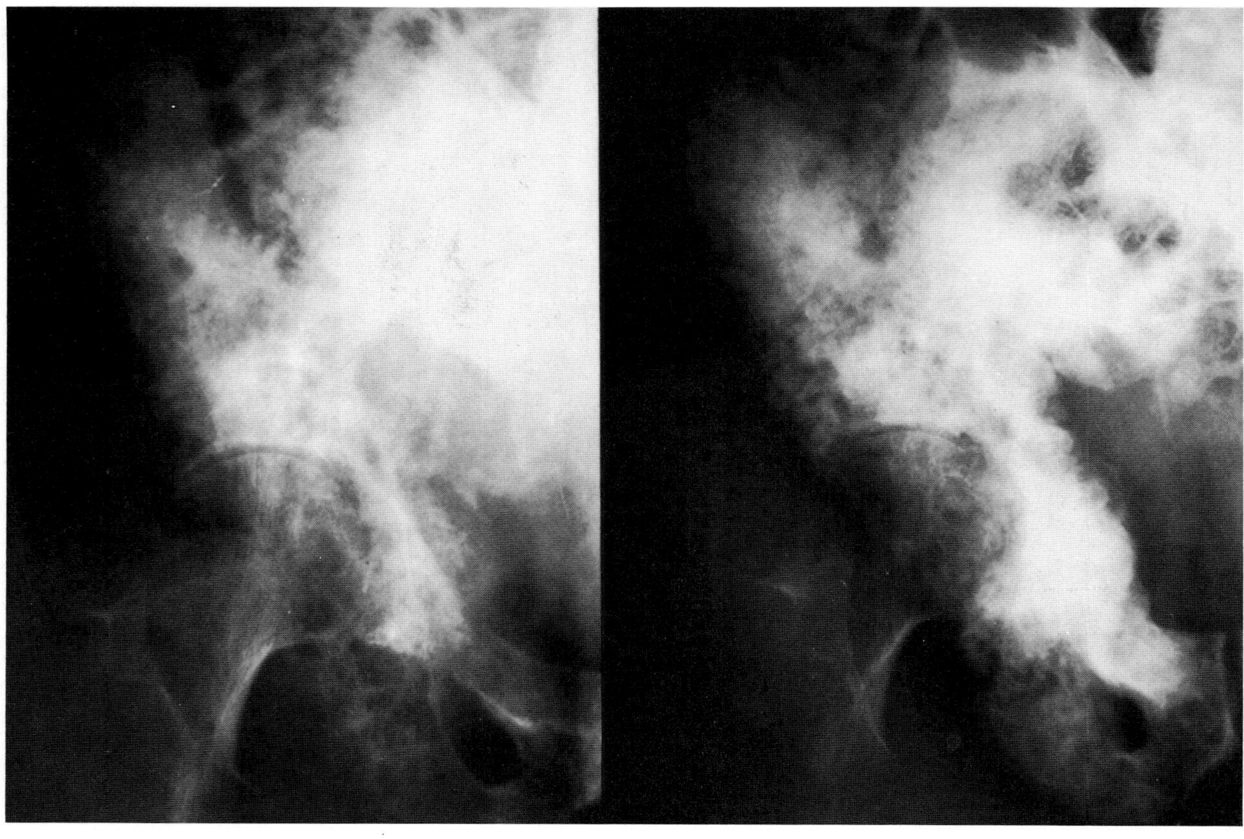

This man's pain was initially attributed to the mild degenerative changes present in the right hip joint. The sclerosis above the right acetabulum was thought to be part of this process, but it is far too extensive, involving most of the ilium, and should have been viewed with suspicion. Bone scintigraphy probably would have suggested the correct diagnosis.

Serial films above show progressive sclerosis in the right hemipelvis. Further investigation, including cystoscopy and a skeletal survey, revealed a prostatic carcinoma and extensive bony metastases.

Carcinoma of the prostate has the highest prevalence of any carcinoma to metastasize to bone. The pelvis or sacrum is involved in 85 per cent, the spine in 60 per cent and the femora in 35 per cent. Skull involvement is rare.

Sclerotic metastases are very common in carcinoma of prostate and carcinoid tumours, but are found less frequently in tumours such as mammary, gastro-intestinal, bronchial and vesical carcinomas, osteosarcoma and lymphoma.

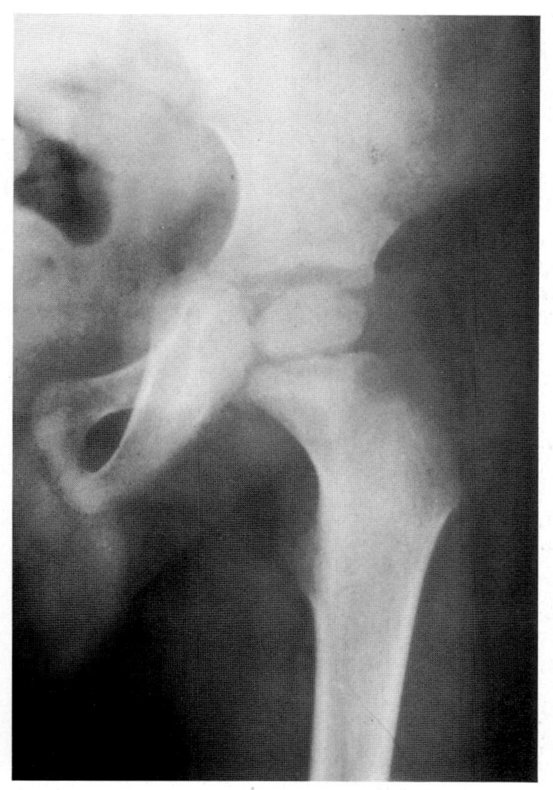 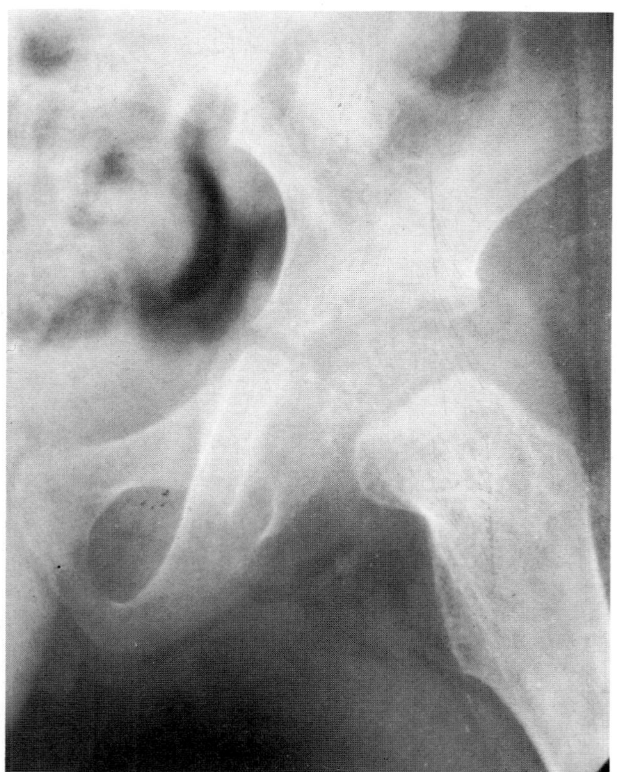

This 3-year-old child presented with a painful limp. The left film was obtained at presentation, the right film nine months later.

- Would you consider a differential diagnosis?

- What is the usual radiological outcome of this condition?

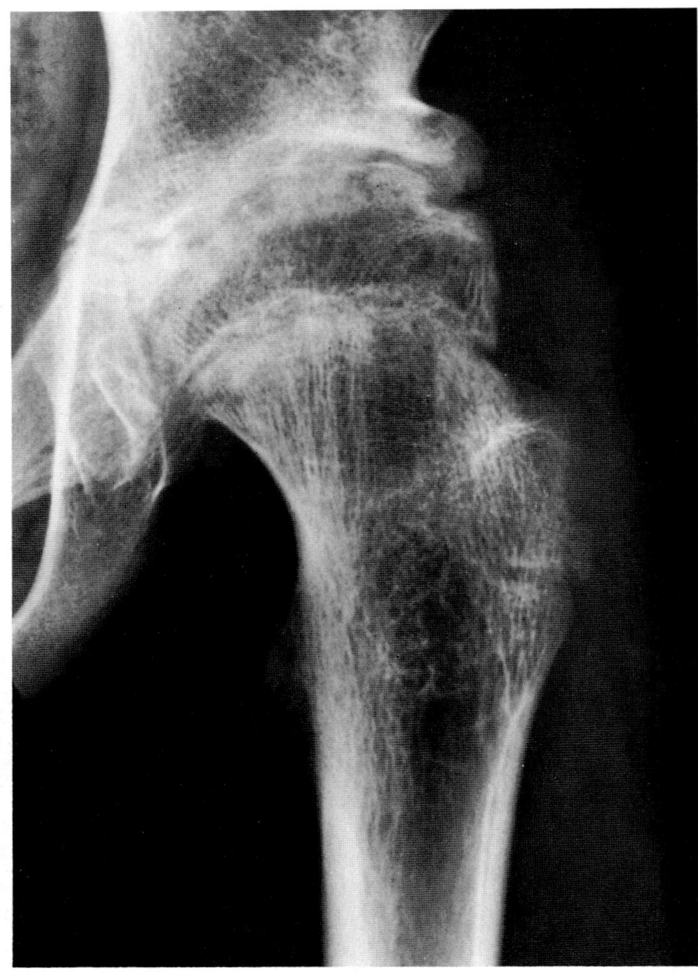

The initial film shows periarticular osteoporosis and marginal erosions around the left hip but no loss of the articular cartilage. The osteoporotic and erosive changes would be in keeping with an inflammatory or septic arthritis but these conditions are almost always associated with an early loss of joint space. Preservation of the joint space in this patient is strongly suggestive of **tuberculous synovitis**, although differentiation from monarticular chronic arthritis of childhood (Still's disease) can be difficult. Culture of aspirated joint fluid is essential.

Anti-tuberculous treatment was started. Nine months later, the bony trabecular pattern had coarsened due to prolonged osteoporosis, but the bony density was starting to improve. The bony articular surfaces had become irregular, while the left capital epiphysis was smaller than the right.

The appearances eight years later are shown above. The abnormal bone texture persists. The capital epiphysis has become wide and flattened (coxa magna luxans) and incomplete ankylosis has developed at the hip joint. These are all typical features of tuberculosis of the hip, the most frequently affected joint. The peak incidence at this site is in the 3-10 year age group.

Reference

Chapman, M., Murray, R. O. and Stoker, D. J. (1979) Tuberculosis of the bones and joints. *Semin. in Roentgenol.*, **14**, 266-282.

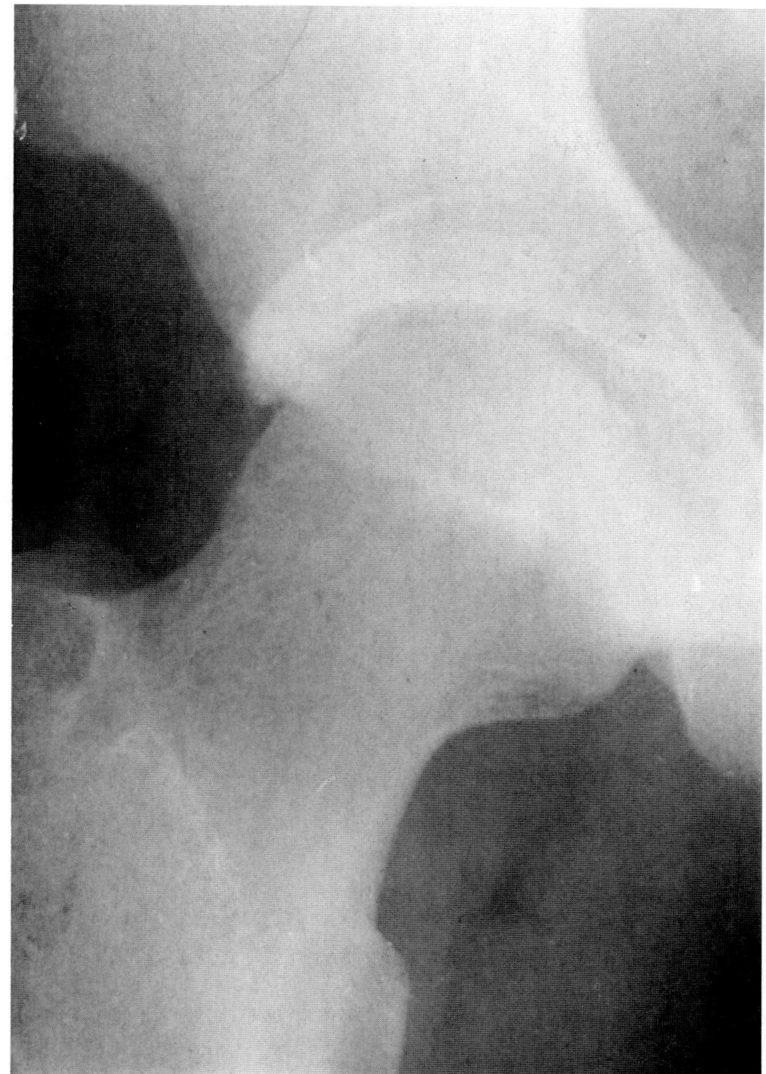

This young man was a front seat passenger involved in a road traffic accident. He was not wearing a seat belt. On examination his right leg was internally rotated and adducted.

- Describe the radiological appearance.

- What is the probable diagnosis?

- Suggest another view to confirm this.

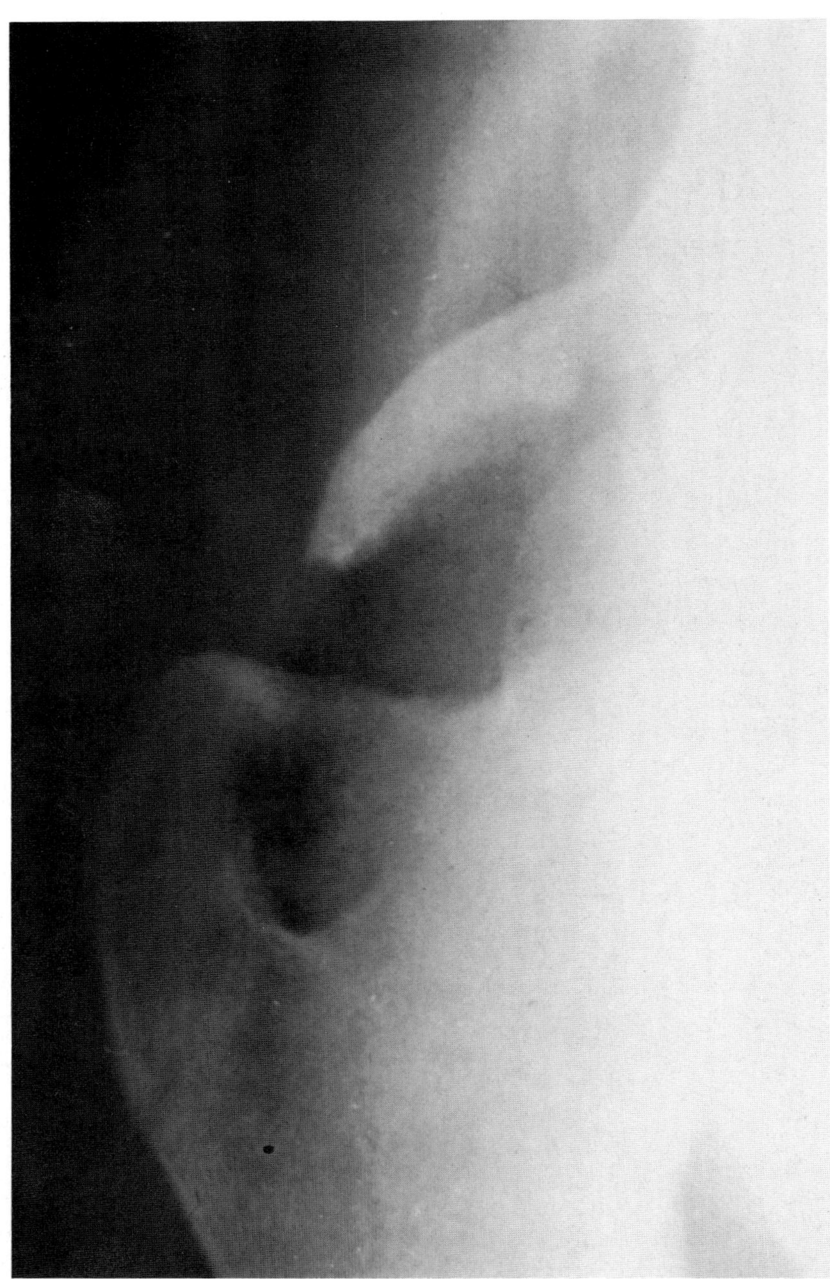

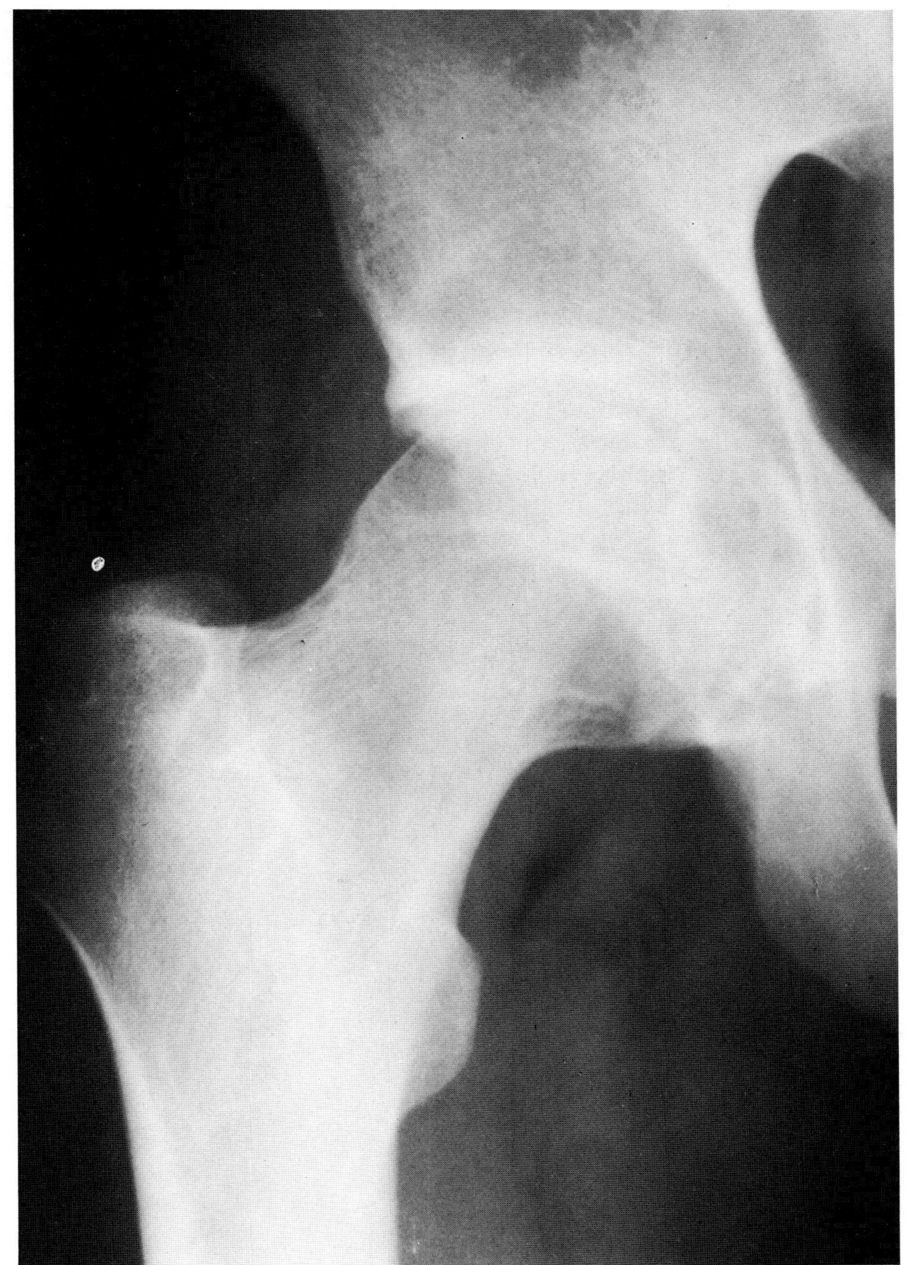

A34

The AP view of the right hip shows a reduction in the superior joint space and a double density projected over the acetabular roof. The appearances are due to a direct posterior dislocation of the femoral head with an associated fracture of the posterior wall of the acetabulum. An oblique view (see page 84) confirms the diagnosis and demonstrates the fracture.

The diagnosis of a posterior dislocation may not always be easy on an AP projection. In most cases the femoral head is displaced out of the acetabulum in a postero-superior direction and the femur is rotated medially so that the lesser trochanter is less visible than normal. However, if the head is dislocated or subluxated directly posteriorly, it may appear to lie within the acetabulum; the only diagnostic clues may be the lack of congruity of the joint margins seen in this patient and/or persisting internal rotation of the femur. Oblique views will usually show both the dislocation and the associated acetabular fracture.

Approximately 85 per cent of hip dislocations and fracture-dislocations are posterior. They occur when an anterior force is applied to the knee while the hip is flexed, e.g. when the knee of a car passenger hits the dashboard. Most patients over 30 will have an associated posterior acetabular fracture and, in younger patients, fracture is more likely to occur if the femur is also abducted. Fractures of the femoral head and shaft also may occur.

Long term complications may arise; a radiograph taken two years after reduction in this patient (see page 85) shows early degenerative change at the hip joint. Avascular necrosis of the femoral head is also a well recognised complication, particularly in the very young and the elderly.

The value of CT in assessment of acetabular fractures is inestimable; small fragments of bone remaining within the hip joint can often only be identified by this imaging technique.

Reference

Whitehouse, G. H. (1978) Radiological aspects of posterior dislocation of the hip. *Clin. Radiol.*, **29**, 431-441.

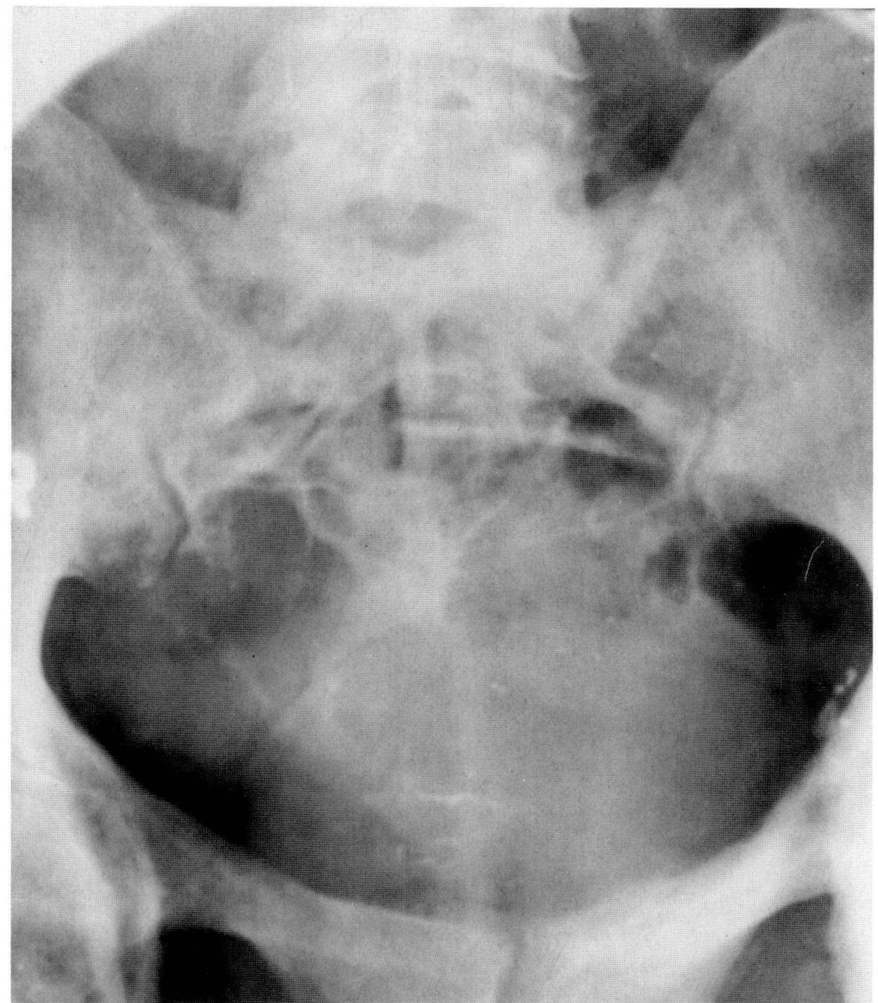

This elderly man complained of low back pain and constipation.

- What abnormalities can you see?
- What is the most likely diagnosis?

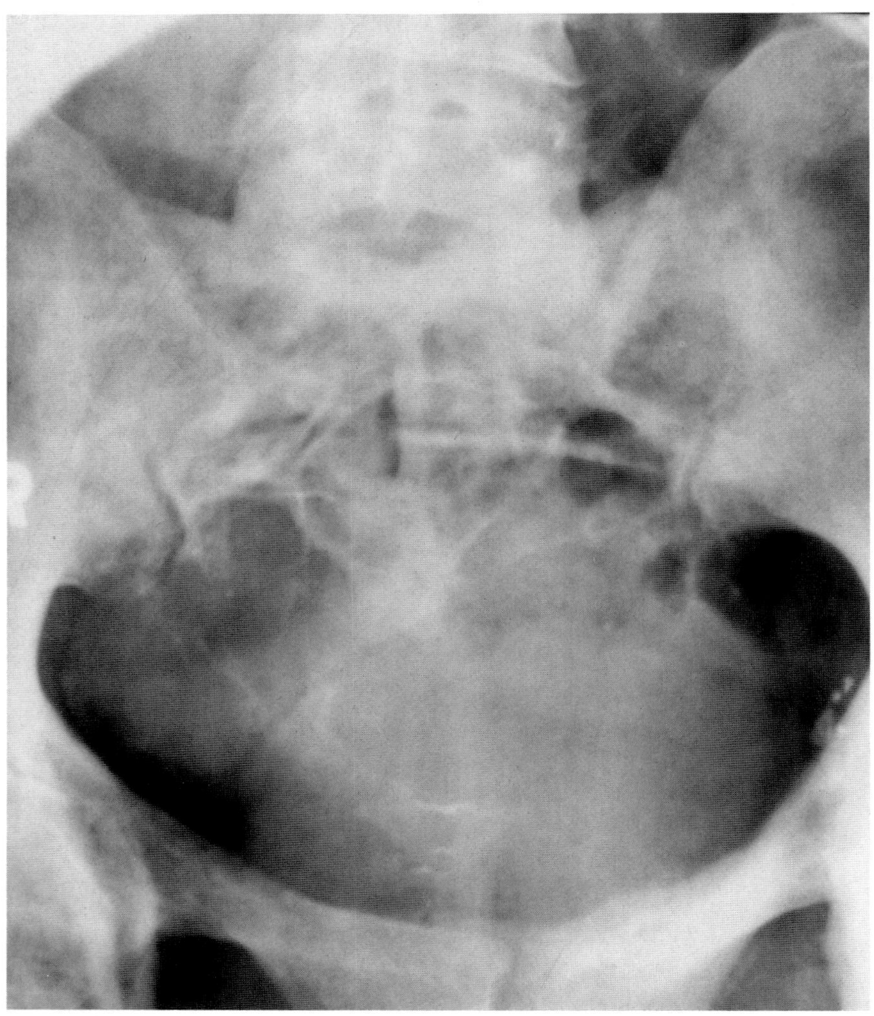

A lytic lesion has destroyed the lower segments of the sacrum. The margins are indistinct with evidence of cortical destruction and a contiguous soft tissue mass. The site and appearances are typical of a chordoma.

This slow-growing, locally aggressive tumour arises in midline structures from ectopic remnants of the notochord. Although no age group is entirely exempt, most of those affected are adults, with the greatest incidence between 40 and 70 years. Favoured sites are the sacrococcygeal region (over half the cases), the clivus (basisphenoid) and the first two cervical vertebrae. The tumour spreads by local extension and is usually fatal, although metastases are rare. The extent of the lesion and its soft tissue extension are best recorded by computed tomography. Sacrococcygeal chordomas show calcification in only a minority of cases on the plain radiograph.

In this patient the thickening of the right iliopectineal line and sclerotic enlargement of the left superior pubic ramus are due to incidental Paget's disease and should not be mistaken for metastatic spread.

Reference

Sundaresan, N. (1986) Chordomas. *Clin. Orthop.*, **204**, 135-142.

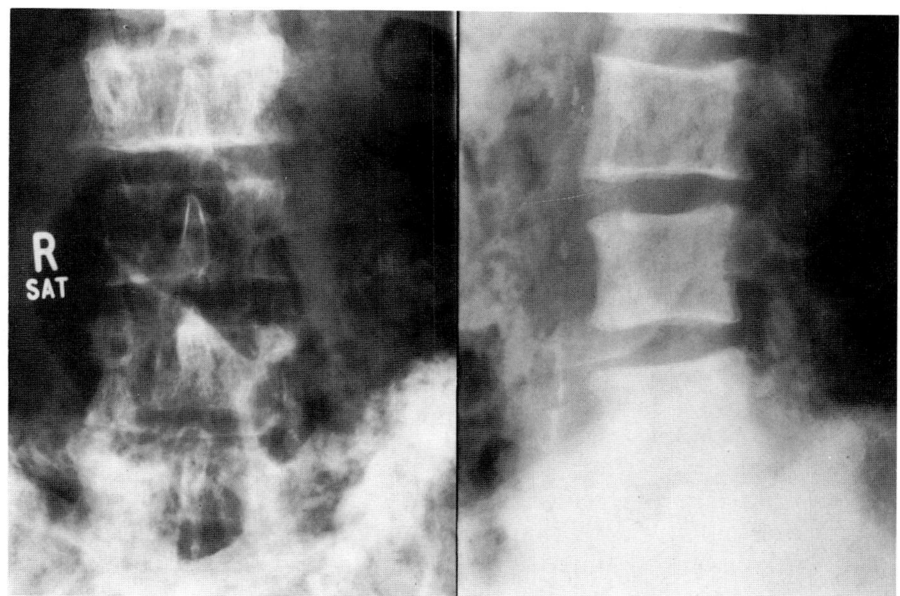

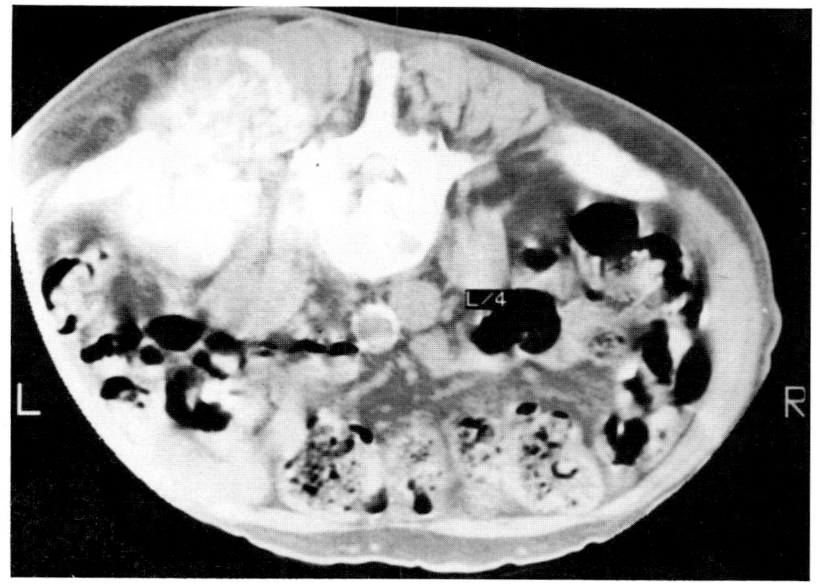

This 70-year-old man was admitted for investigation of painful proptosis of three months duration. While in hospital, he developed low back pain.

- What is the cause of his back pain?

- How might the proptosis be related?

A36

The plain radiographs show the enlargement, sclerosis and coarse trabeculation of the lumbar vertebral bodies typical of Paget's disease. Florid sclerosis is present in the left ilium and the iliac crest is also dense and irregular.

The recent onset of pain raised the suspicion of sarcomatous change in the Pagetic bone and a CT scan was performed. This shows an expanding, destructive lesion in the left iliac crest and body of L4 with an associated soft tissue mass containing new bone formation. Biopsy of this area and of an orbital mass showed osteosarcoma at both these sites.

Although the prevalence of sarcomatous change in Paget's disease reported in the literature varies from 1 to 10 per cent, many series are highly selective and it is likely that the true prevalence of sarcomatous change is well below one per cent. Most sarcomas occur in the femur, pelvis and humerus and comprise osteosarcomas (50-60 per cent), fibrosarcomas (20-25 per cent) and chondrosarcomas (10 per cent). The clinical signs indicating malignant change are soft tissue swelling and pain. Multiple sarcomas may be present, as in this patient. They are thought to be independent in origin and not due to metastatic spread.

Little firm evidence exists to suggest that the incidence of sarcomatous change is related to the extent of involvement of the skeleton by the pre-existing Paget's disease.

Reference

Greditzer, H. G., McLeod, R. A., Unni, K. K. and Beabout, J. W. (1983) Bone sarcomas in Paget disease. *Radiology*, **146**, 327-333.

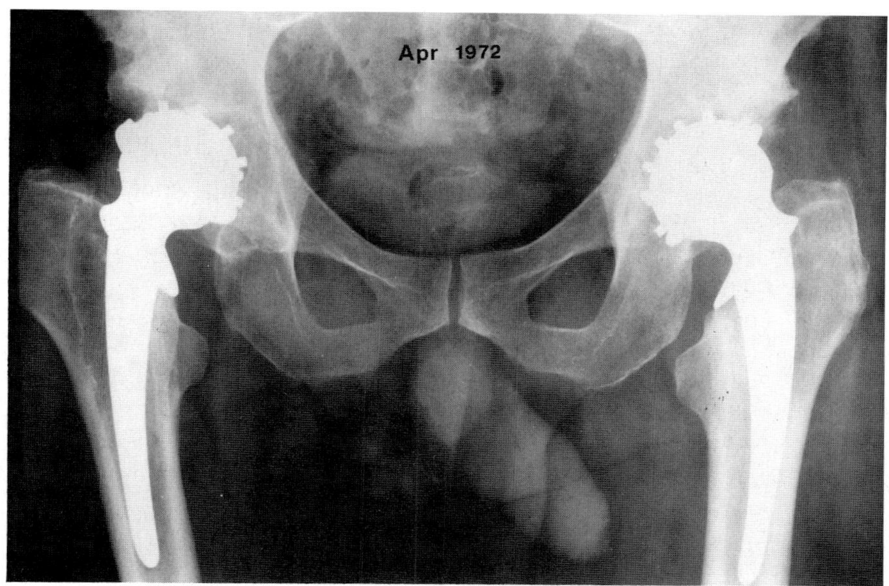

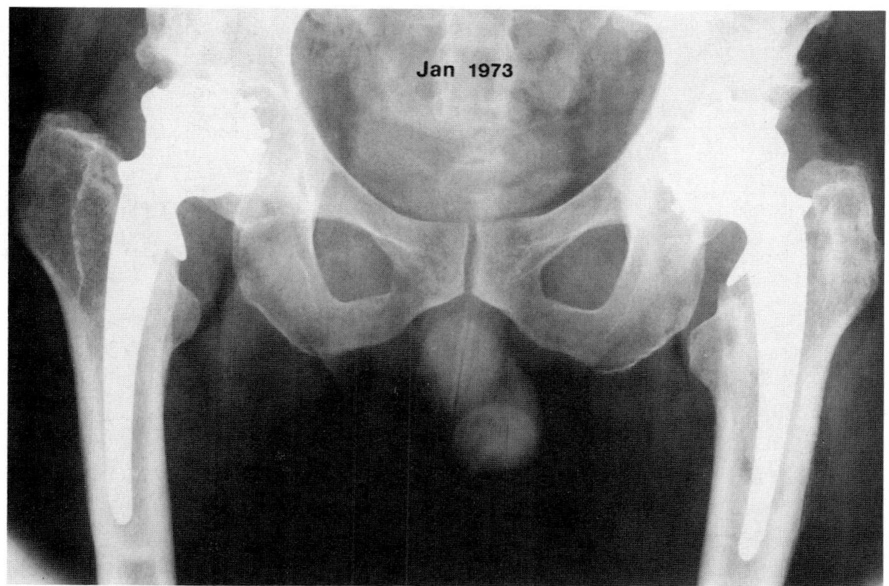

This 52-year-old man complained of pain in his left hip and discharge from the operative wound 15 months after a total hip replacement for osteoarthritis. A film taken at this time (January 1973) is shown with an earlier film for comparison.

- What is the cause of his pain?

- What radiological technique may be used to confirm the diagnosis?

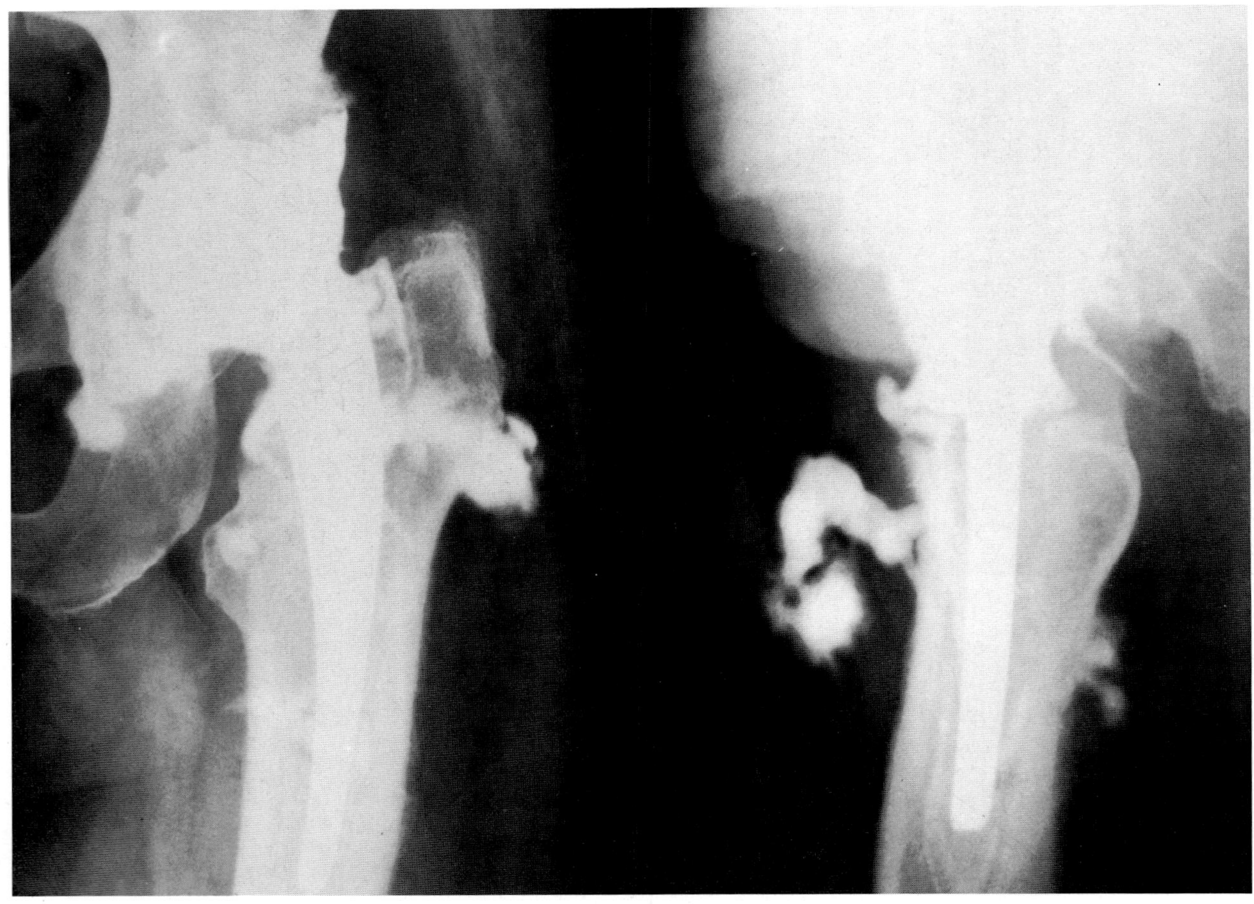

The earlier film shows the normal post-surgical appearances of the bilateral McKee-Farrar total hip replacements. Eight months later, lucencies have appeared in the left femur adjacent to the prosthesis, suggesting loosening and/or infection. A sinus discharging through the skin incision supports the possibility of infection. An arthrogram was performed; loosening of the femoral component was confirmed by the tracking of contrast alongside it, at the bone-cement interface. Contrast also outlined the sinus track, demonstrating communication with the joint space.

Following hip replacement, regular serial films are obtained to check the position of the acetabular and femoral components and assess any possible subluxation, loosening or infection, especially when painful symptoms appear. The prostheses shown are held in position with methyl methacrylate, a radiolucent cement sometimes rendered opaque with barium. Initially, no gap is demonstrable between the methacrylate and bone, but the formation of a fibrous reaction often results in the appearance of a fine 1-2 mm radiolucent line, usually within one year. Any increase in the width of this line, development of new focal lucencies, or change in position of the prosthesis suggests loosening. Serial films are desirable as subtle changes may only be detected by comparison with earlier films. Scintigraphy may prove to be another helpful investigation in these circumstances.

Reference

Freedman, M. D. (1979) *The Radiology of the Postoperative Hip.* John Wiley & Sons, London.

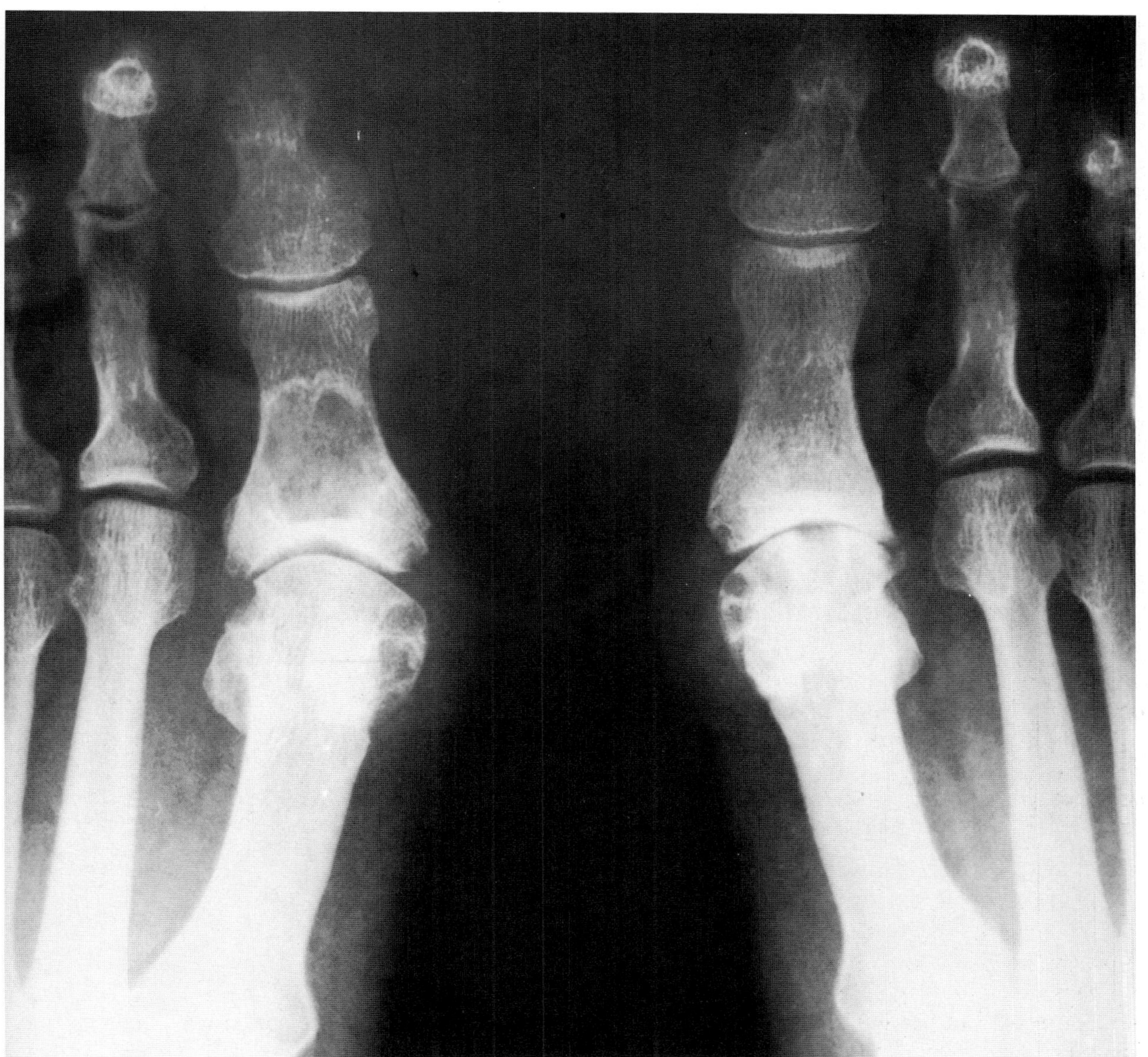

This man suffered from painful feet.

- What is the diagnosis?
- Is the condition of recent origin?

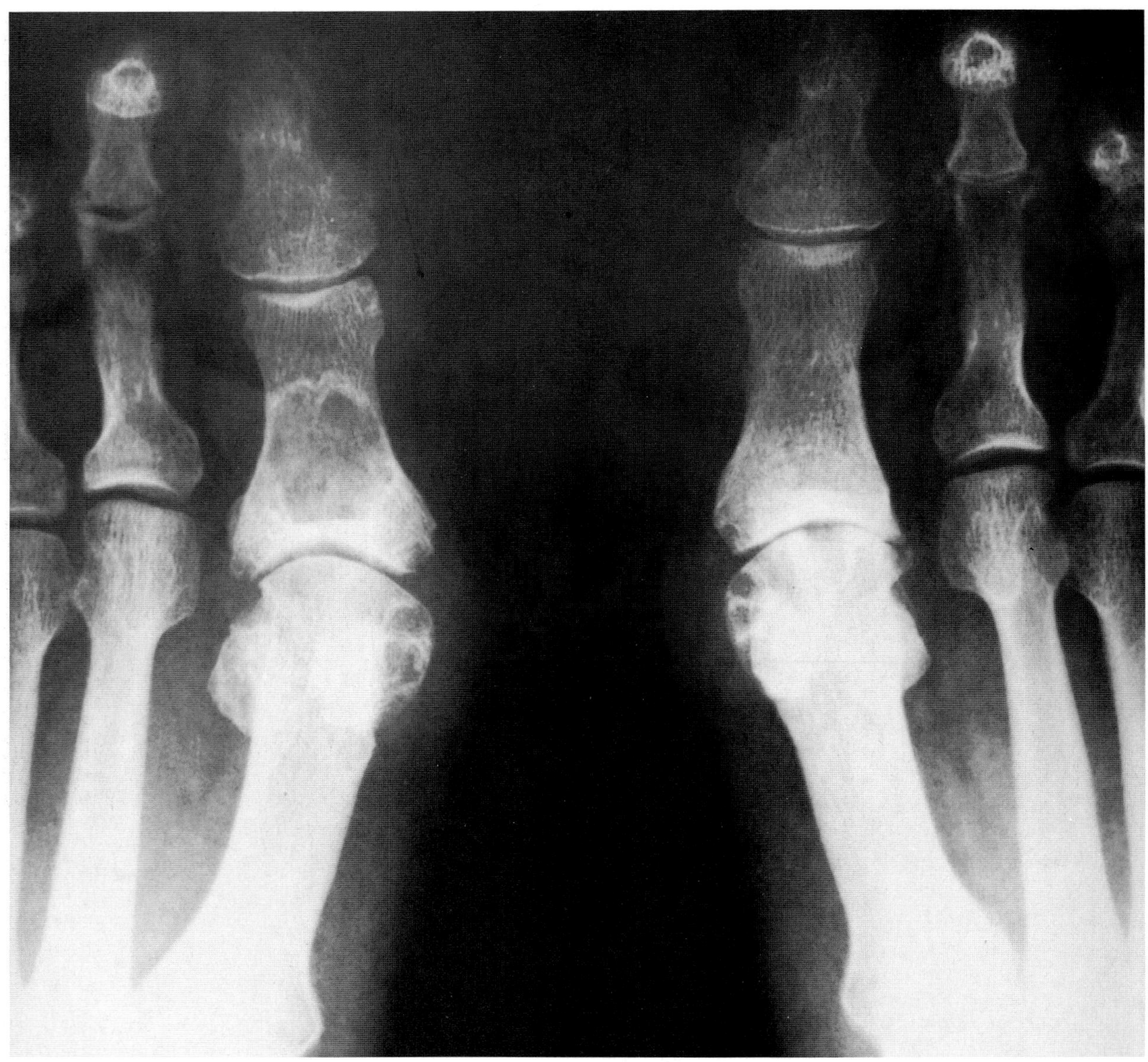

The punched-out erosions of varying sizes around the first metatarsophalangeal joints and the normal bony density are typical features of gout (Podagra). The joint space in gout tends to be preserved until late in the disease; the narrowing in this case suggests longstanding disease and, indeed, the patient had suffered from gout for 18 years. Features to be observed in this case are the intraosseous tophus of the proximal phalanx of the left great toe and the erosion of the central subchondral bone of the right first metatarsal.

The first metatarsophalangeal joint is often the initial site of involvement and is ultimately affected in 75-90 per cent of patients. During the first episodes of gout, no radiological bony changes may be present. Erosions often only appear after years of intermittent arthritis.

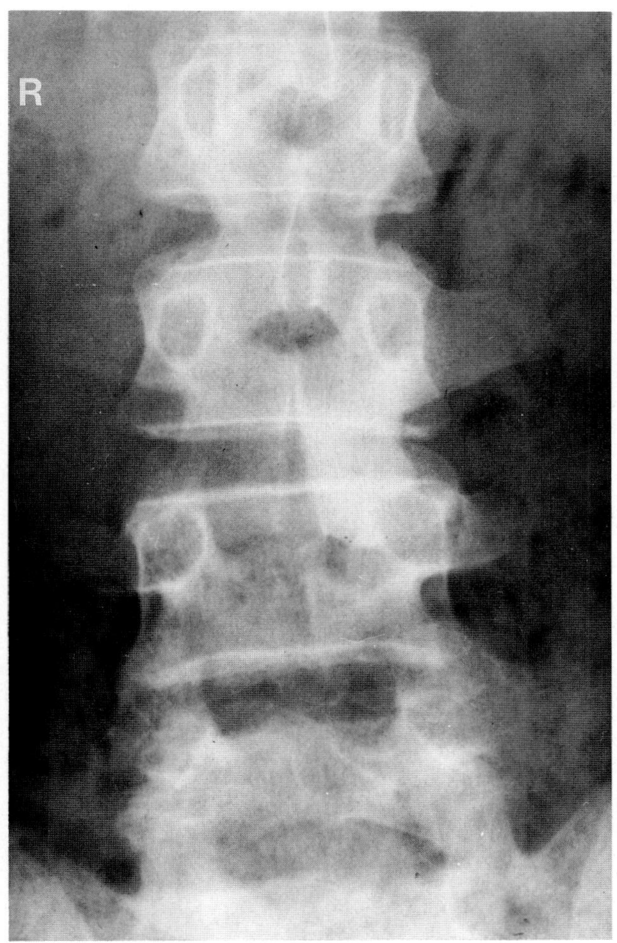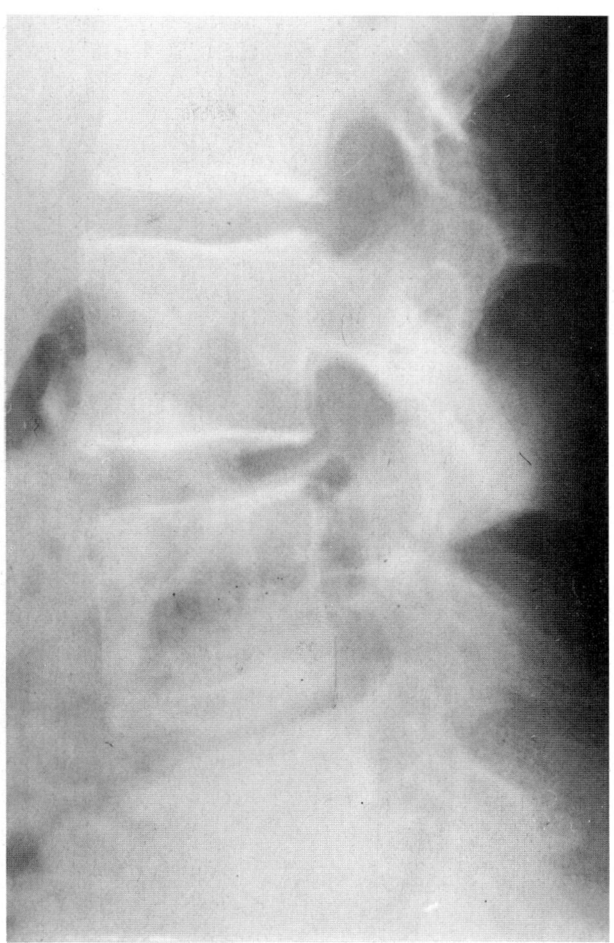

This 16-year-old boy gave a one-year history of low back pain. Examination revealed a mild scoliosis and an area of localised tenderness in the lumbar spine.

- What diagnosis can you suggest?
- Are the findings typical?

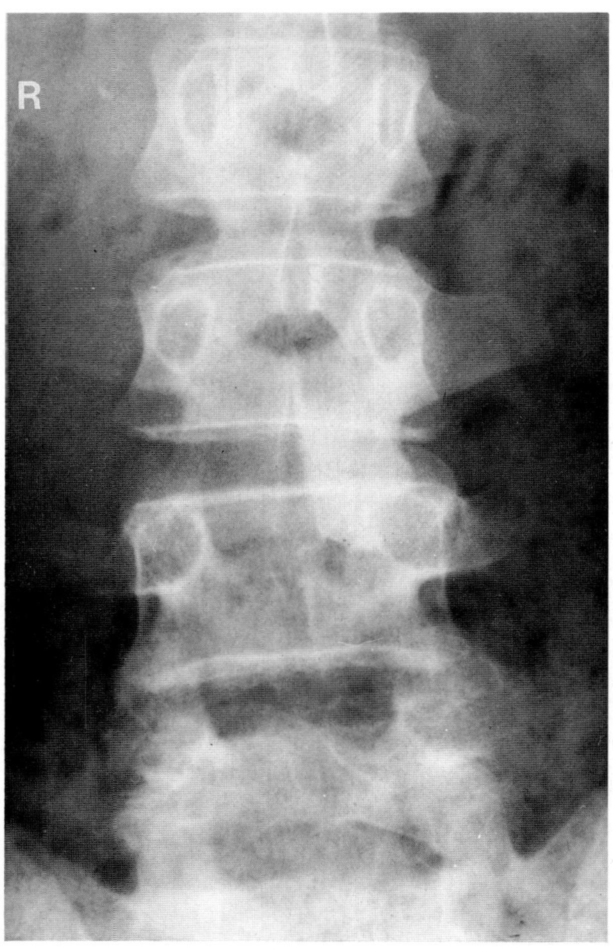

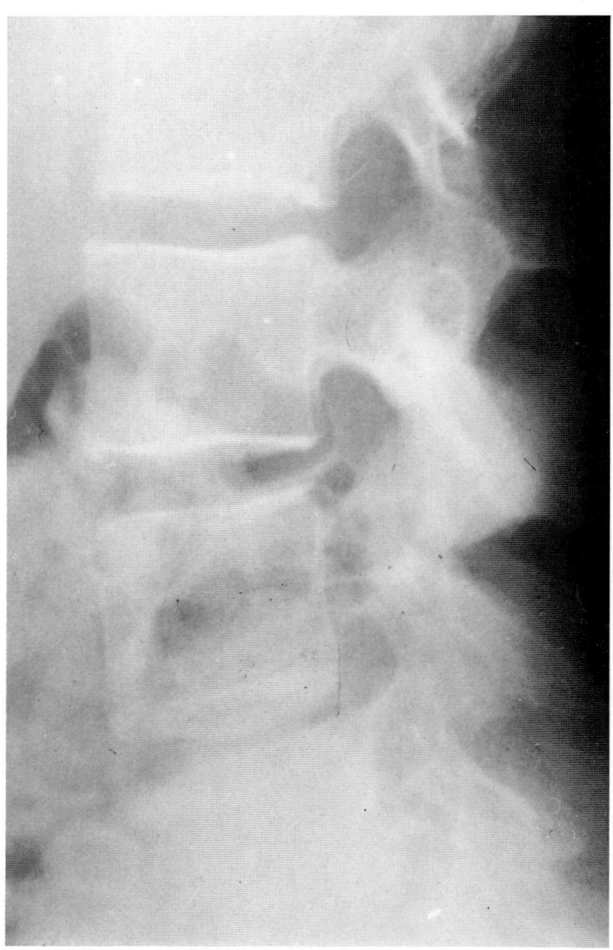

A mild right-sided scoliosis is centred at the L3/4 level with increased density of the left lamina of L3. The appearances are consistent with the presence of an osteoblastoma, a benign neoplasm which, in the spine, is usually accompanied by a scoliosis due to painful muscular spasm. Osteoid osteoma may produce a similar appearance.

Osteoblastomas are histologically similar to osteoid osteomas but larger, and not usually as painful. Thirty to forty per cent occur in the spine, most frequently in the posterior elements. The peak incidence is in the second and third decades and the mode of presentation in this patient is typical.

Reference

Marsh, B. W., Bonfiglio, M., Brady, L. P. and Enneking, W. F. (1975) Benign osteoblastoma: range of manifestations. *J. Bone Joint Surg.*, 57-A, 1-9.

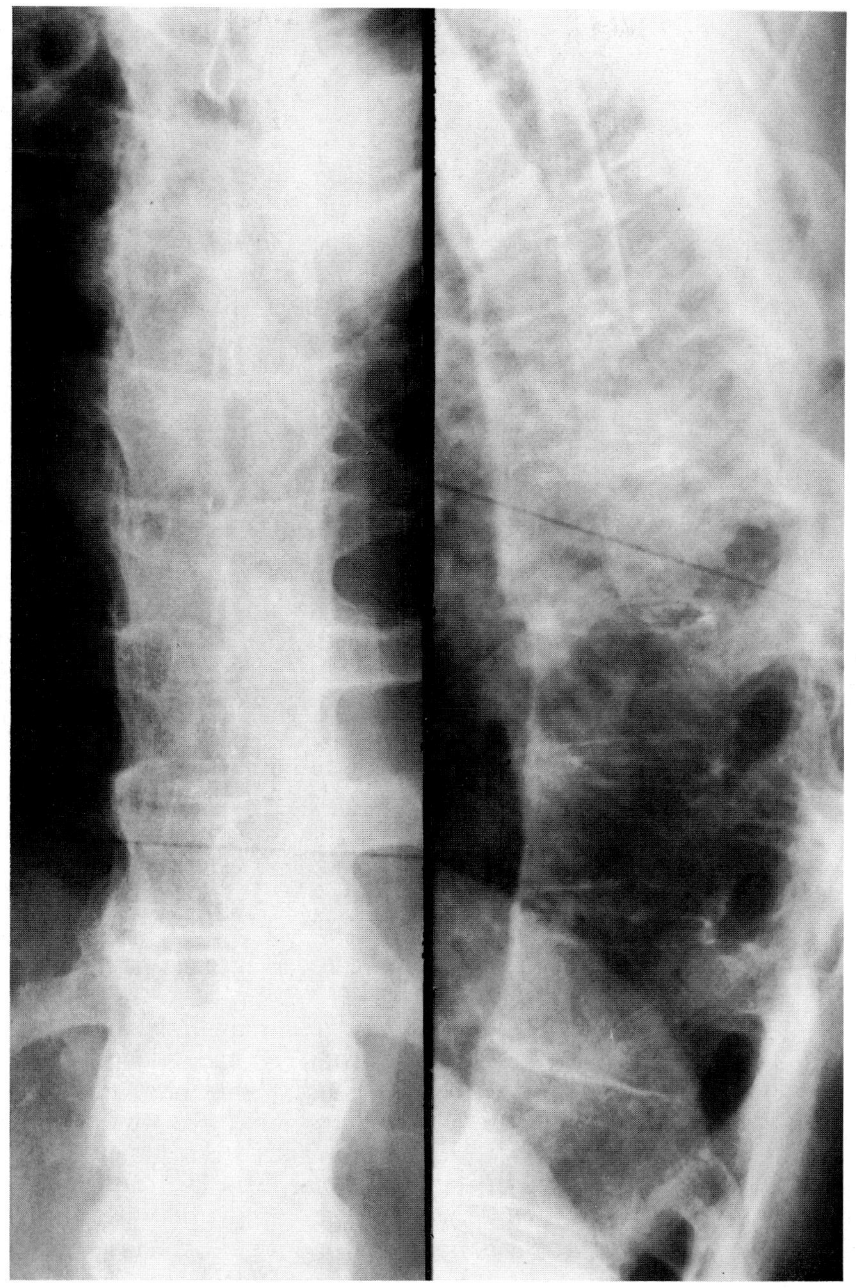

This 60-year-old man complained of back pain following a fall in the street.

- What abnormalities can you see on the radiographs?

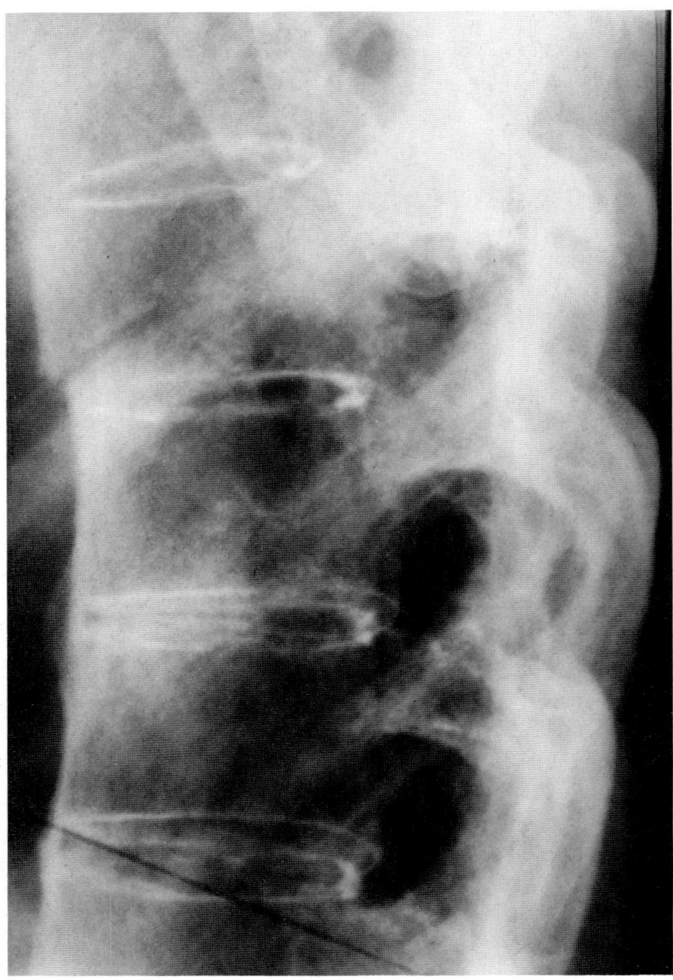

This man has ankylosing spondylitis and his pain is due to a fracture-dislocation through the body of T7.

In ankylosing spondylitis, ossification of the superficial fibres of the anulus fibrosus of the intervertebral discs results in fine vertical bony spurs (syndesmophytes), which span the disc and become continuous with the margins of the vertebral bodies. Further ossification in the paraspinal ligaments and ankylosis of the apophyseal joints combine to produce a rigid 'bamboo' spine. Note the calcification of the intervertebral disc in association with ankylosis.

The increased incidence of spinal fractures in ankylosing spondylitis, especially in the cervical spine, is related to the rigidity and co-existing osteoporosis. Fractures often follow minor hyperextension or hyperflexion injuries and are most frequent in the lower cervical spine. Despite the relatively trivial radiological abnormality in association with an undisplaced fracture, all such fractures involve the vertebral body and arch and are essentially unstable fractures or fracture-dislocations.

Reference

Harding, J. R., McCall, I. W., Park, W. M. and Jones, B. F. (1985) Fracture of the cervical spine in ankylosing spondylitis. *Brit. J. Radiol.*, 58, 3-7.

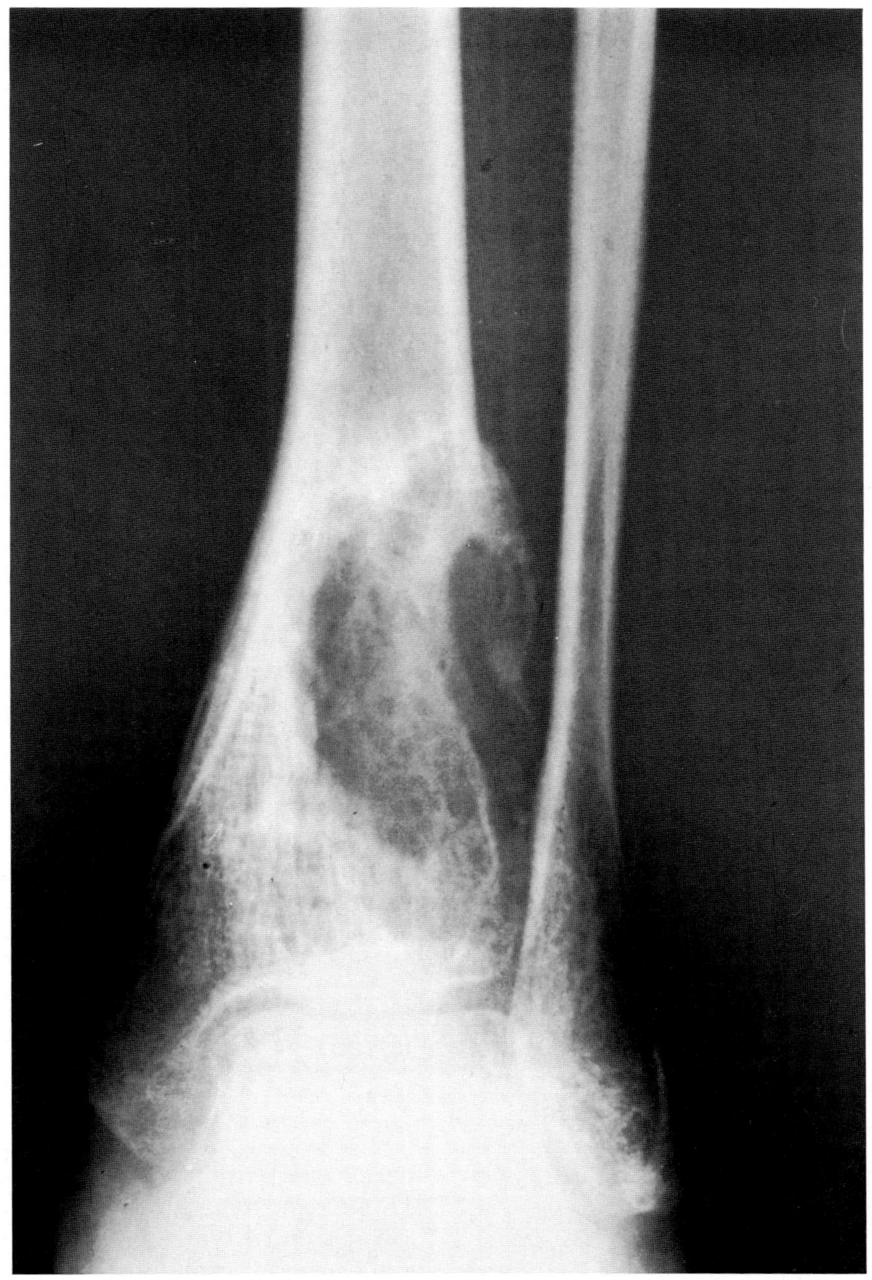

This 19-year-old girl presented with a tender swelling above the ankle.

- Describe the appearances shown in the radiograph.

- What is the most likely diagnosis?

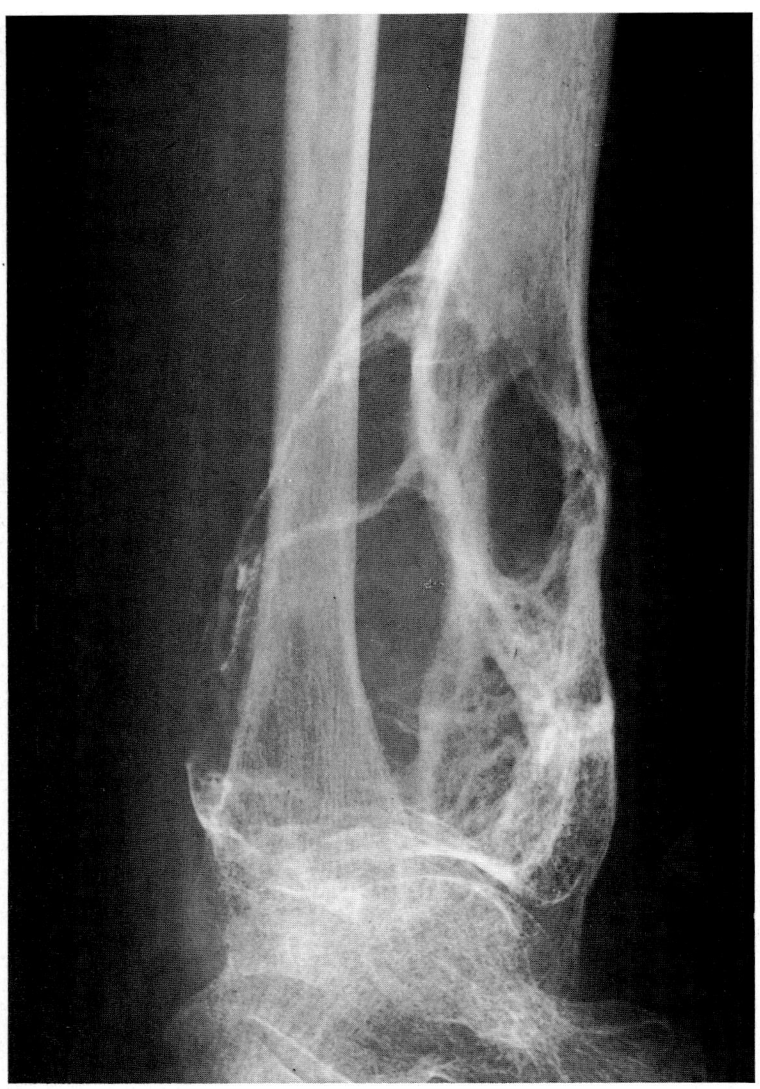

An eccentric, expanded lesion in the distal tibia shows a narrow zone of transition and gives the impression of being septate. It has caused thinning of the cortex medially. No soft tissue extension or calcification of the matrix is present.

The most likely cause for these appearances is an **aneurysmal bone cyst**, but other locally aggressive lesions such as giant-cell tumour and fibrous dysplasia cannot be excluded radiologically. The diagnosis was proven by biopsy. Despite radiotherapy the lesion progressed over two years and a film at this time (above) shows the classical features of this lesion—marked expansion, septation, extreme cortical thinning and a narrow zone of transition.

Aneurysmal bone cysts are neither aneurysms nor cysts but rapidly growing lesions whose septated cavities contain blood. Seventy per cent occur before the age of 20, and 50 per cent are found in the long bones, usually towards the ends. The posterior elements of the vertebrae are also commonly involved.

Reference

Bonakdarpour, A., Levy, W. M. and Aegerter, F. (1978) Primary and secondary aneurysmal bone cysts. A radiological study of 75 cases. *Radiology*, **126**, 75-83.

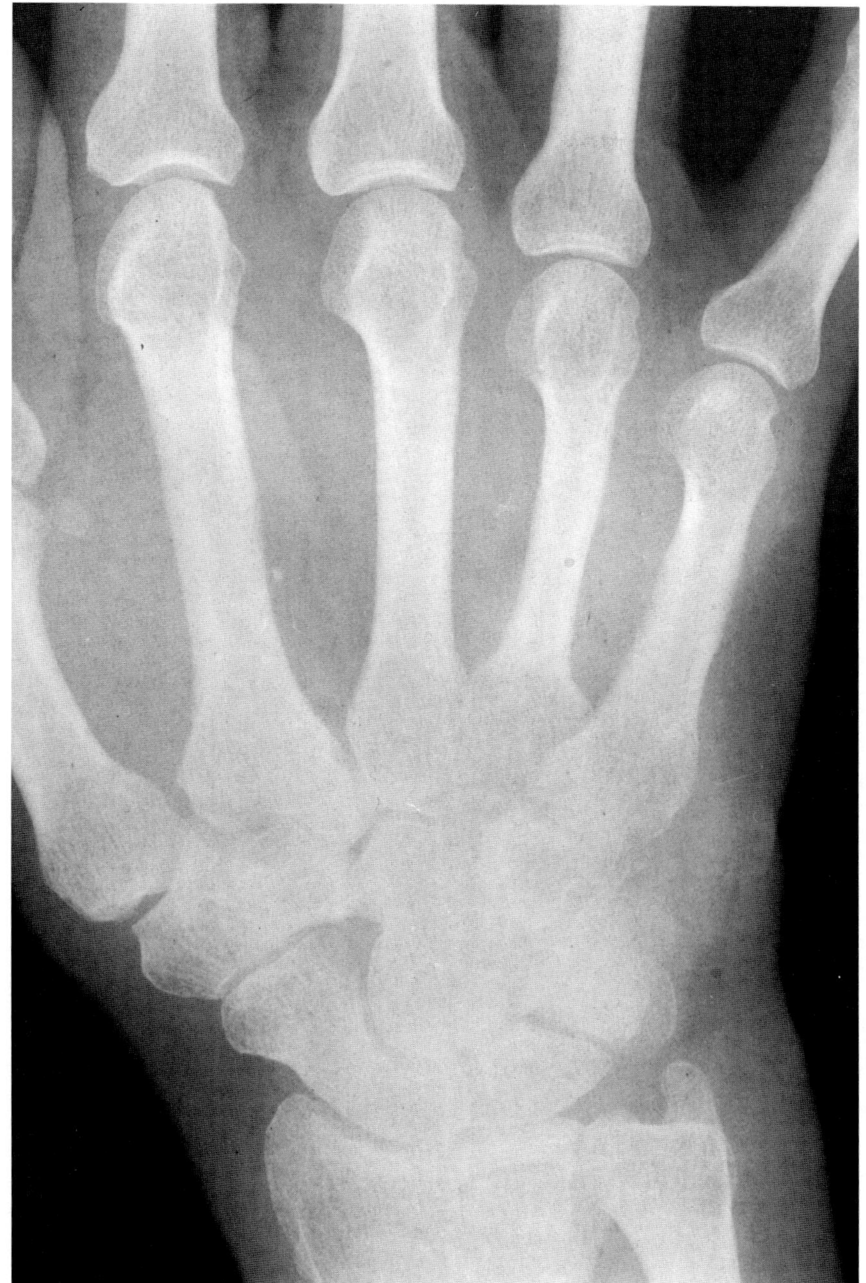

A man aged 51 with a one-year history of joint
pains.

- Describe the important radiological features.
- What is the probable diagnosis?

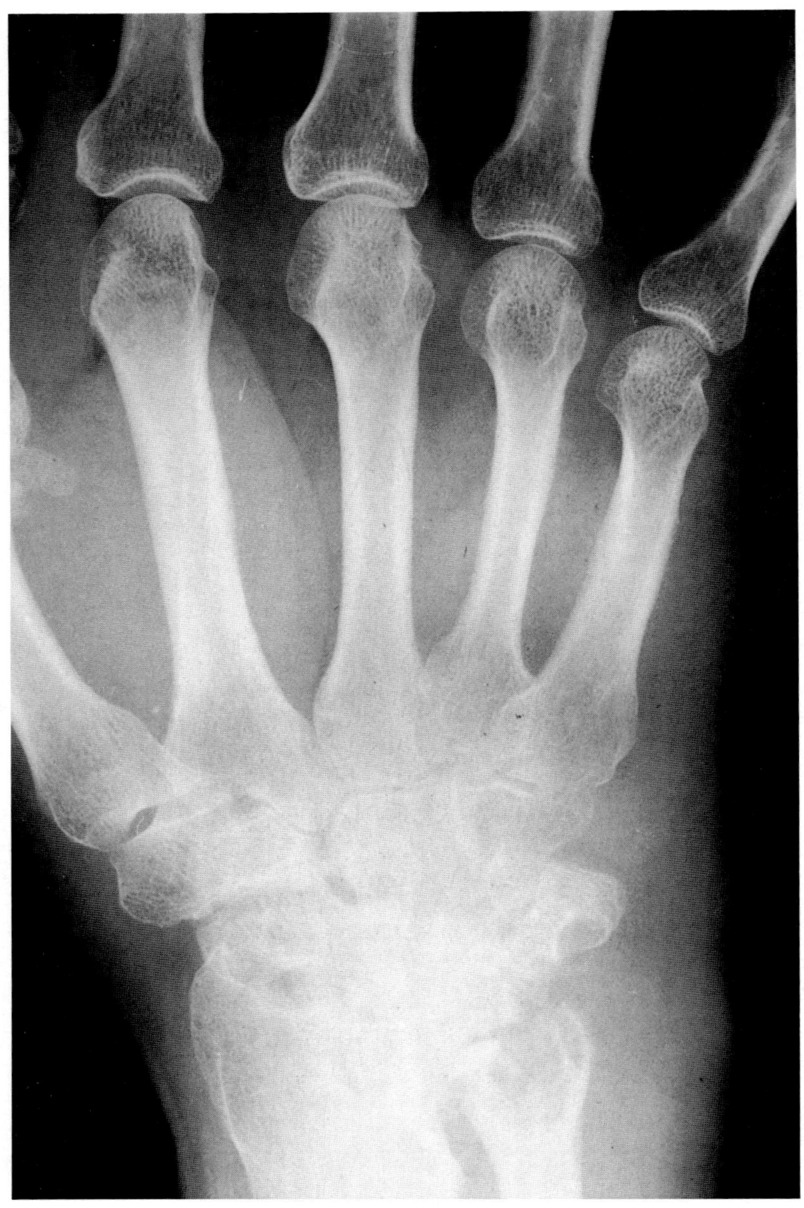

The initial film shows a mild periarticular osteoporosis, soft tissue swelling overlying the ulnar styloid and separating the distal ends of the second and third metacarpals. These are subtle early radiological changes of rheumatoid arthritis; the film above, obtained five years later, shows how the disease has progressed. The ulnar styloid has been destroyed and severe erosive changes affect the distal radio-ulnar joint and proximal row of carpal bones. Erosions are also present at the proximal and distal ends of the second and third metacarpals.

Reference

Martel, W., Hayes, J. T. and Duff, I. F. (1965) The pattern of bone erosion in the hand and wrist in rheumatoid arthritis. *Radiology.* 84, 204-214.

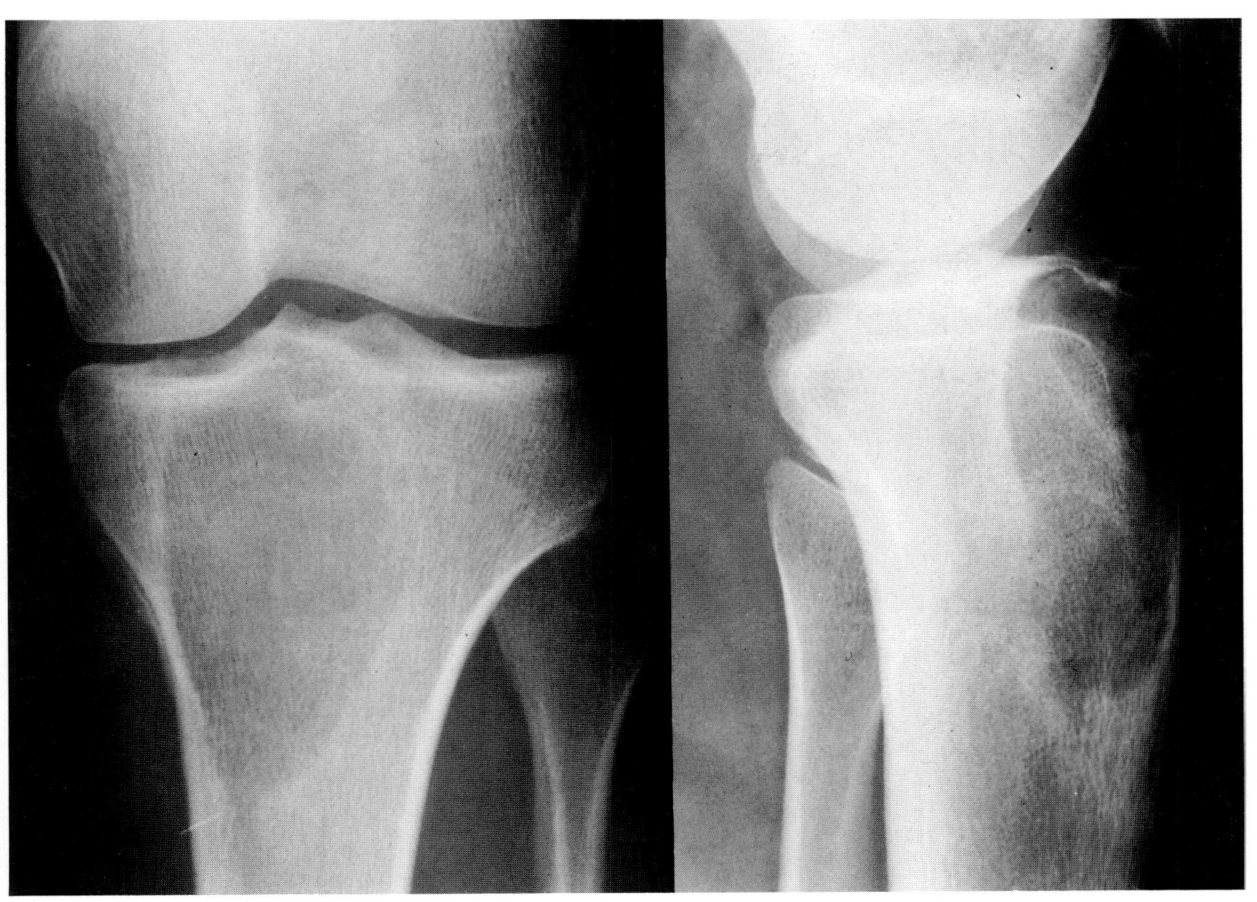

This 19-year-old woman complained of a painful knee one year after a fall.

- What differential diagnosis would you consider?

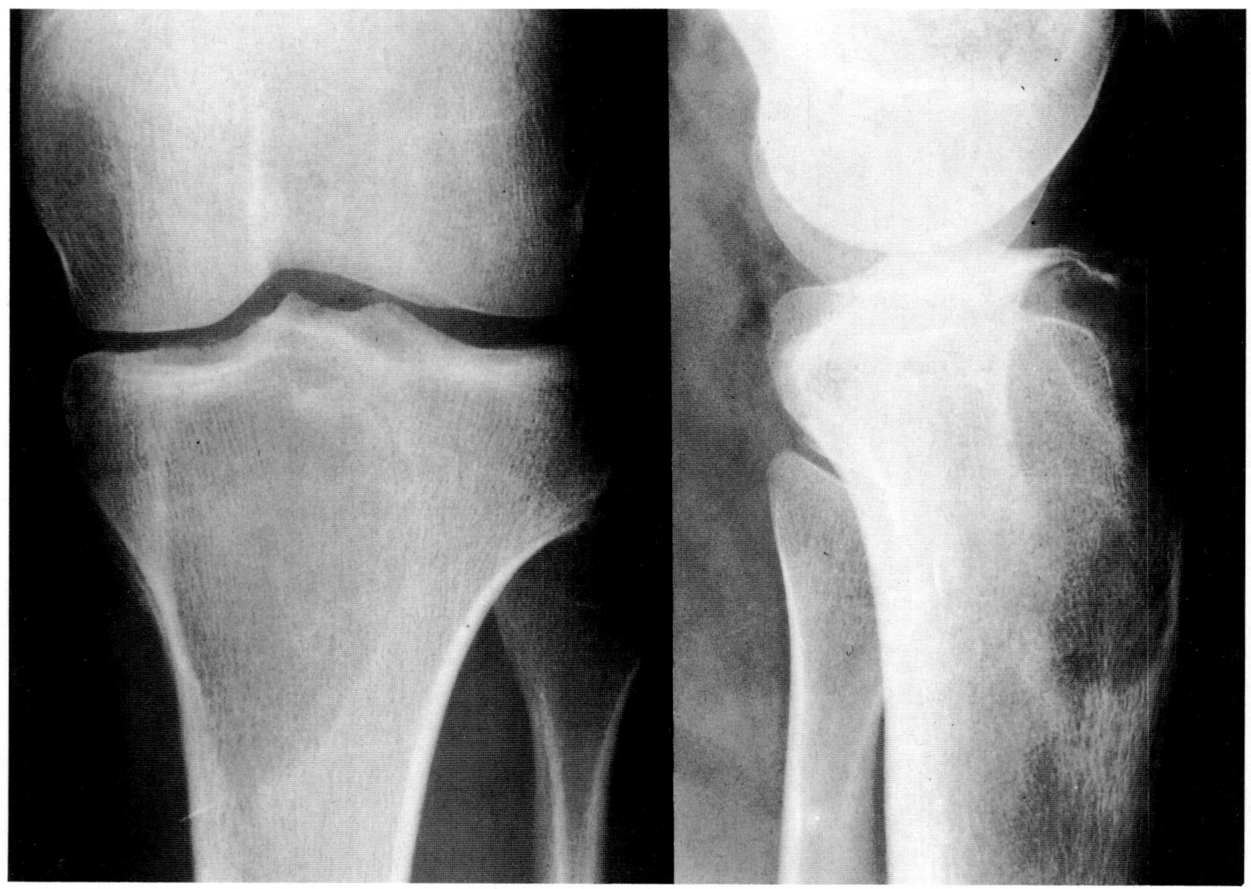

A well-defined lytic lesion is present, lying anteromedially in the proximal end of the tibia and extending to the articular margin. The lesion has thinned the cortex anteriorly and the periosteal reaction seen on the anteroposterior view suggests that it may even have been breached.

The lytic appearance, subarticular site, and age of the patient favour the diagnosis of a giant-cell tumour. An aneurysmal bone cyst is less likely as it would be expected to produce a greater degree of expansion. A biopsy confirmed the diagnosis of a giant-cell tumour. These locally aggressive neoplasms comprise about five per cent of all primary bone tumours and have a peak incidence in young and middle-aged adults. Over 80 per cent present between the ages of 18 and 45 years, and occurrence in childhood is rare. Fifty to sixty per cent are found on one or other side of the knee.

Reference

Eckardt, J. J., Cooper, K. L., Unni, K. K. and Sim, F. H. (1980) Benign giant cell tumor of bone. *Orthopedics*, 3, 1142-1152.

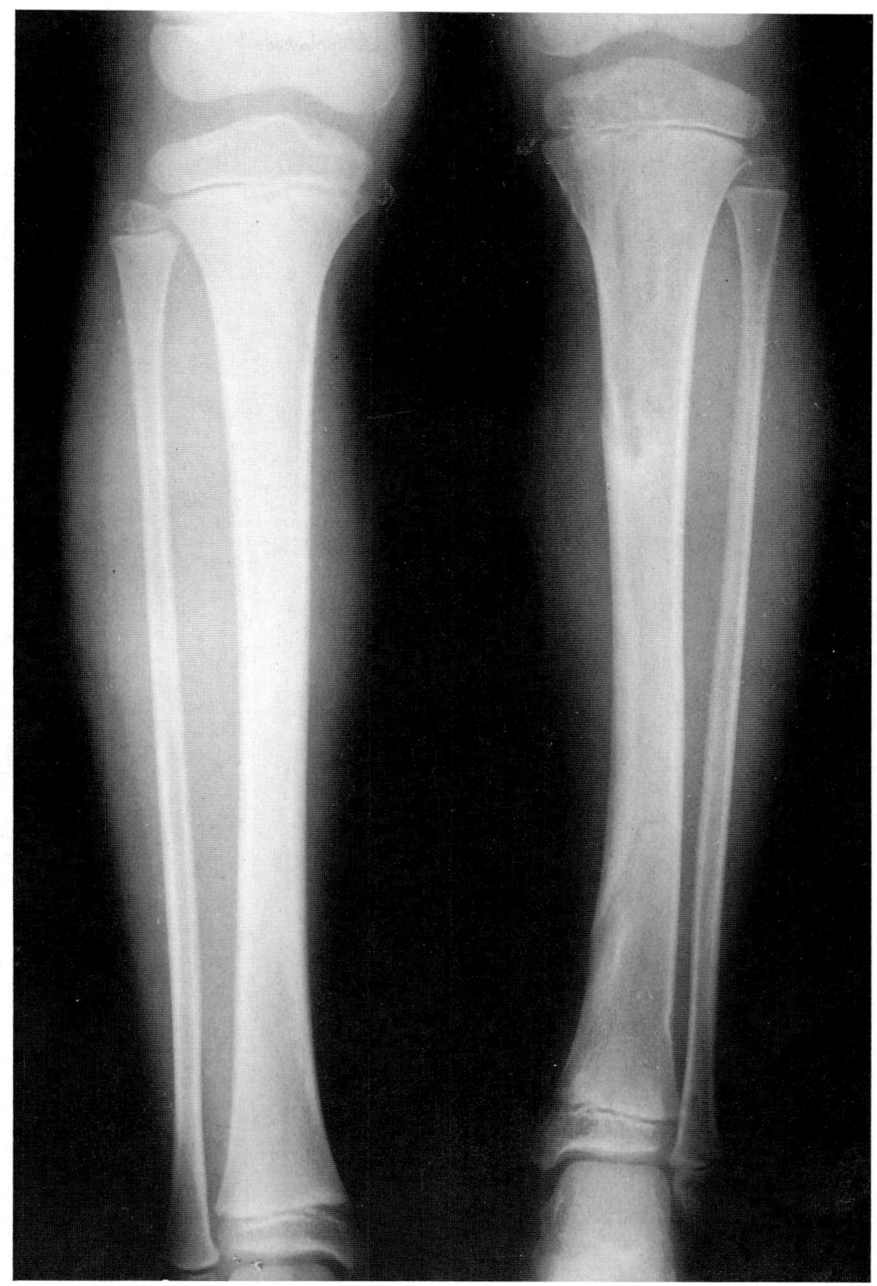

This child presented with legs of unequal length.

- Describe the appearances and suggest the diagnosis.

- What serious complication has been reported in this disorder?

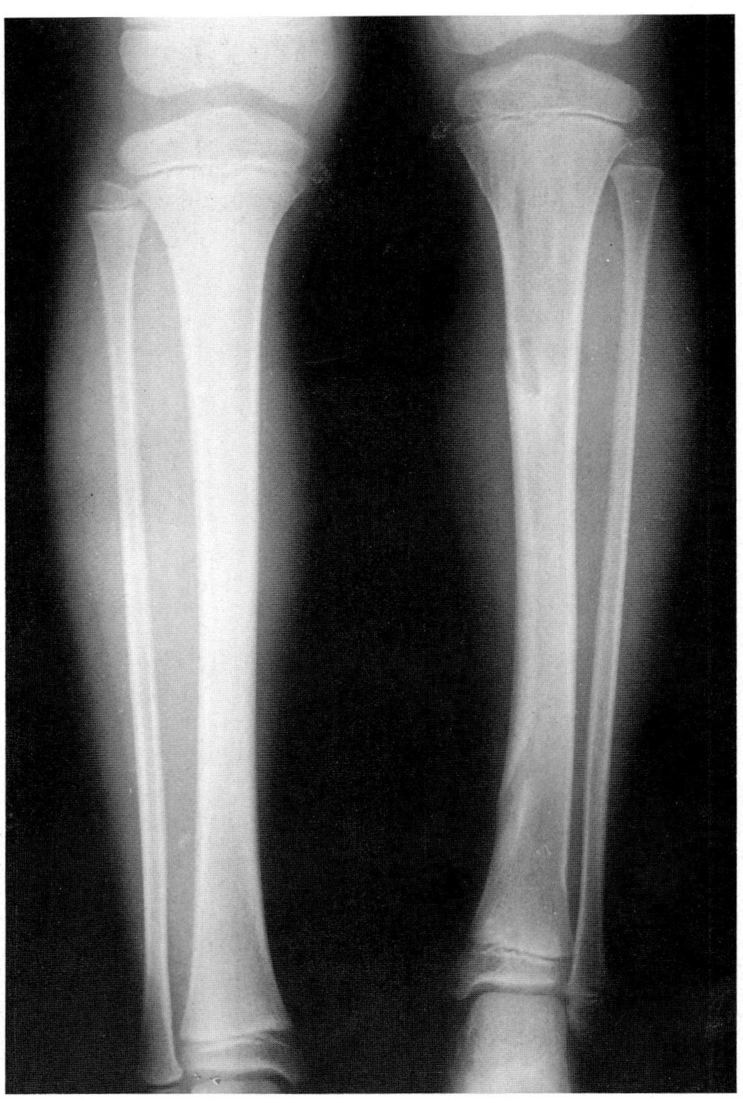

Linear radiolucencies are present in the proximal and distal metaphyses of the left tibia and these extend from the growth plate into the diaphysis. They are due to the persistent cartilaginous tissue found in the non-hereditary condition, enchondromatosis (Ollier's disease).

The distribution is often monomelic (affecting one limb) and asymmetrical within the limb. Impairment of metaphyseal growth in the affected bone often results in unequal limb length, as in this case. Lesions may be expansile, particularly in the hands, and be confused with fibrous dysplasia. Although malignant change is reported in over 20 per cent of cases in some series, these have often been highly selective and the incidence is probably much lower. The incidence of malignancy is higher in the presence of associated soft tissue haemangiomas, when the condition is termed Maffucci's syndrome.

Louis Ollier (1830-1900), a surgeon in Lyons, France, who played an important role in the development of orthopaedic surgery, published the description of a single case of 'dyschondroplasia' in 1889.

Angelo Maffucci (1845-1903) was an Italian physician who described the disorder in 1881.

Reference

Mainzer, F., Minagi, H. and Steinbach, H. (1971) Variable manifestations of multiple enchondromatosis. *Radiology,* 99, 377-388.

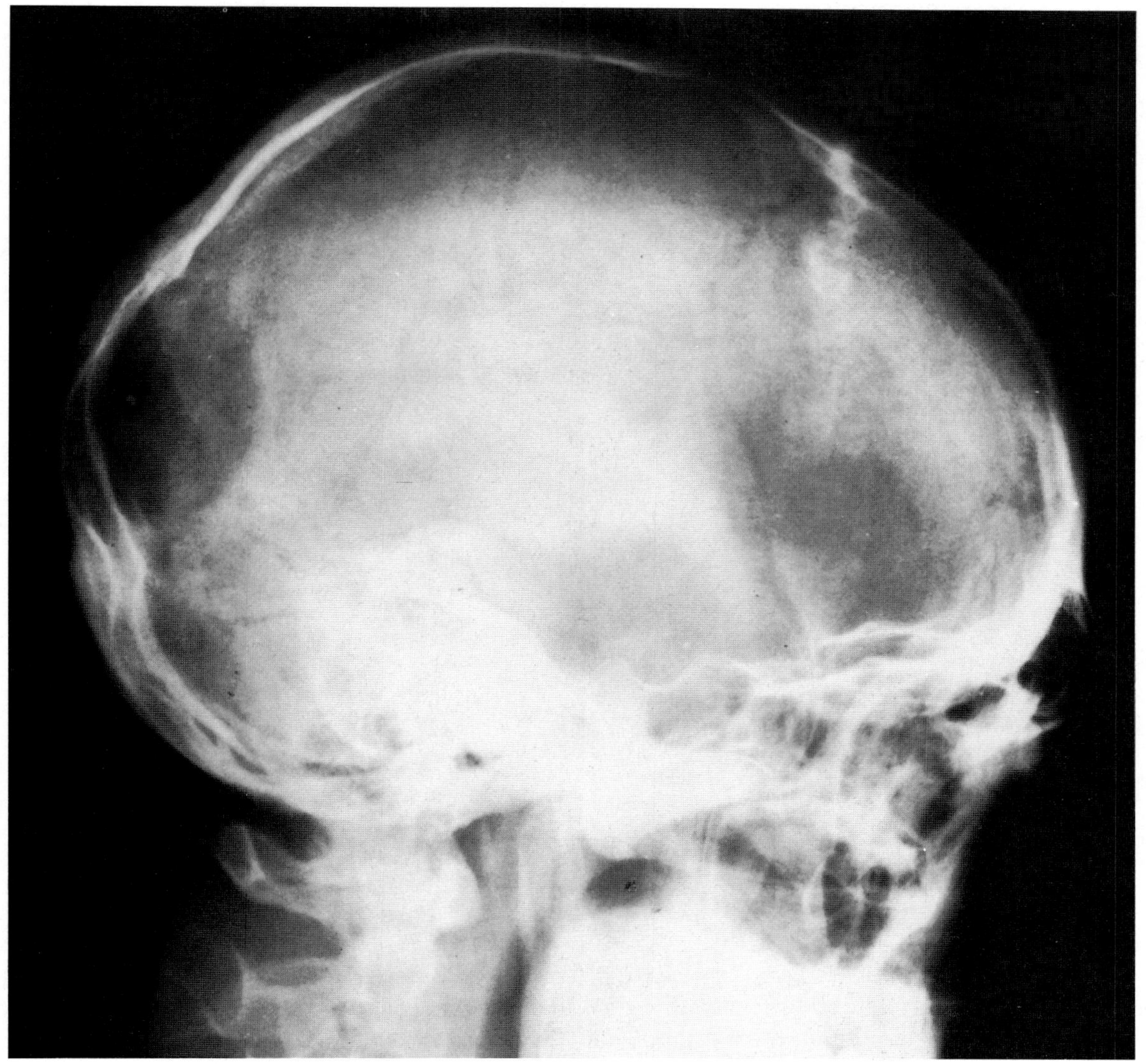

This patient was involved in a road traffic accident.

- How was this view obtained?
- What does it show?

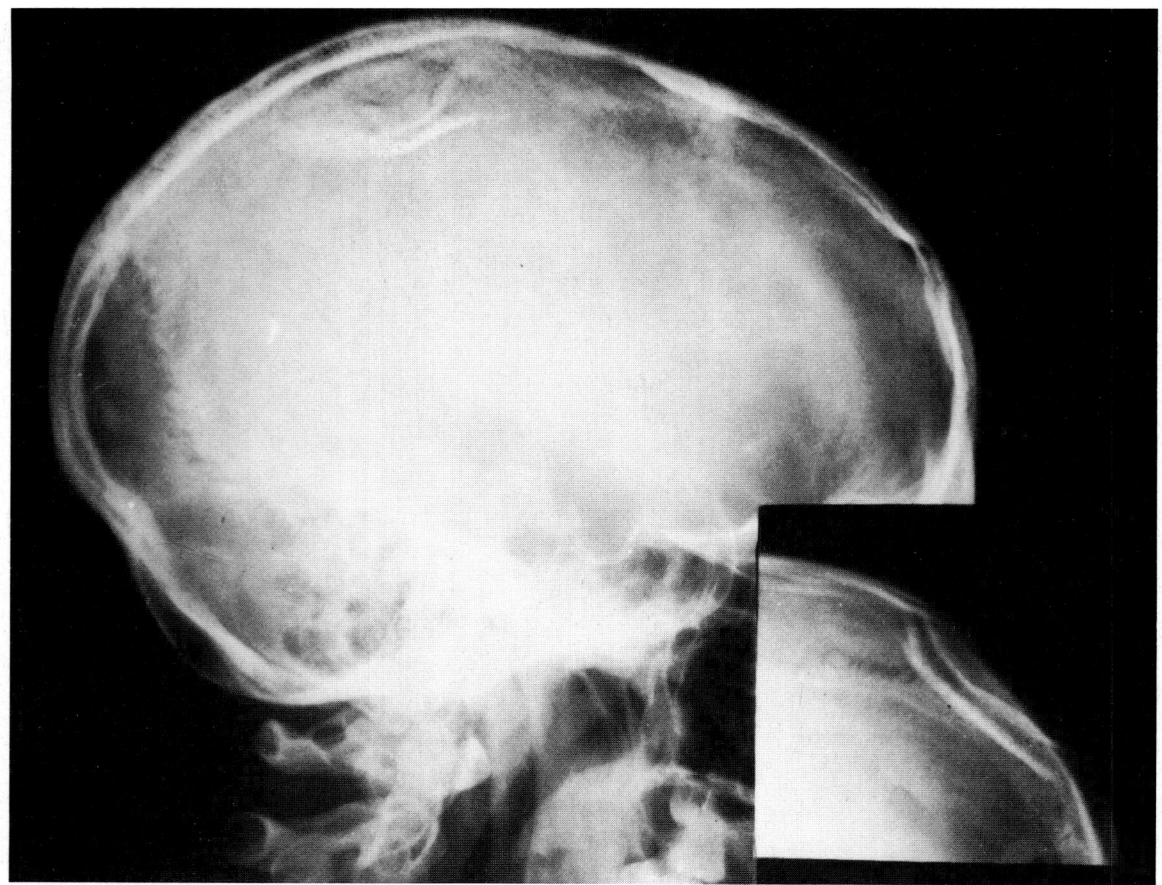

The brow-up horizontal beam lateral projection of the skull shown on page 107 reveals air-fluid levels in the sphenoidal and maxillary sinuses.

Although suggestive, an air-fluid level in the maxillary sinus is not always the result of an antral wall fracture and may be caused by fluid from a nasal haemorrhage or sinusitis. In contrast, opacification or an air-fluid level in the sphenoidal sinus is a reliable indicator of a basal skull fracture; a fracture will be demonstrated in approximately 75 per cent of these patients if tomography is employed. A CT scan in this patient confirmed the presence of both basal and antral fractures.

In another patient (shown above), two linear densities in the parietal area are due to the depressed fracture seen in profile on the tangential view. Depressed fractures comprise 15 per cent of all skull fractures; approximately one-third of these are associated with dural tears. Any area of increased density on the radiograph of a skull following injury should be considered as a possible depressed fracture and tangential views obtained.

Reference

Robinson, A. E., Meares, B. M. and Goree, J. A. (1967) Traumatic sphenoid sinus effusion: an analysis of 50 cases. *Amer. J. Roentgenol.*, **101**, 795-801.

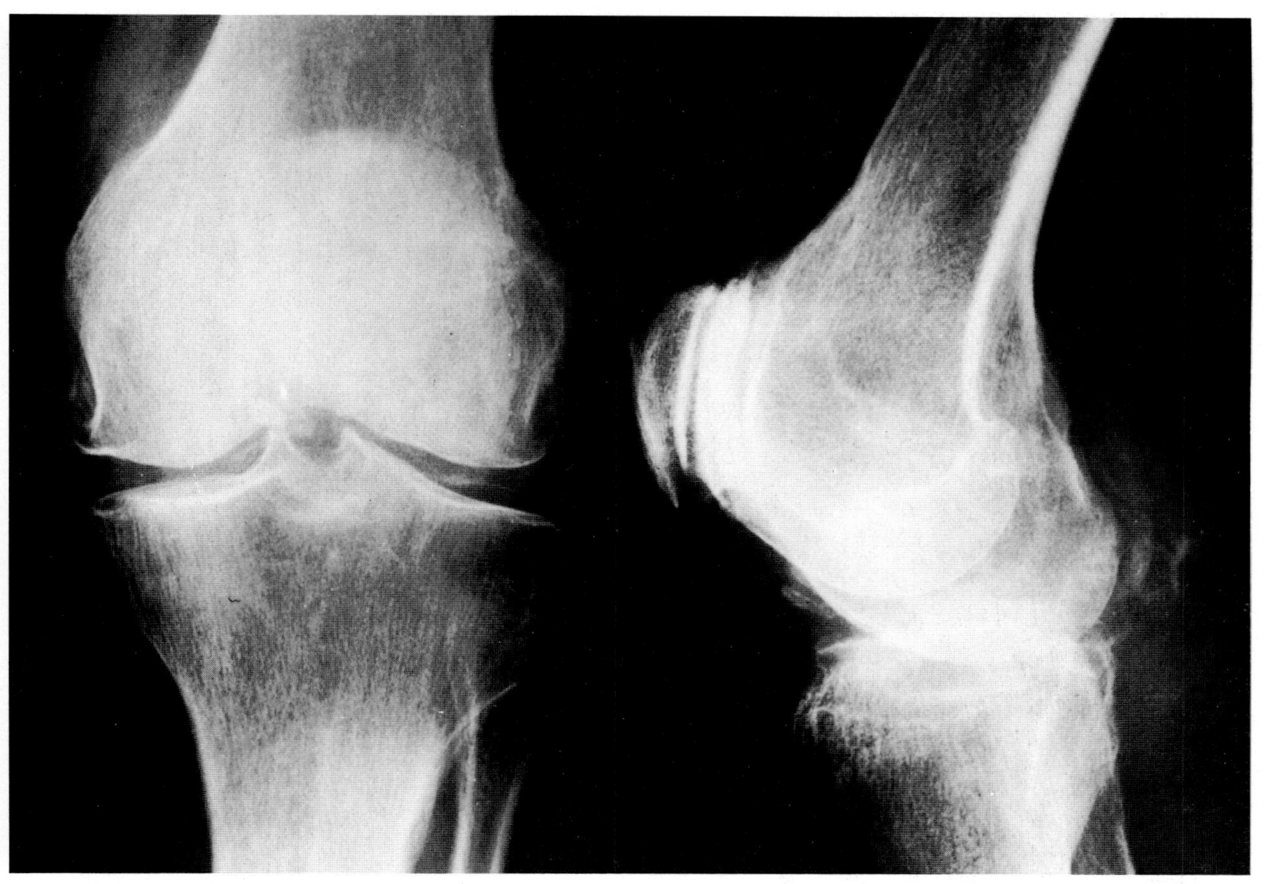

A clinical diagnosis of rheumatoid arthritis was made in this 74-year-old woman.

- Do the radiological findings support the diagnosis?

- What alternative diagnosis should be considered?

- How may this be confirmed?

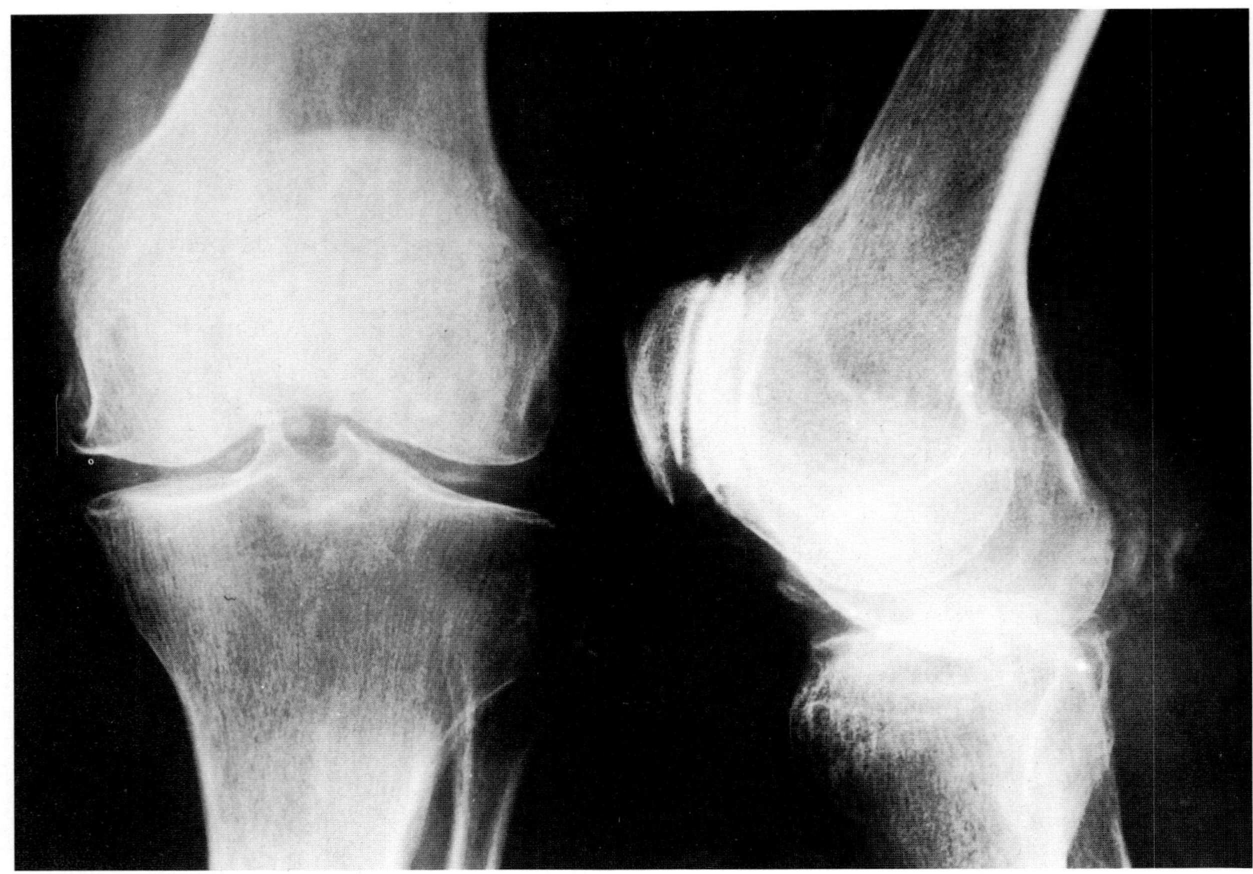

Despite the clinical diagnosis of rheumatoid arthritis, the patient was seronegative and had an ESR of only 17 mm/hour. The chondrocalcinosis, synovial and joint capsular calcification, and the isolated severe osteoarthritic change at the patellofemoral joint are more like calcium pyrophosphate deposition disease (CPPD). The erosion of the anterior aspect of each femur is due to recurrent or persistent enlargement of the suprapatellar synovial pouch. The diagnosis was confirmed by the finding of calcium pyrophosphate crystals at synovial biopsy.

CPPD resembles osteoarthritis superficially but has a different articular and intra-articular distribution. It most commonly affects the knees, wrists and elbows, and in particular the patellofemoral and radiocarpal articulations. Calcification of intra- and extra-articular structures is typical. A progressive, destructive pyrophosphate arthropathy may occur.

Reference

Resnick, D., Niwayama, G., Goergen, T. G., Utsinger, P. D., Shapiro, R. F., Haselwood, D. H. and Wiesner, K. B. (1975) Clinical, radiographic and pathological abnormalities in calcium pyrophosphate dihydrate deposition disease (CPPD): pseudogout. *Radiology*, **122**, 1-15.

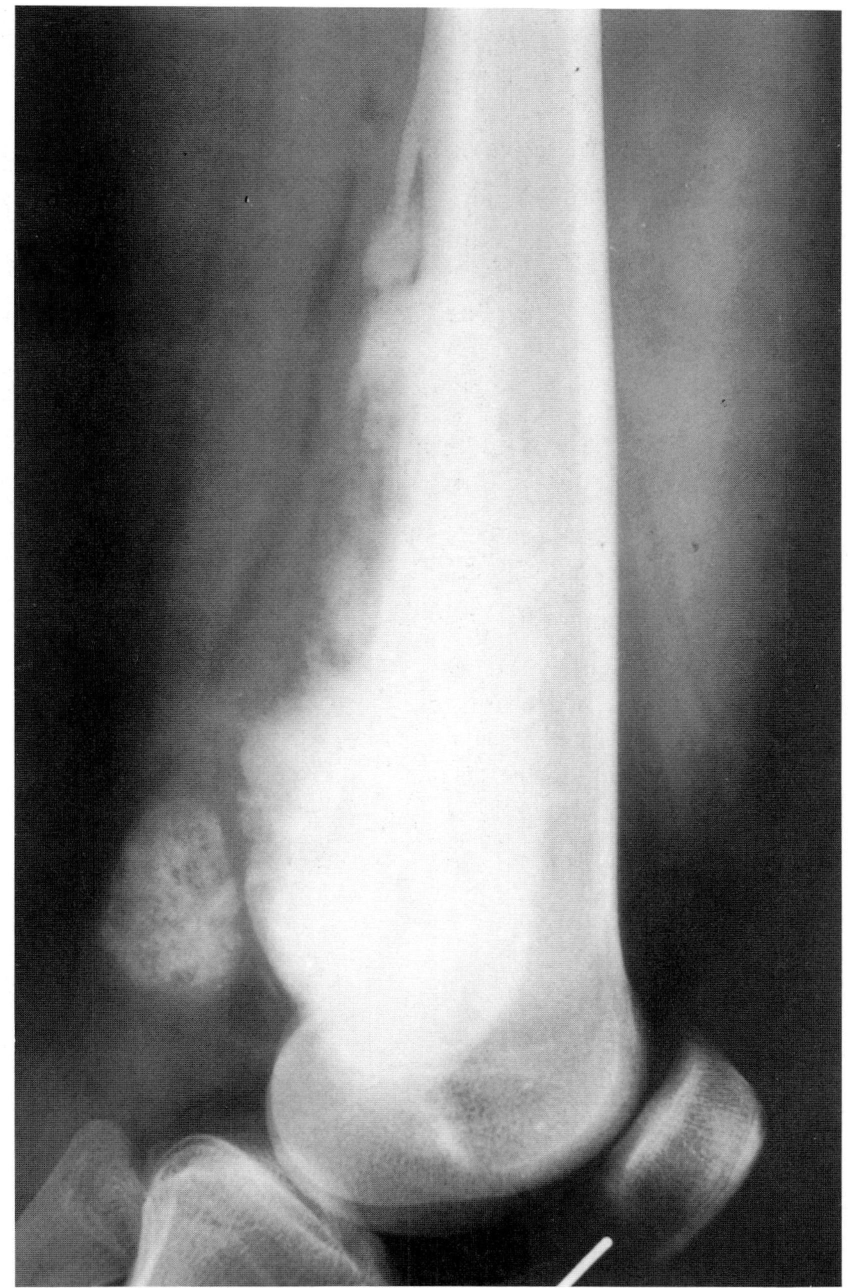

This 18-year-old girl complained of a slightly tender swelling behind her left knee.

- What is your differential diagnosis?
- What is the likely diagnosis?

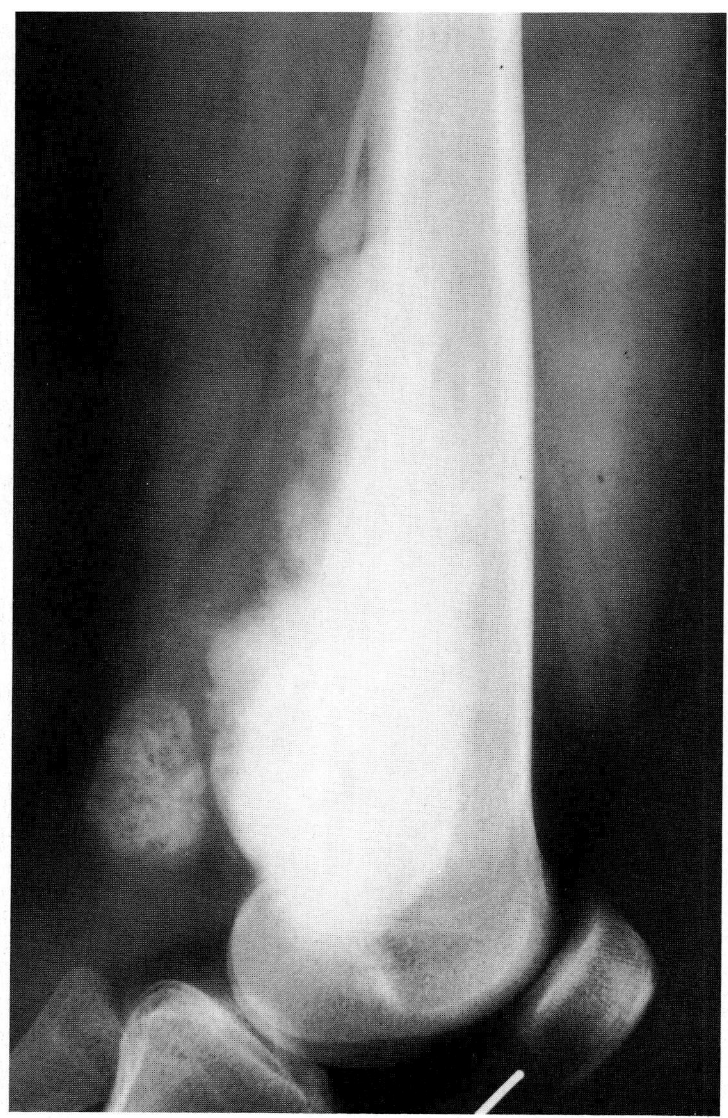

Dense new bone surrounds the posterior aspect of the distal femur obscuring the underlying bone. The new bone is most dense centrally as it tends to wrap itself around the femoral shaft.

The main differential diagnosis lies between a parosteal osteosarcoma and post-traumatic myositis ossificans. The latter is unlikely as the appositional new bone is altogether too extensive and applied too closely to the femur; the density of bone would also tend to be greater at the periphery of the lesion.

This was a biopsy-proven parosteal osteosarcoma, a low-grade malignant tumour which probably originates in the periosteum and extends into the soft tissues. The peak age of incidence is higher than that of osteogenic sarcoma; the majority of patients are over the age of 20.

Although a few will progress rapidly, the prognosis is generally good, with a ten-year survival exceeding 60 per cent.

Reference

Lorentzon, R., Larsson, S.-E. and Boquist, L. (1980) Parosteal (juxtacortical) osteosarcoma. *J. Bone Joint Surg.*, **62-B**, 86-92.

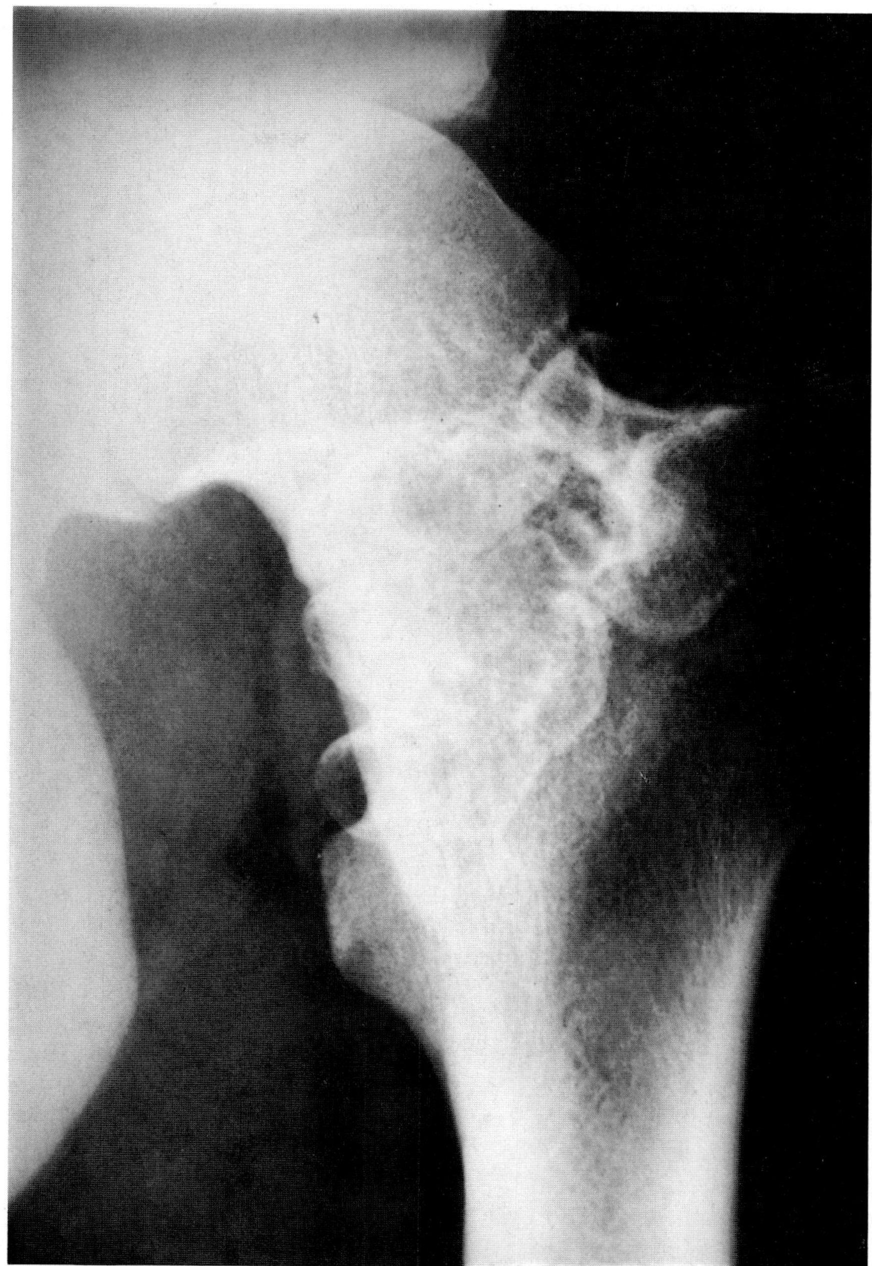

(by courtesy of Dr. Philip Jacobs, Birmingham)

This 29-year-old man had had a painful hip for 18 months.

- What might account for the appearances?
- What further projection is essential?

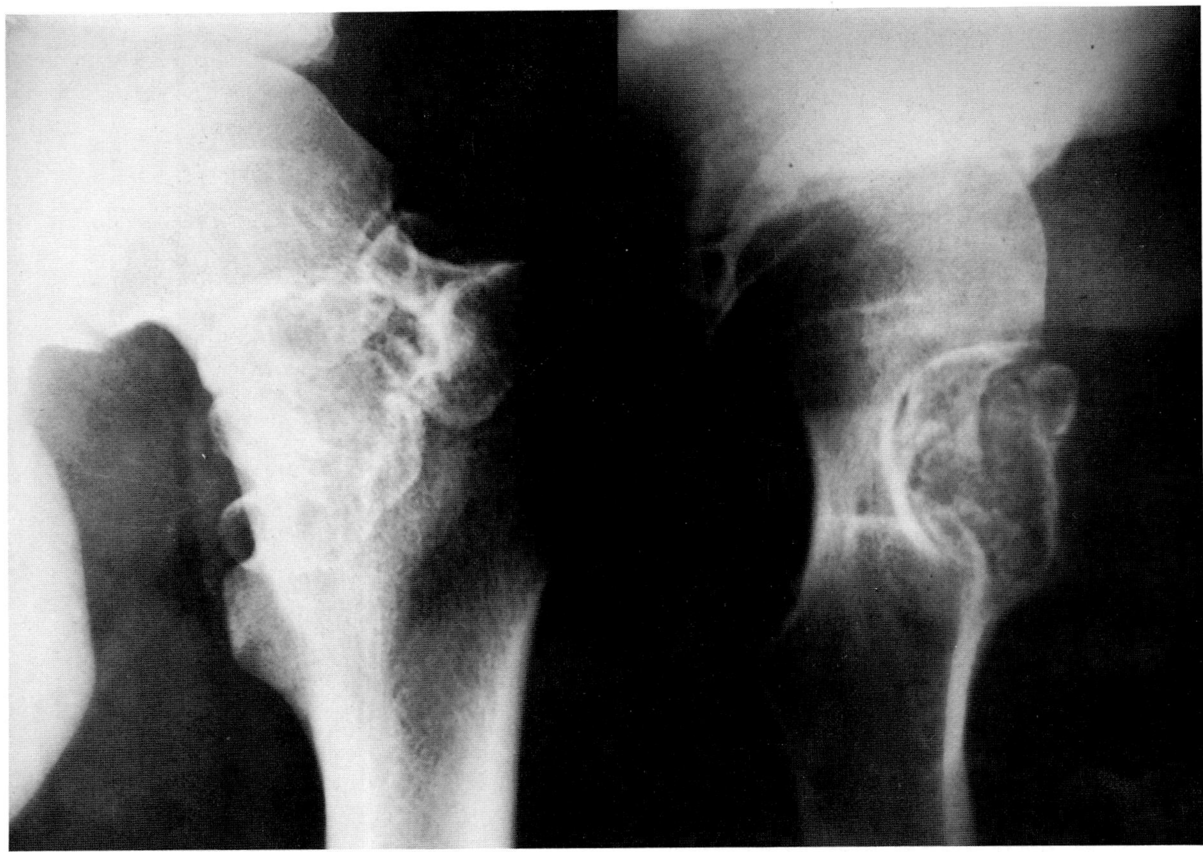

The radiograph of the proximal femur shows a well-defined and lobulated bony lesion causing pressure erosion of the adjacent femoral neck. This appearance could be due to multiple osseous loose bodies within the capsule and synovial space, as in synovial osteochondromatosis. The nature of the lesion is revealed in the lateral projection, which shows the stem of an osteochondroma arising from the distal end of the femoral neck.

Outward growth of the benign tumour has been prevented by tightness of the joint capsule and it has been forced against the anterior aspect of the femoral neck, causing progressive pressure erosion. Reduction in thickness of the femoral neck puts the patient at risk from a fracture.

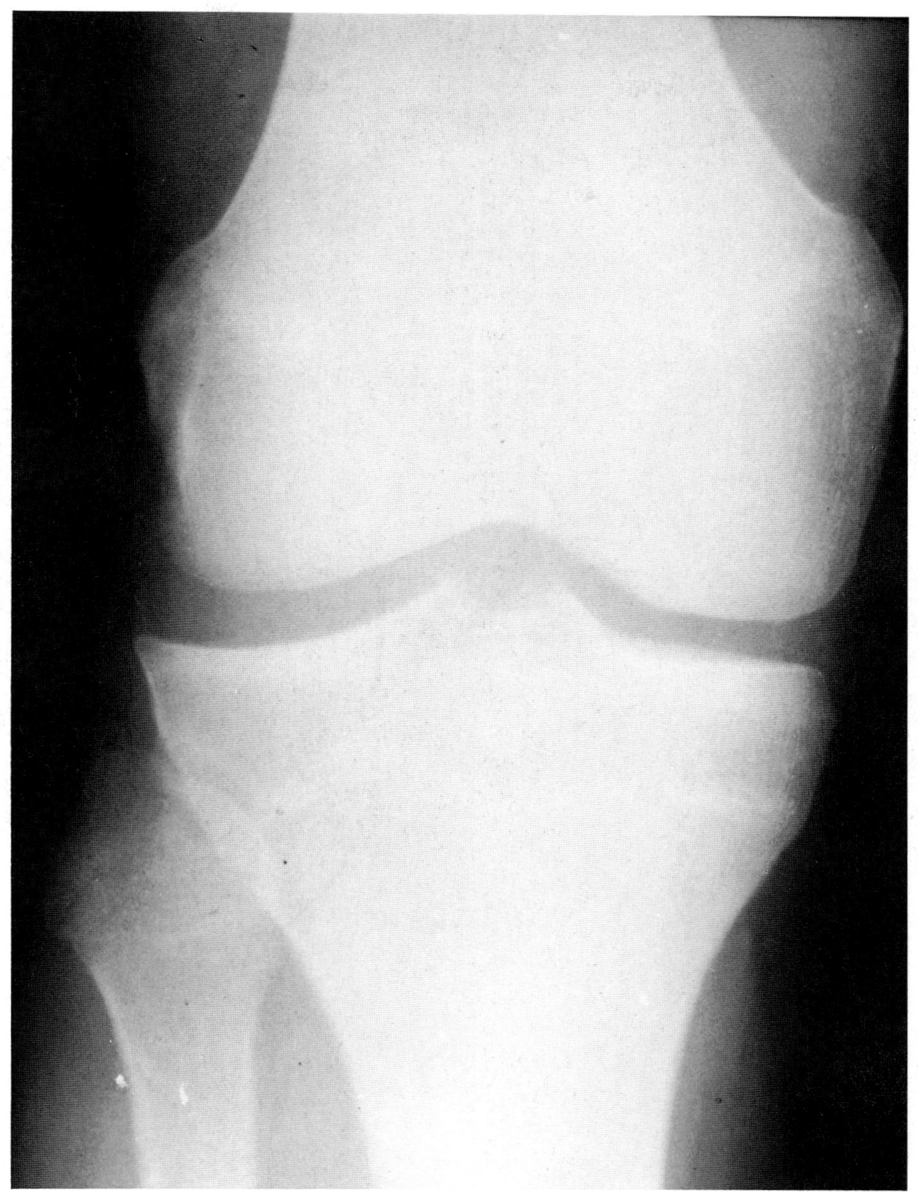

This child complained of a clicking knee.

- What abnormality would you expect at arthrography?
- What complication commonly occurs?

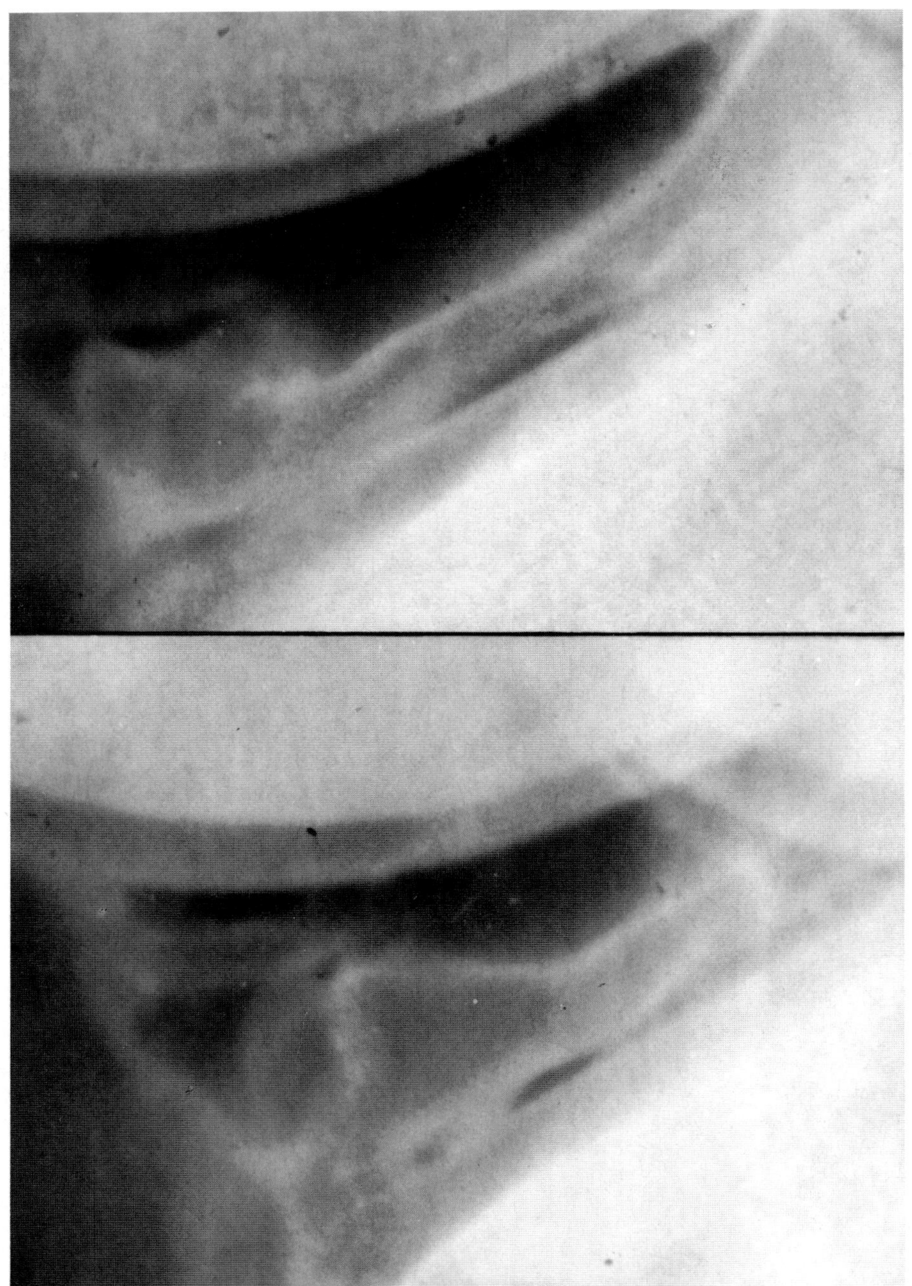

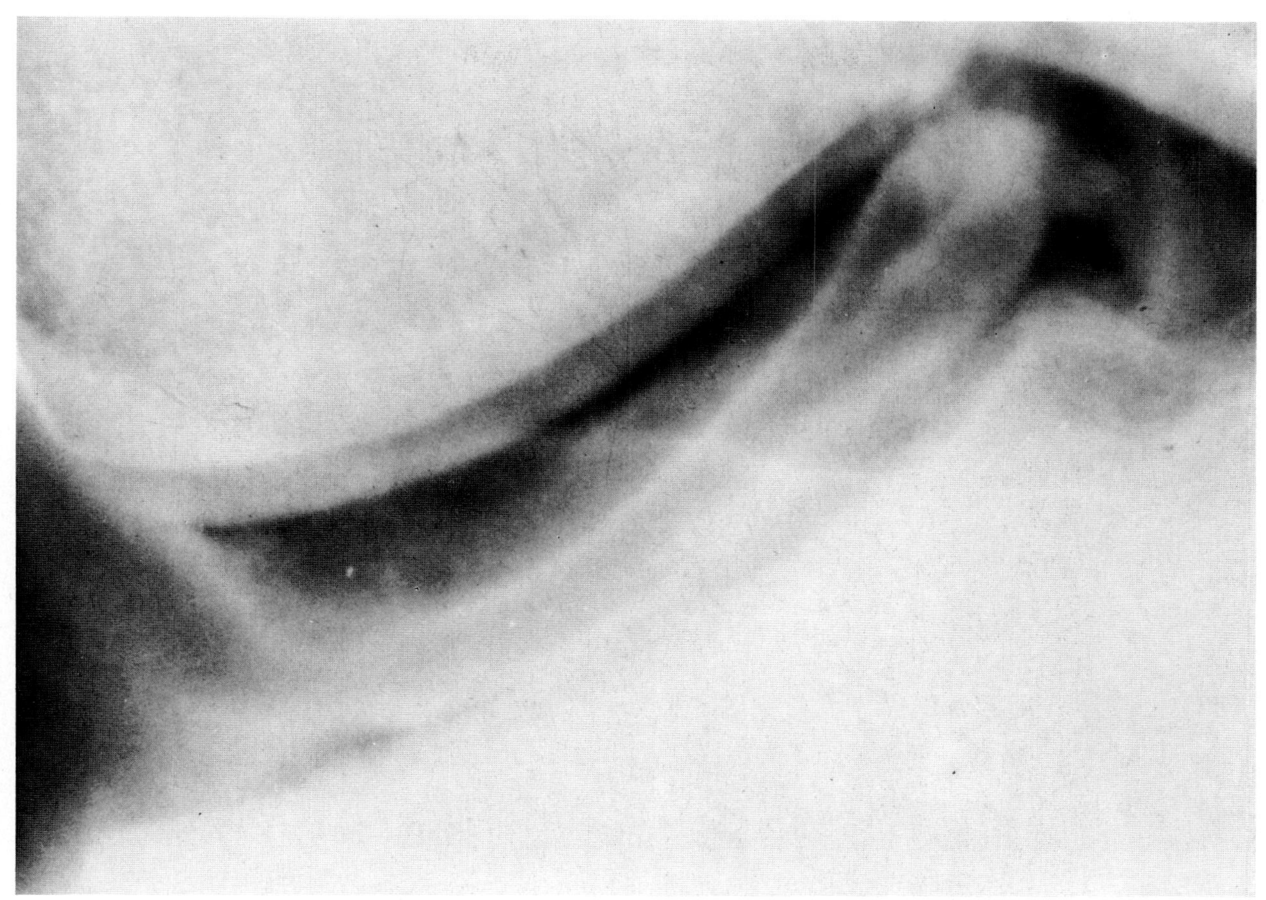

The height of the lateral compartment of the right knee is abnormally large, suggesting the presence of a discoid lateral meniscus. The diagnosis was confirmed by arthrography (see left and above), where the lateral meniscus is not its usual wedge shape, but has parallel surfaces and a bulbous end instead. The meniscus is very wide, extending to the intercondylar notch.

Discoid menisci are thicker and wider than normal and may be attached to the medial femoral condyle by the meniscofemoral ligament; their posterior horns lack the normal attachment to the tibial plateau. The abnormality almost always involves the lateral meniscus and is more common in females. Discoid menisci are prone to tear at an early age. An intact discoid meniscus, as in this example, typically causes a clicking knee, sometimes producing an audible noise on flexion and extension.

Reference

Stoker, D. J. (1980) *Arthrography*. Chapman & Hall, London, pp. 82-85.

Q50

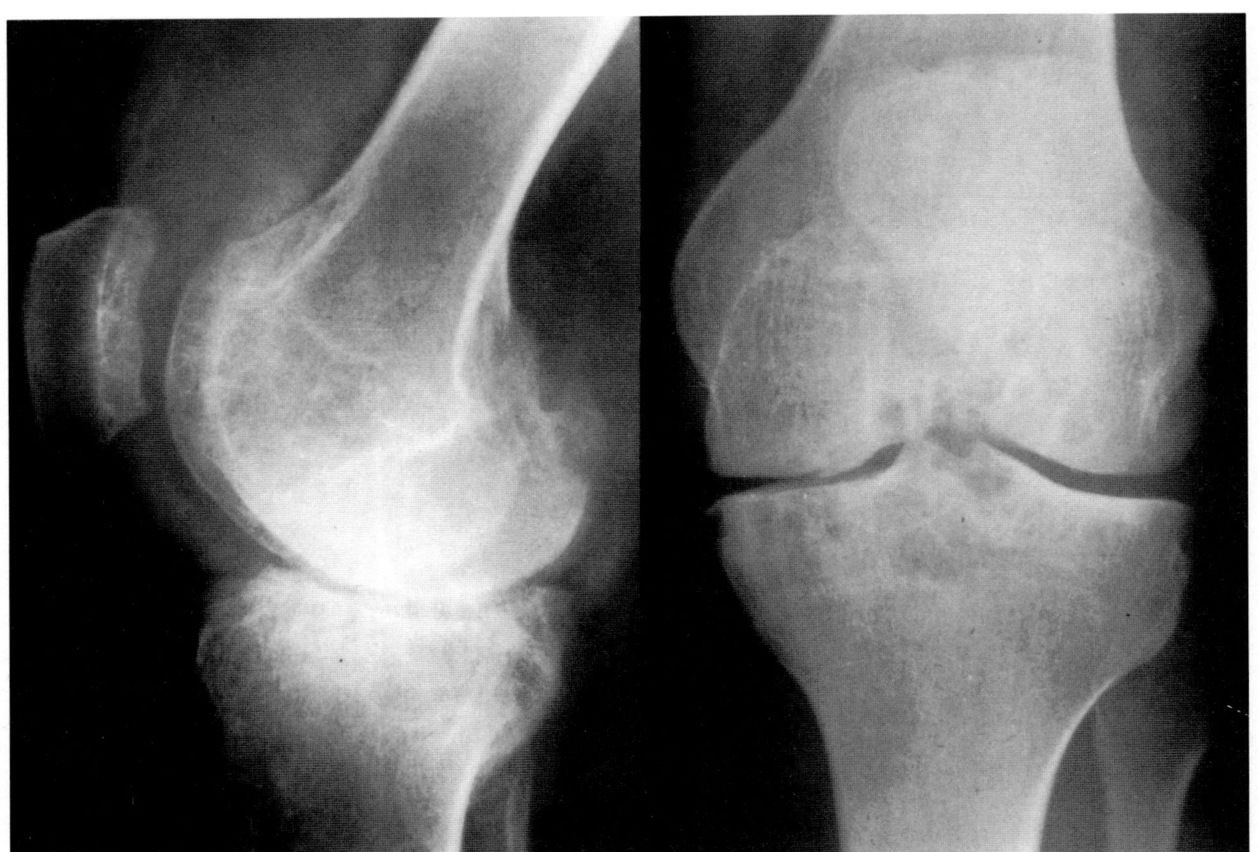

This 19-year-old man presented to Casualty with a painful swollen knee. There was no history of trauma.

- What treatment was he given?

- How do the radiological manifestations of this condition develop?

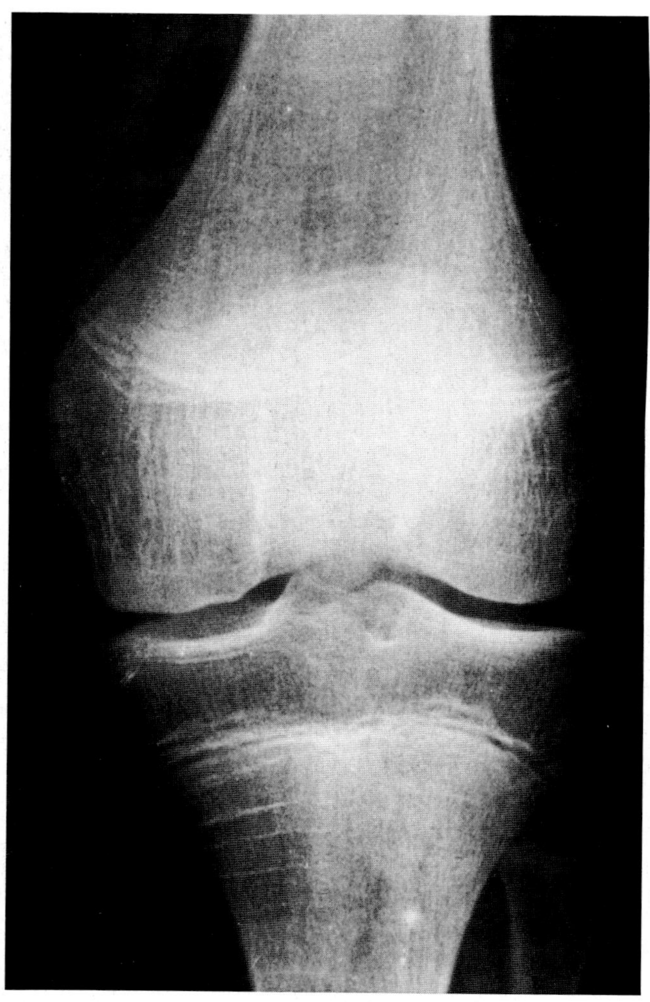

The joint capsule of the knee is distended and diffusely opaque due to a combination of synovial hypertrophy and an acute haemarthrosis. The very dense areas in the soft tissues are caused by deposits of haemosiderin within the thickened synovium. Coarse trabeculation and enlargement of the ends of the long bones, joint space narrowing and degenerative subchondral cysts are also present. The appearances follow repeated bleeds into the joint of a haemophiliac.

Treatment with Factor VIII was given to control active bleeding. Intra-articular bleeds in haemophilia begin in early childhood and permanent osseous changes result from the effects of hyperaemia and disuse on the developing skeleton. Recurrent haemarthroses cause the production of an active synovial pannus, similar to that in rheumatoid arthritis, which destroys the articular cartilage and leads to premature degenerative joint disease. Ankylosis was common before the use of Factor VIII in treatment.

The film above is of the patient aged ten years. Hyperaemia has caused epiphyseal enlargement, coarsening of the trabecular pattern in the epiphyses due to chronic osteoporosis, and accelerated fusion of the growth plate. Numerous growth arrest lines are visible in the tibia.

Reference

Petterson, H. and Gilbert, M. S. (1985) *Diagnostic Imaging in Haemophilia*. Springer Verlag, Berlin.

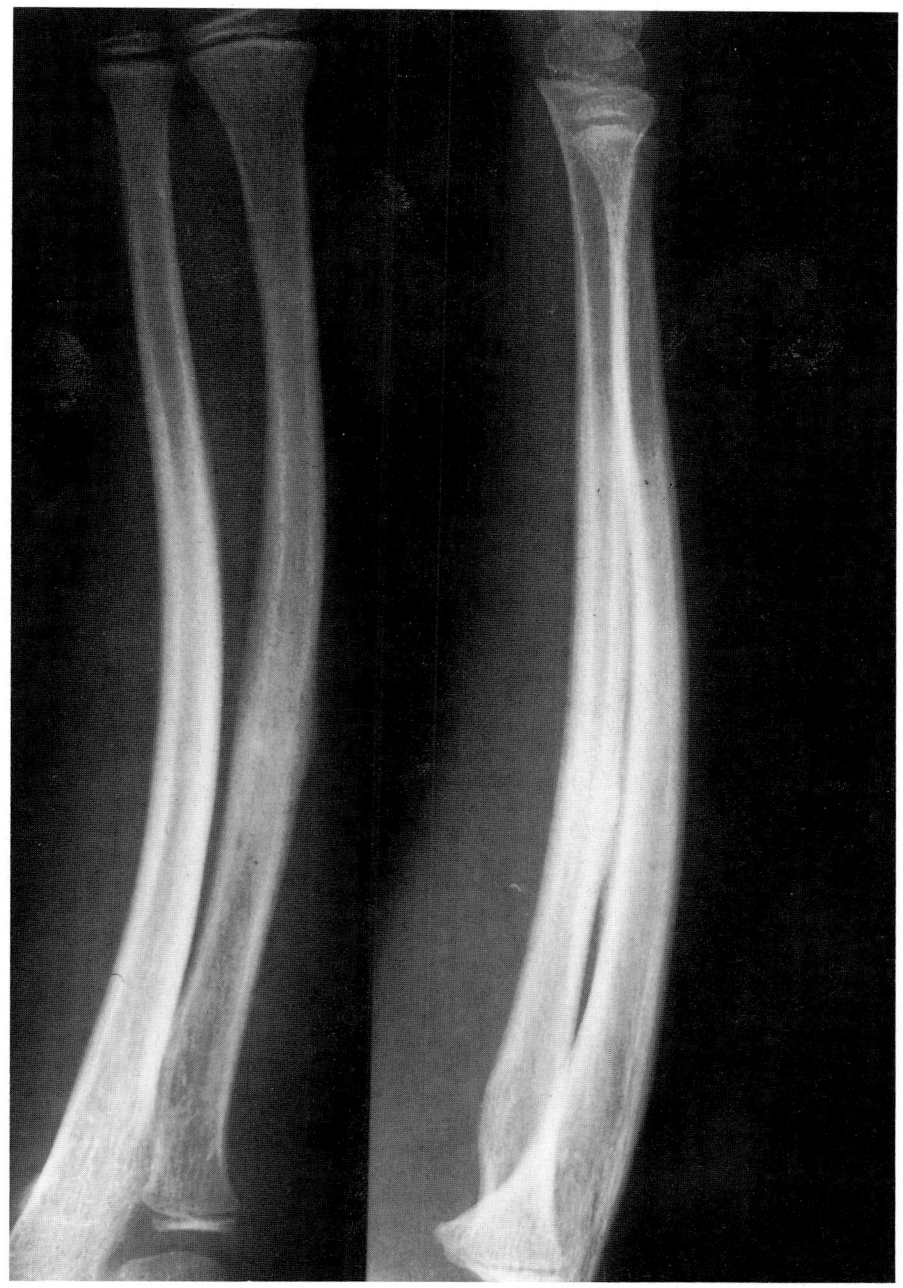

This child fell off her bicycle.

- What is the injury?
- How does it occur?

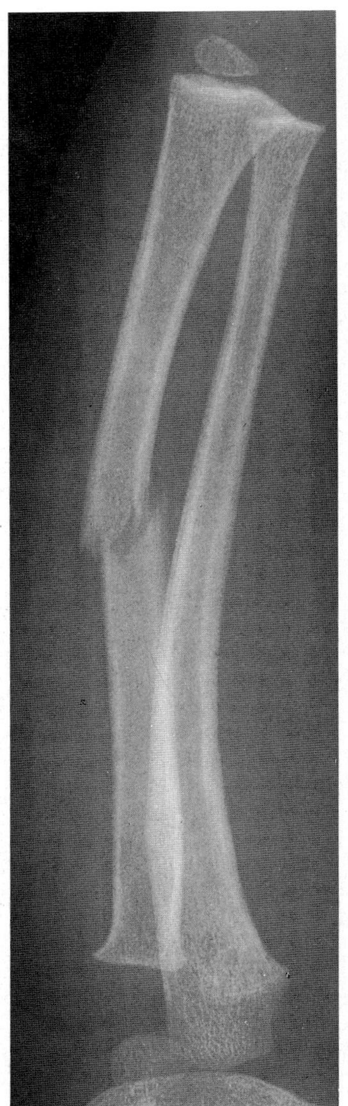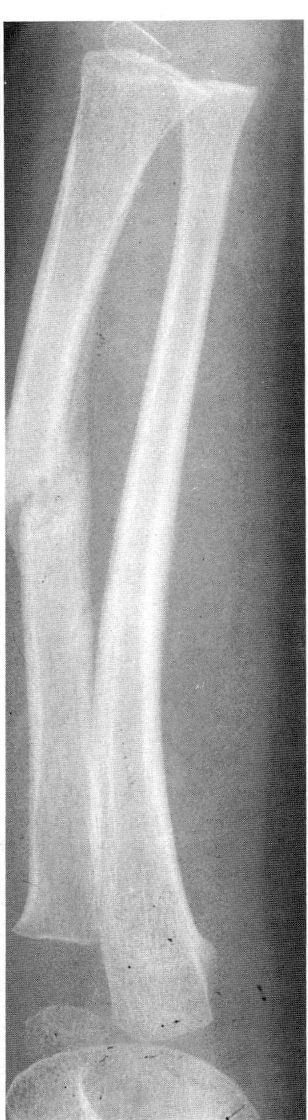

Both forearm bones are bowed laterally and a small periosteal reaction follows the concavity of the curve in the radius. The deformities are due to bowing fractures, which are a form of greenstick fracture most commonly seen in the forearm in the 3-13 age group. They result from longitudinal compressive forces which are not strong enough to produce an obvious fracture, but are sufficient to cause bowing and microfractures on the convex side of the curve. An associated periosteal reaction is common.

In the majority of cases, bowing only occurs in one of the paired bones and is associated with an angulated fracture of the other, as in a second example shown above. Bowing of both bones, or bowing of one bone with dislocation of the other, occurs much less frequently.

Failure to reduce the bowing may result in permanent deformity at the site of any associated fracture.

Reference

Crowe, J. E. and Swischuk, L. E. (1977) Acute bowing fractures of the forearm in children: a frequently missed injury. *Amer. J. Roentgenol.*, **128**, 981-984.

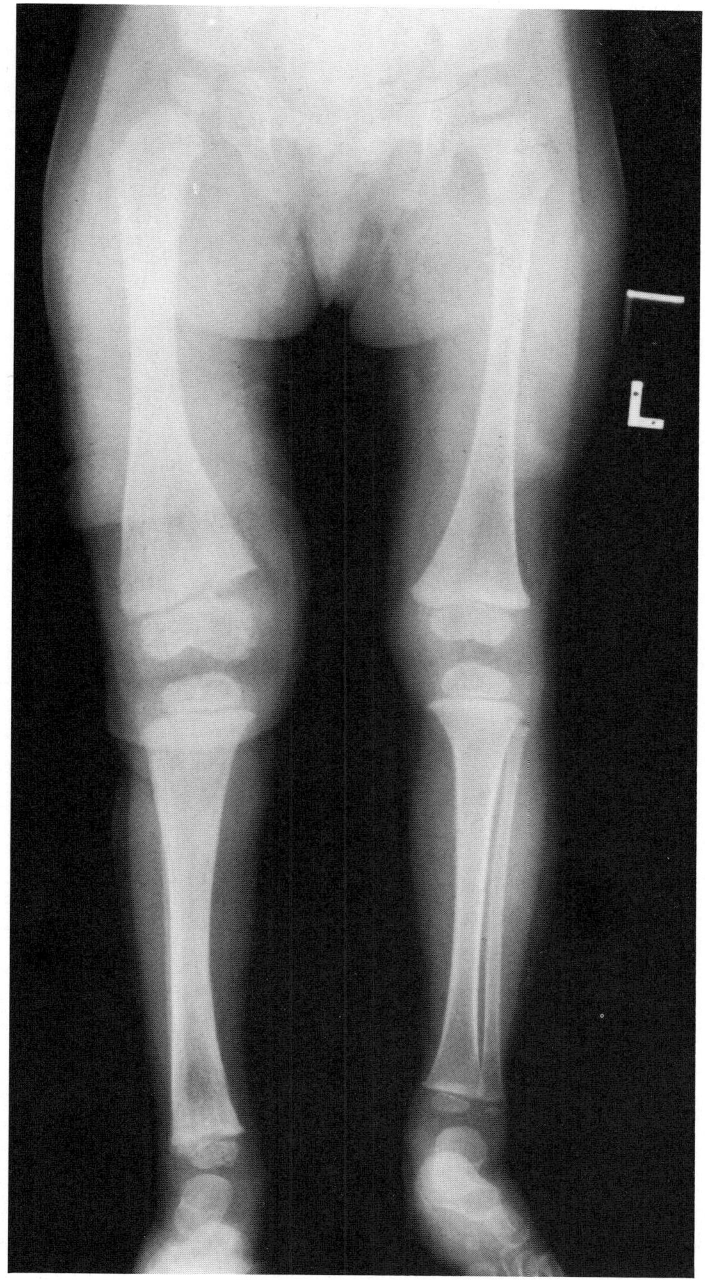

This child was referred with an enlarged lower limb.

- Describe the abnormalities.
- Why was the child's skin examined?

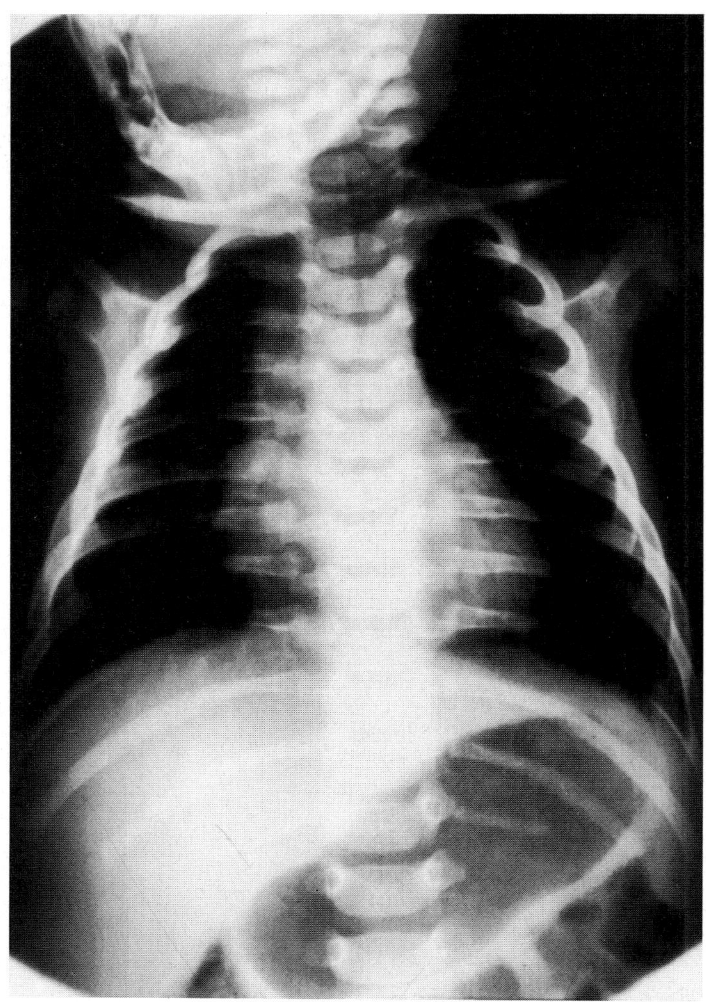

Bony and soft tissue hypertrophy in the right lower limb has resulted in limb lengthening. Abnormal modelling and bone texture are also seen.

The child had multiple cafe au lait spots and a palpable soft tissue mass on the back overlying the right seventh and eighth ribs, which at biopsy proved to be a neurofibroma. The chest film above shows hypertrophy of the underlying ribs.

Soft tissue hypertrophy of all of part of a limb is a well-recognised manifestation of neurofibromatosis and may be accompanied by under- or overdevelopment of the bones. The soft tissues frequently contain a lymphangiomatous or haemangiomatous component and plexiform neuromas are common. Any increase in length of a bone is usually related to an increase in blood supply. Abnormal modelling may result from organisation of an associated subperiosteal haematoma.

Other conditions associated with enlargement of all or part of a limb include arteriovenous malformations and macrodystrophia lipomatosa.

Friedrich von Recklinghausen (1833-1910) was Professor of Pathology in Strasbourg. Although not the first to describe the disorder (Robert Smith of Dublin had described it in 1849), his description in 1890 is considered the definitive one.

Reference

Klatte, E. C., Franken, E. A. and Smith, J. A. (1976) The radiographic spectrum in neurofibromatosis. *Semin. in Roentgenol.*, **11**, 17-33.

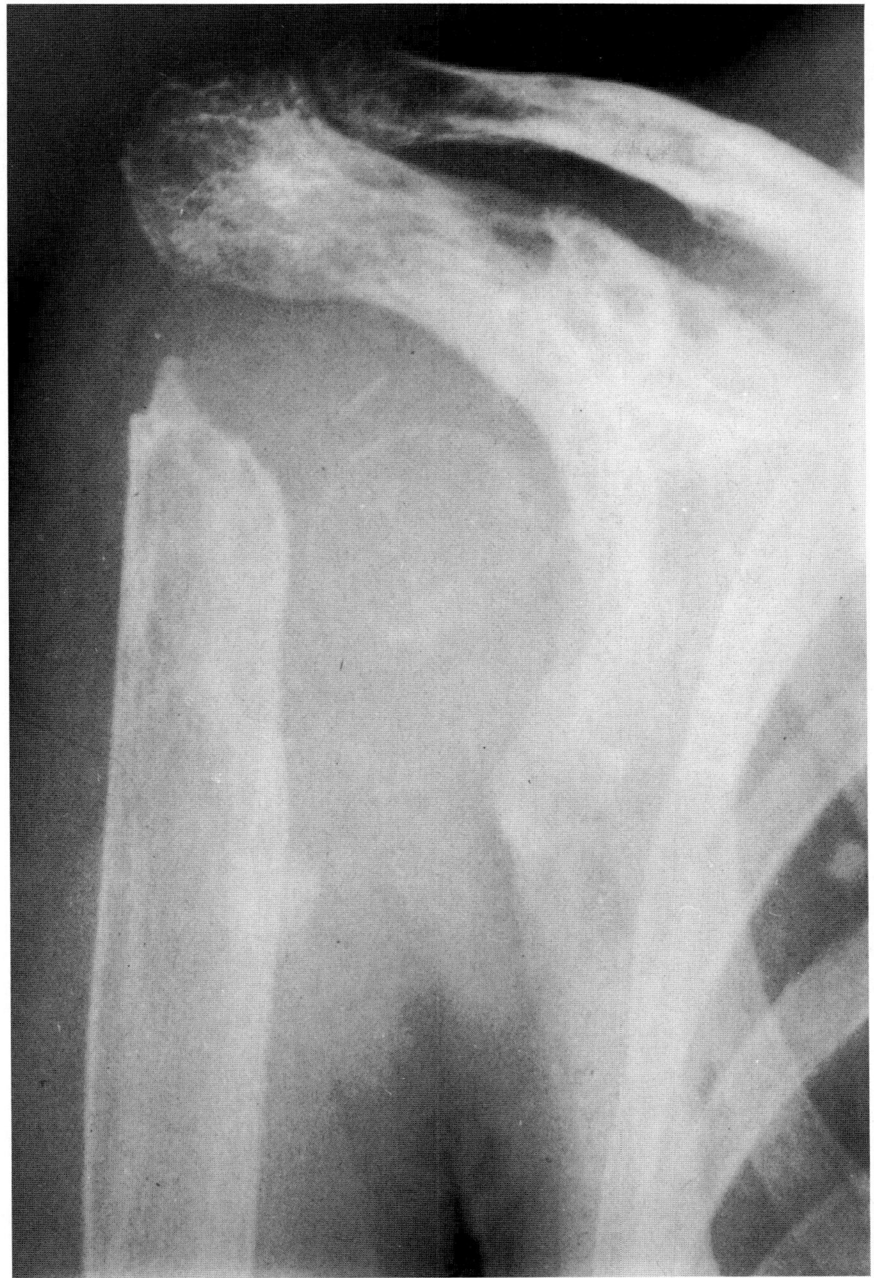

This elderly woman complained of a painful shoulder. She had been treated for a serious illness several years before.

- Describe the abnormalities.

- What was her previous complaint likely to have been?

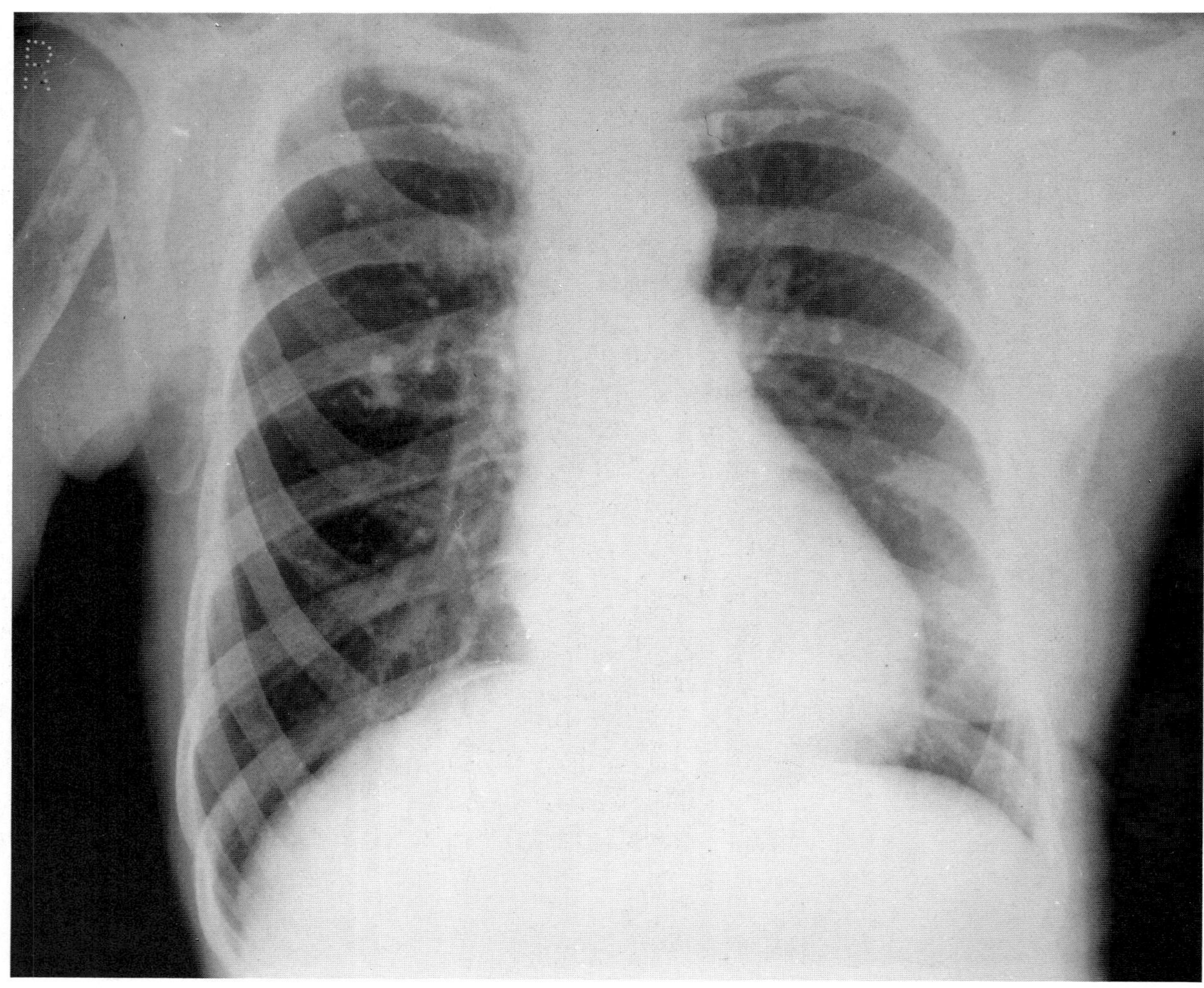

The pathological fractures of the humeral neck and glenoid fossa, and the osteopenia, coarse trabeculation and cortical thickening of the bones around the shoulder are radiological manifestations of radiation osteonecrosis. The patient had been treated for breast carcinoma with a mastectomy and radiotherapy six years earlier.

The calcification in the soft tissues medial to the humeral shaft is a common finding in radiation osteonecrosis, particularly in the shoulder region. Soft tissue calcification is also seen in radiation-induced osteosarcomas but these are almost always accompanied by soft tissue swelling. Osteosarcomas occur 5 to 15 years or sometimes longer after irradiation; radiological evidence of radiation osteonecrosis tends to appear earlier than this.

Reference

Bragg, D. G., Shidnia, H., Chu, F. C. H. and Higinbotham N. L. (1970) The clinical and radiographic aspects of radiation osteitis. *Radiology*, 97, 103-111.

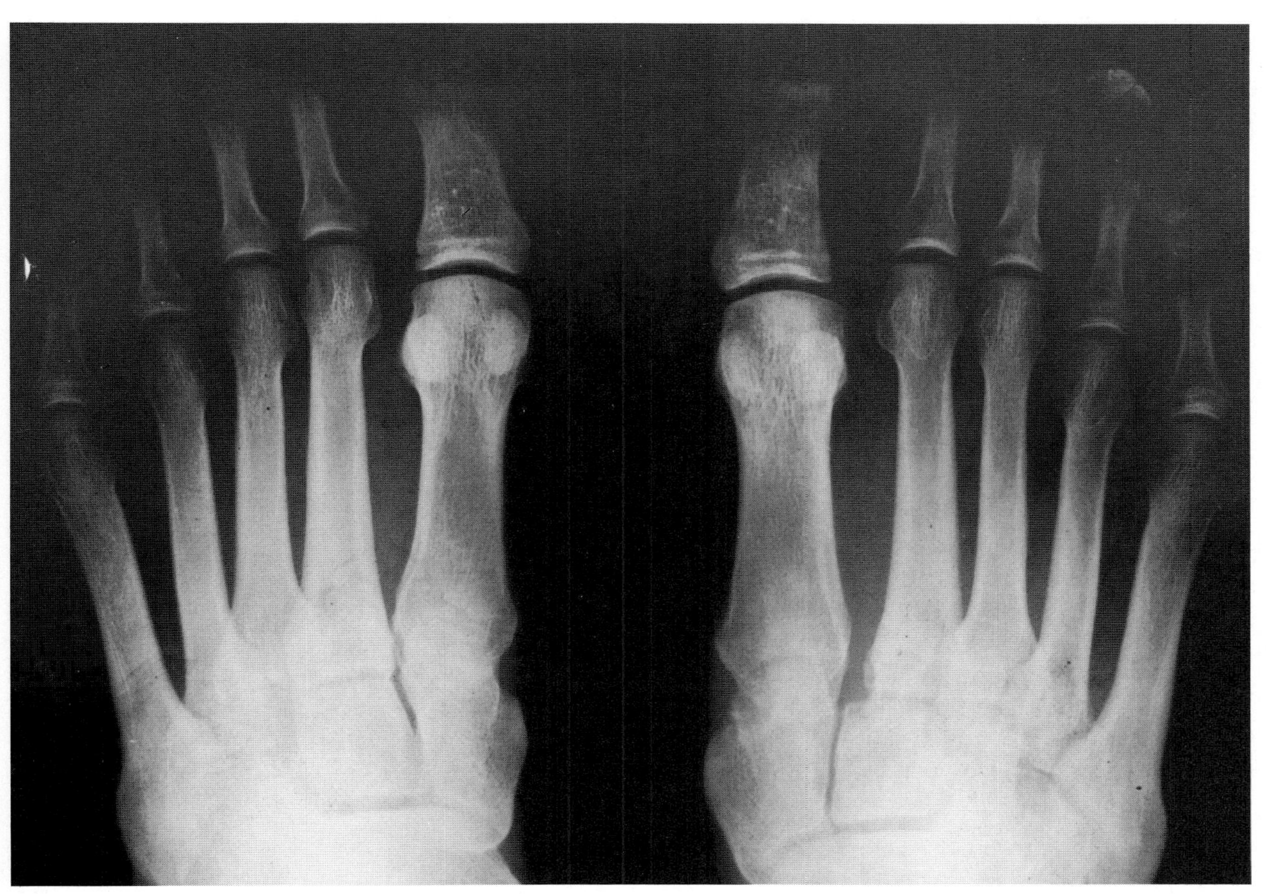

This man fell off a ladder.

- What is the nature of the injury?
- Has there been a fracture?

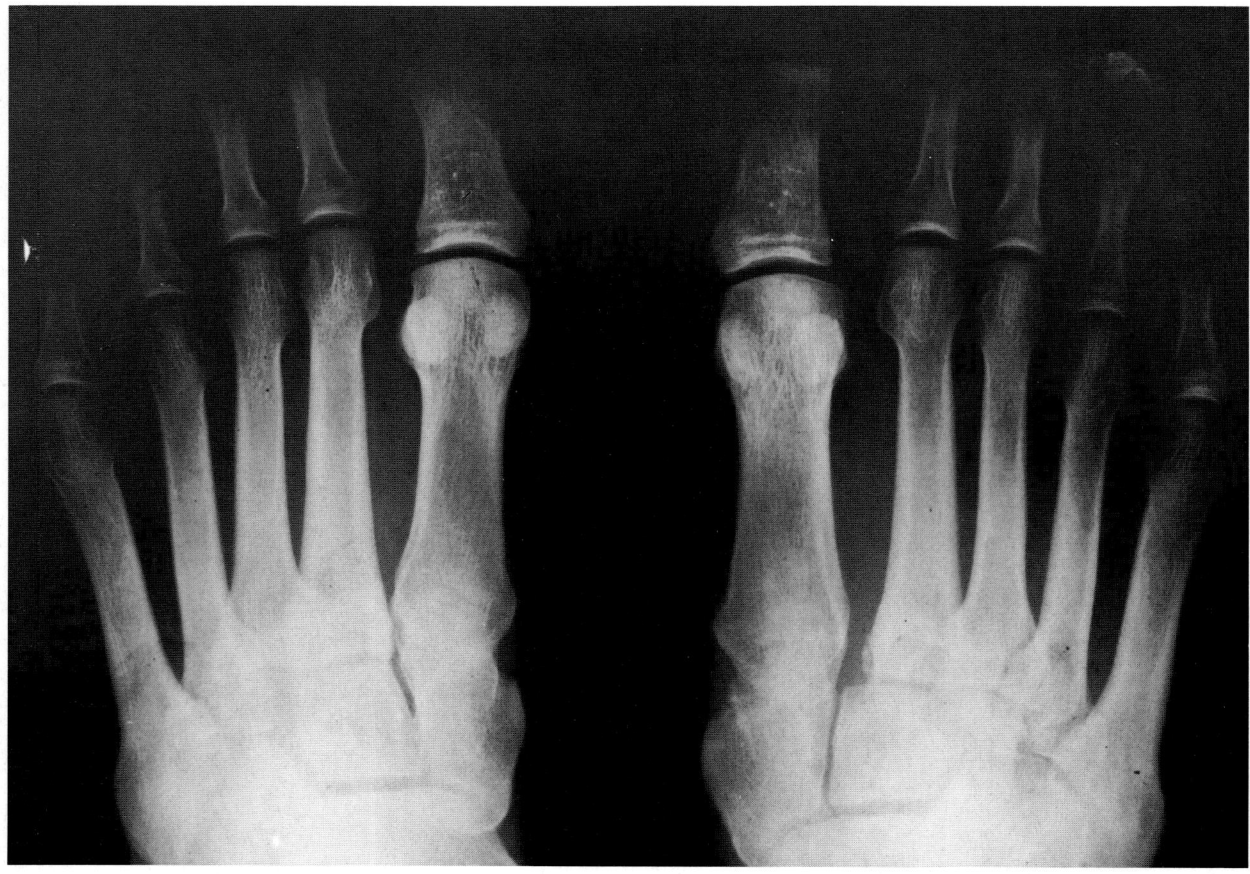

The abnormal separation of the right first and second metatarsals with malalignment of the middle cuneiform and second metatarsal are the radiological manifestations of a Lisfranc fracture-dislocation through the tarsometatarsal joints.

The commonest form of the injury involves lateral and dorsal dislocation of the second to fifth metatarsals. The base of the second metatarsal is held in a recess formed by the cuneiforms and separation of the first and second metatarsals can only take place if the base of the second metatarsal has fractured. As in this case, the fracture line may not be visible.

Jacques Lisfranc (1790-1847) was a military surgeon with Napoleon's armies. He did not describe the fracture but his name is given to the injury as he perfected the technique of amputation through the tarsometatarsal joint without anaesthetic. The operation took him just one minute to perform.

Reference

Foster, S. C. and Foster, R. R. (1976) Lisfranc's tarsometatarsal fracture-dislocation. *Radiology*, **120**, 79-83.

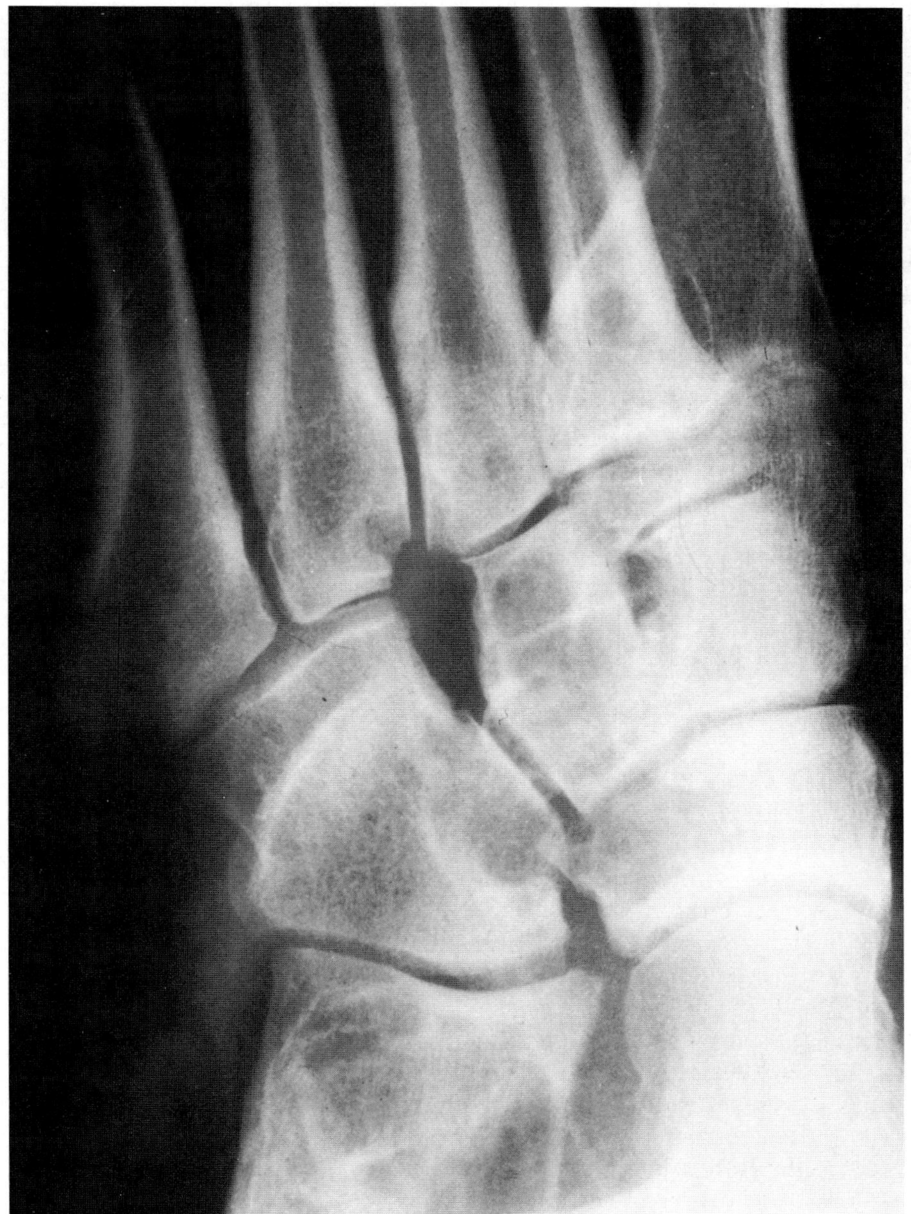

This 48-year-old man presented with a six-year history of gradually increasing pain in the left foot and swelling for two years.

- What does the radiograph show?
- What diagnosis would you suggest?

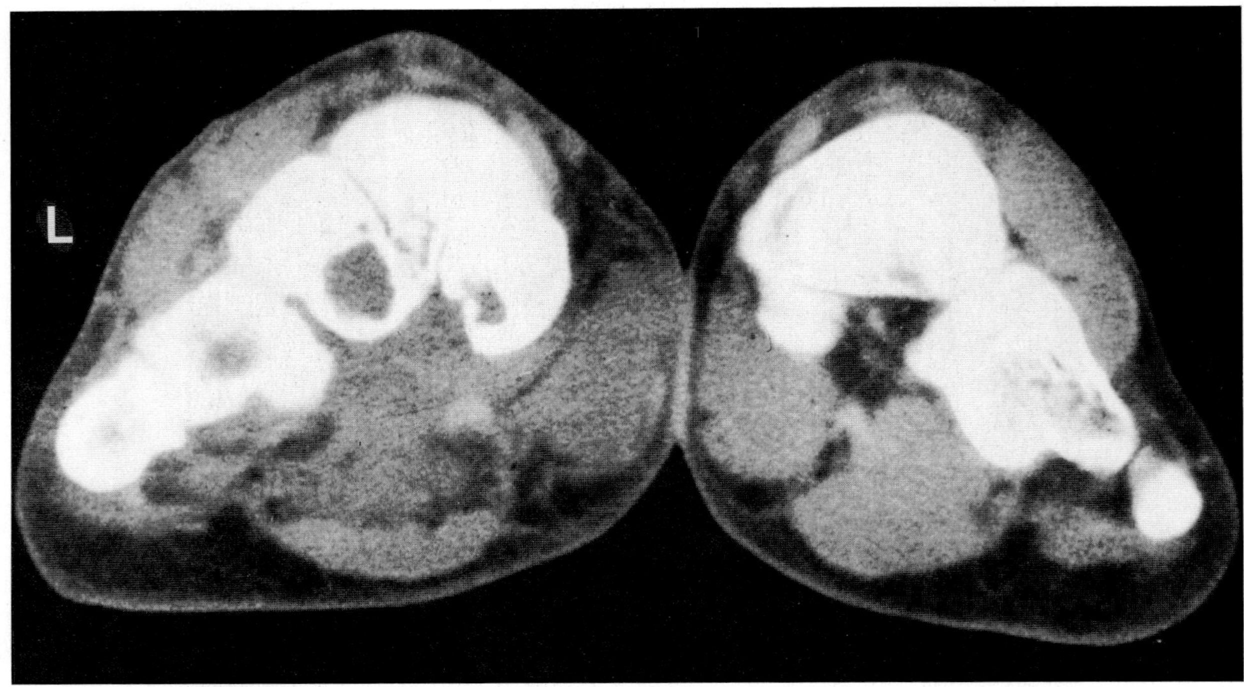

Multiple erosions with sharp sclerotic margins are present in many of the tarsal bones and also the bases of the third and fourth metatarsals of the left foot. In association with widening of the joint space between the cuboid and lateral cuneiform, and normal bone density, the radiological diagnosis is pigmented villonodular synovitis (PVNS).

In this proliferative synovial disorder, the growing soft tissue mass produces erosions in the adjacent bones. These erosions tend to be larger in more tightly encapsulated joints, as in the tarsus. This case illustrates the value of CT in demonstrating both the bony erosions and the soft tissue mass lying inferior to the tarsal bones.

Rheumatoid arthritis, infection and osteoarthritis should be considered in the differential diagnosis of periarticular erosions, but these disorders are all associated with a narrowed joint space and reduction in bone density to some degree. In addition, the distribution of rheumatoid arthritis with particular involvement of smaller joints in the hands and feet, and the presence of osteophytes in osteoarthritis, are important diagnostic features.

The absence of periarticular osteoporosis in most cases of PVNS probably reflects its relatively painless progress so that disuse does not occur.

Reference

Byers, P. D. et al. (1968) The diagnosis and treatment of pigmented villonodular synovitis. *J. Bone Joint Surg.*, **50-B**, 290-305.

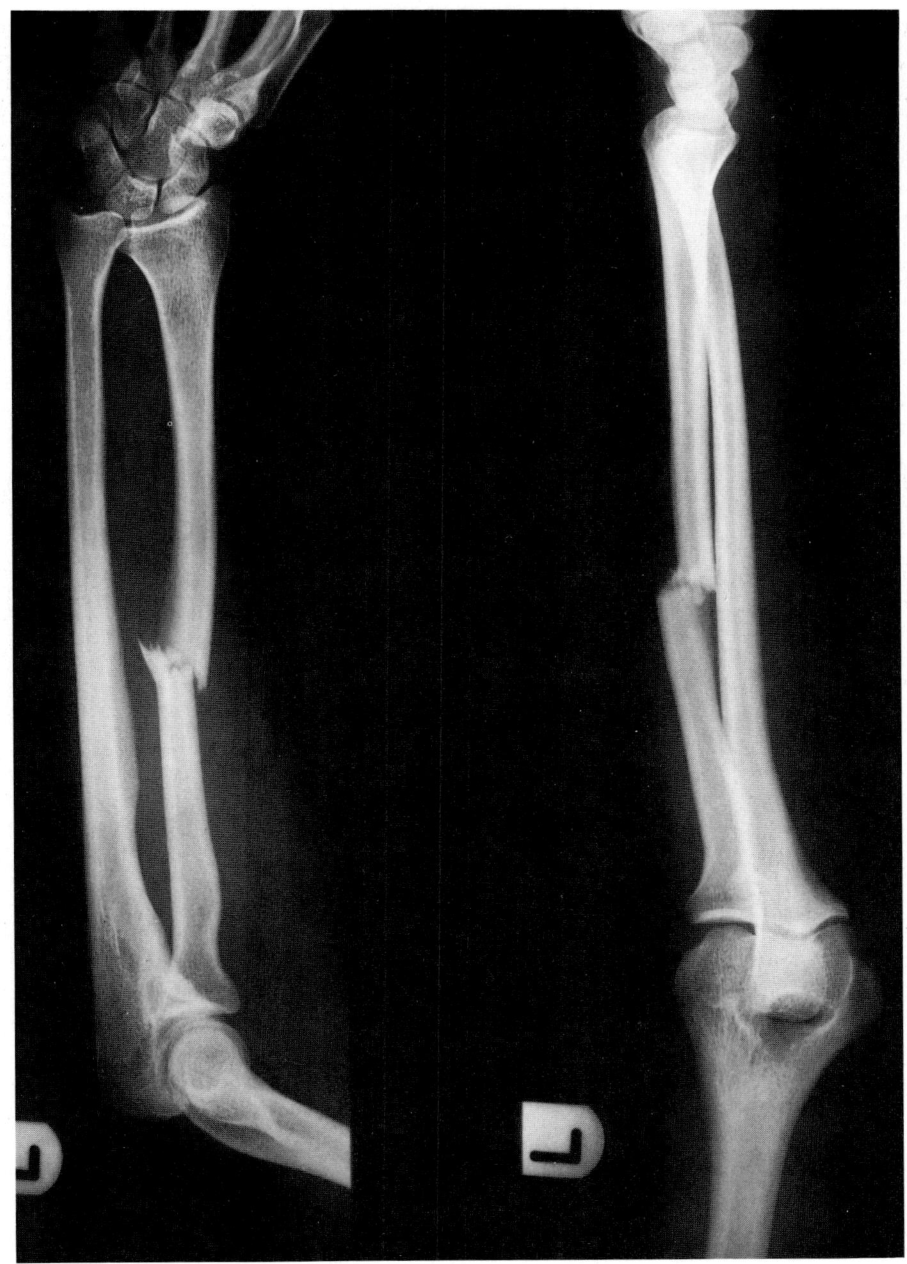

This patient was seen after falling on to her outstretched hand.

- Describe the radiographs.
- What is the name given to this injury?

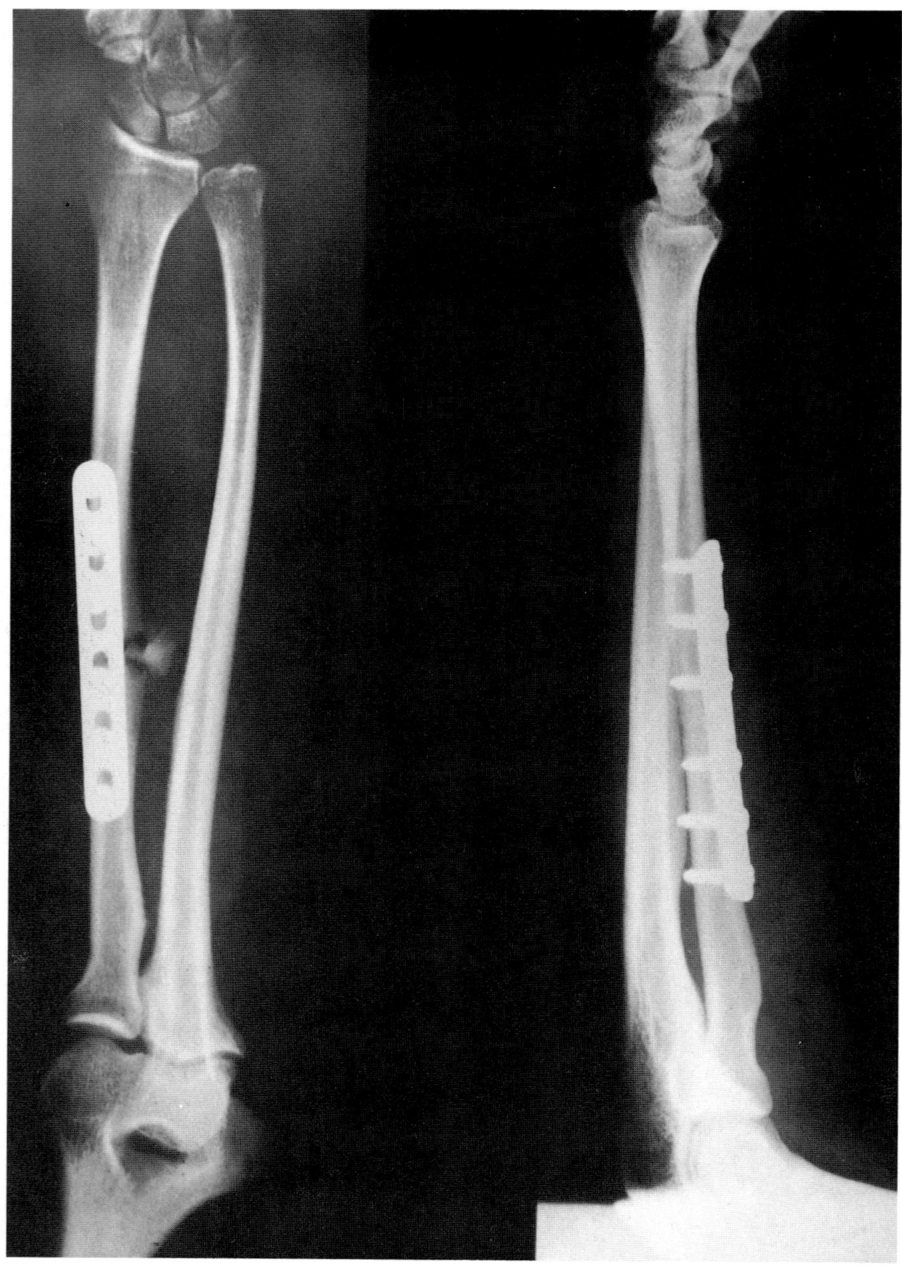

The combination of a fracture through the shaft of the radius and dislocation of the ulna at the distal radio-ulnar joint is termed a Galeazzi fracture-dislocation. An associated injury to the ulnar nerve may occur.

Note the normal relationship at the radio-ulnar joint following internal fixation of the fracture (see above). Successful treatment of the fracture by simple immobilisation is uncommon and internal fixation is usually necessary to prevent deformity.

Ricardo Galeazzi (1866-1952), an orthopaedic surgeon in Milan, described the injury in 1934.

Reference

Mikic, Z. D. (1975) Galeazzi fracture-dislocations. *J. Bone Joint Surg.*, **57A**, 1071-1080.

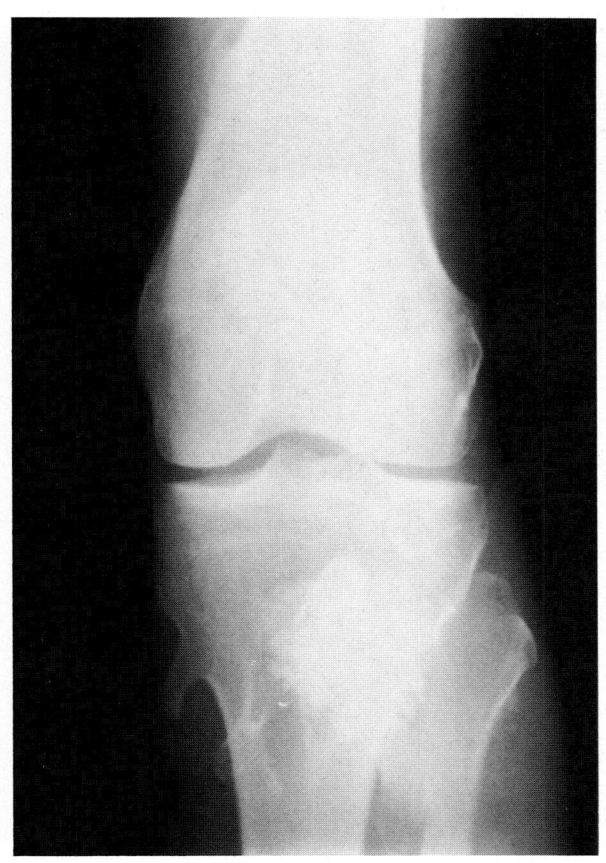 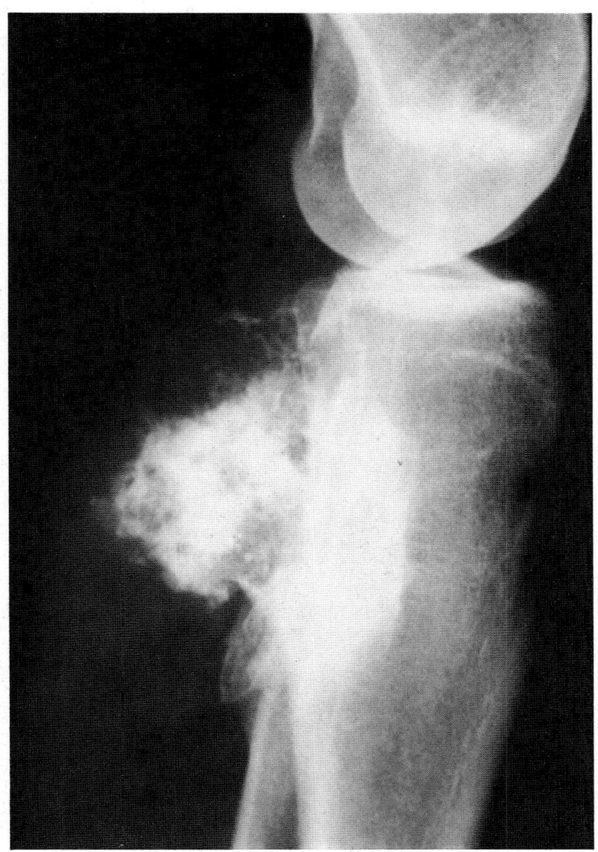

This adult patient complained of a painful swelling behind the knee.

- Describe the appearances and suggest a diagnosis.

- Are any of the radiological features of particular importance in this case?

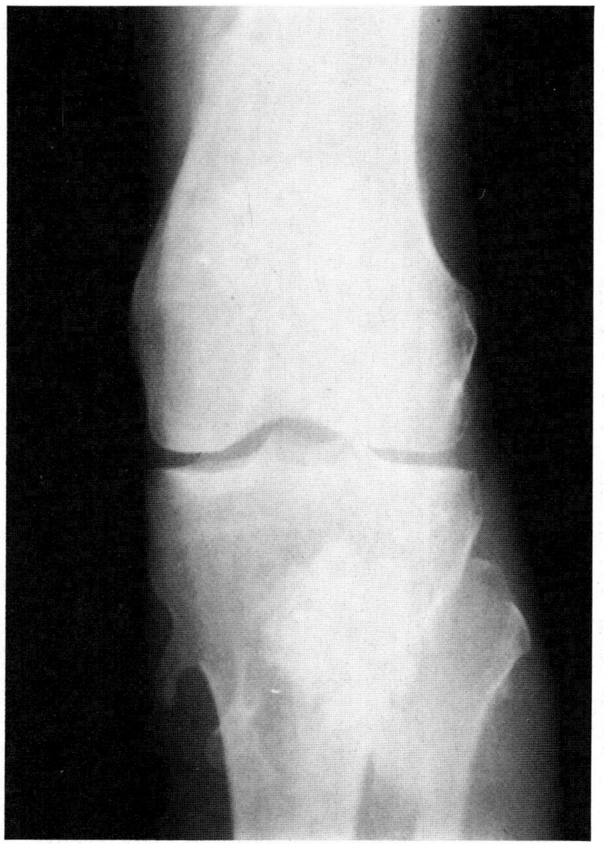
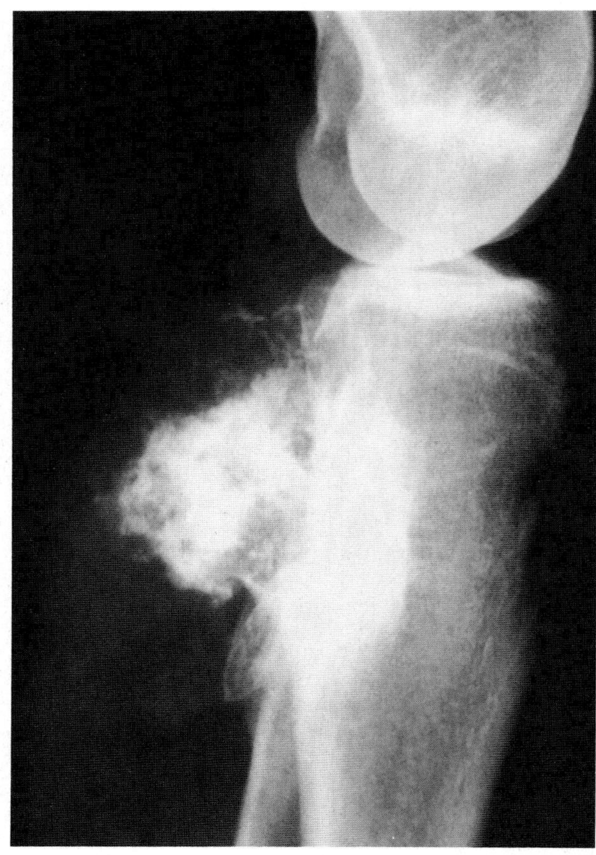

Several exostoses of the 'coat-hanger' type are present in the femoral, tibial and fibular diametaphyses, all directed towards the diaphyses. One on the posterior aspect of the tibia has become enlarged, irregular and sclerotic, consistent with chondrosarcomatous change in the cartilage cap of the exostosis. The patient's complaint of increased swelling and pain is of great importance in suggesting the presence of this complication.

Diaphyseal aclasis is an autosomal dominant condition presenting in childhood with palpable bony excrescences. The cartilage-capped exostoses occur in the long bones, particularly around the knee, and occasionally in the spine. They may produce symptoms by pressure on nerves and vessels and are often associated with asymmetrical interruption of growth which may result in altered limb length and Madelung's deformity.

Sarcomatous change occurs in a minority of cases, probably rather fewer than the ten per cent incidence reported in some highly selected series.

Reference

Garrison, R. C., Unni, K. K., McLeod, R. A. et al. (1982) Chondrosarcoma arising in osteochondroma. *Cancer*, **49**, 1890-1897.

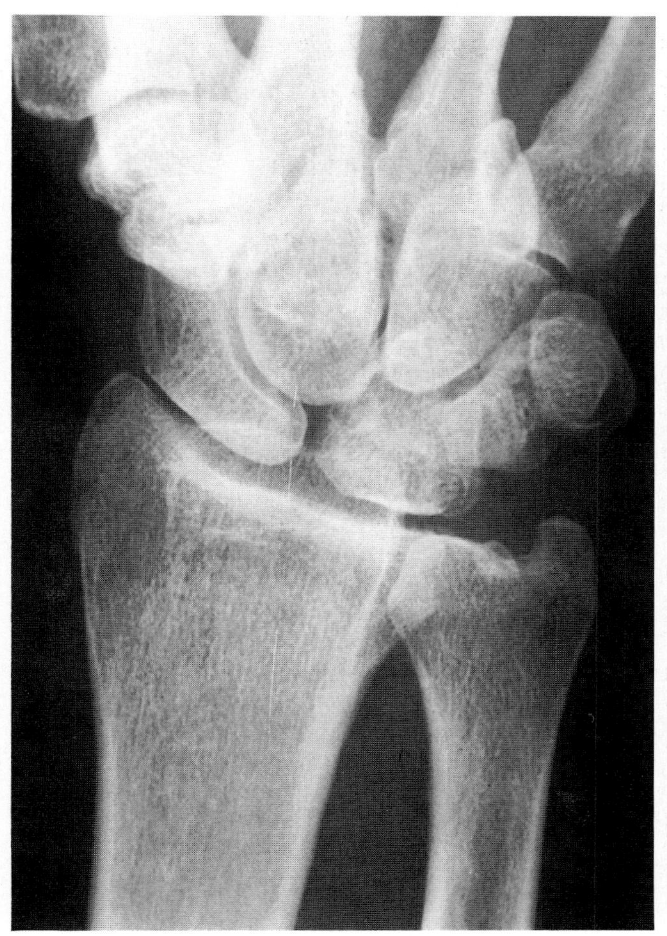 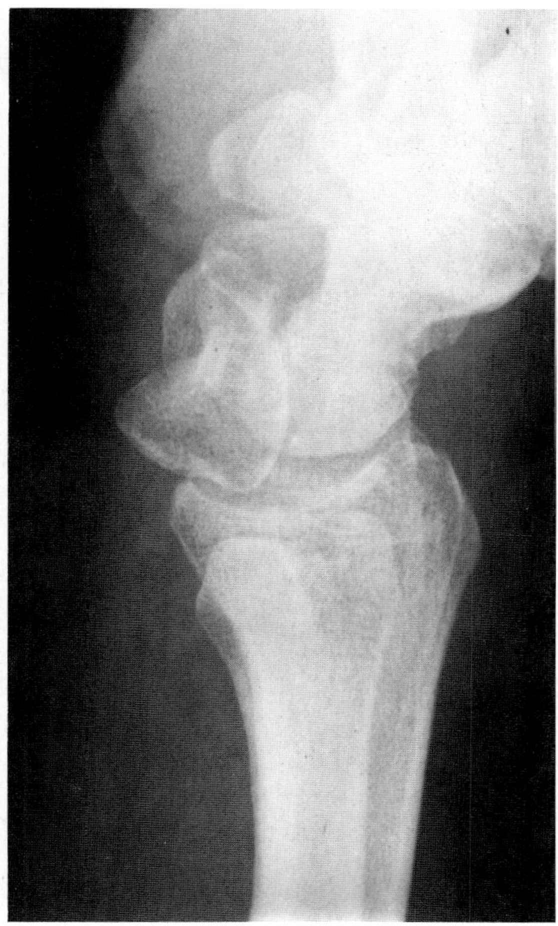

This patient was seen in the Casualty Department following a road traffic accident.

- What is the diagnosis?
- What complication is associated with this injury?

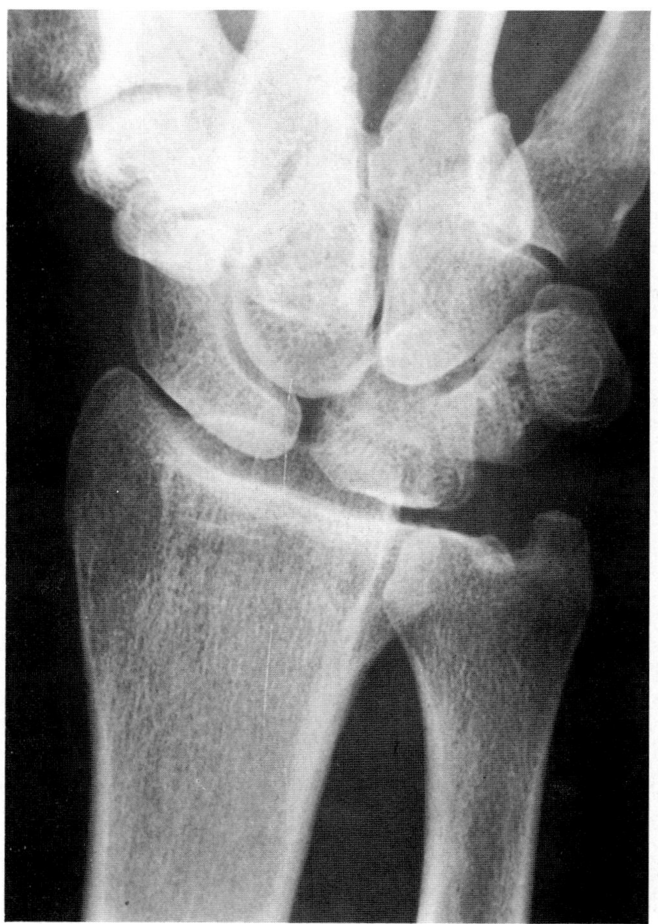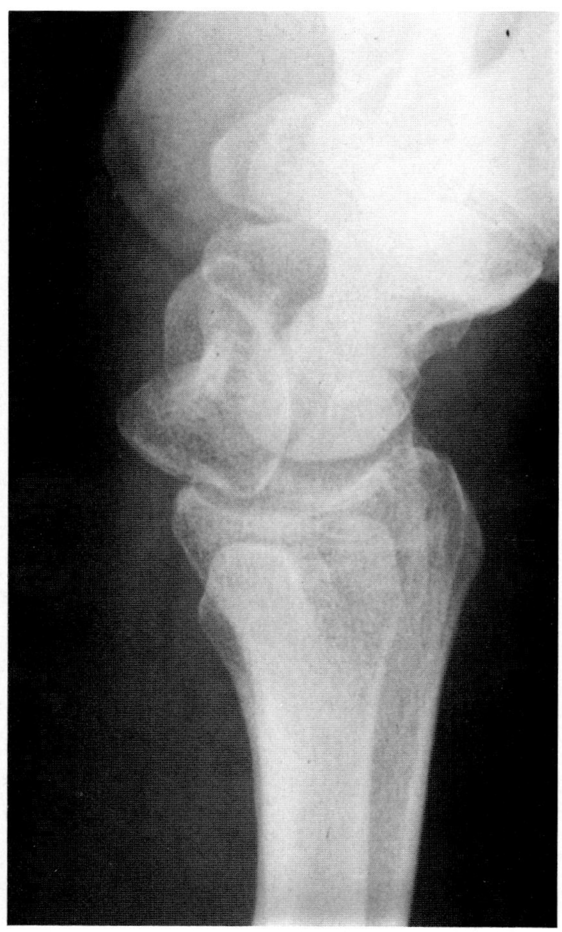

The lateral projection of the wrist shows that the lunate has been displaced in a volar direction while the normal alignment of the articular surface of the radius has been maintained. The capitate has moved proximally to take up the normal position of the lunate in relationship to the radius. In the PA view the lunate does not have its normal quadrilateral shape but is more or less triangular in configuration. These are the appearances of a lunate dislocation.

Early detection is important as the dislocated lunate may compress the median nerve and delayed reduction can result in incomplete recovery of a nerve palsy.

In some instances it may be difficult to decide whether the injury is a volar dislocation of the lunate or a dorsal perilunate dislocation.

Reference

Gilula, L. A. (1979) Carpal injuries: analytic approach and case exercises. *Amer. J. Roentgenol.*, 133, 503-517.

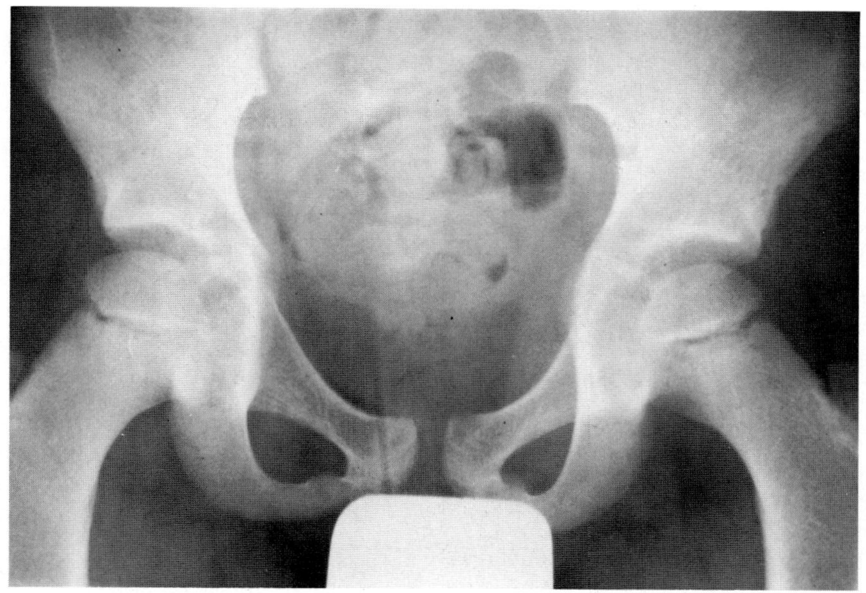

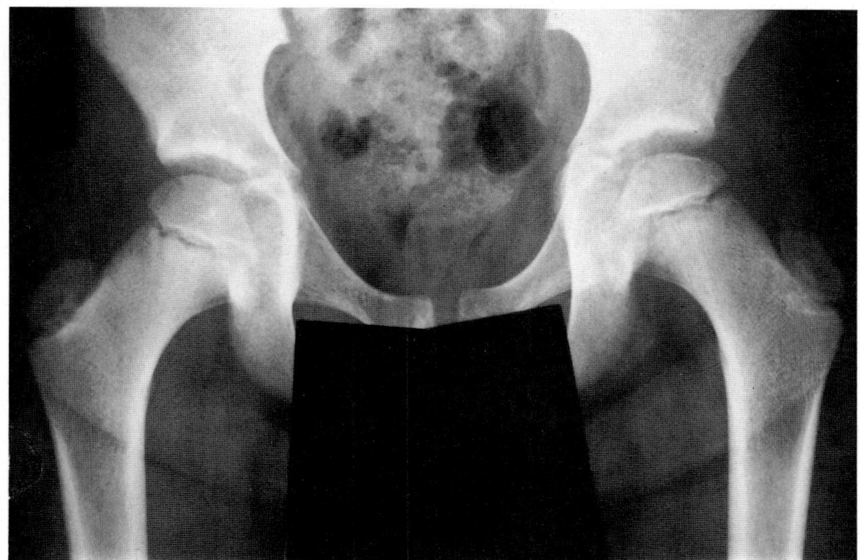

A 7-year-old boy presented with a limp and pain in his left hip.

- Describe the radiographs, the bottom one taken three months later than the top one.

- What diagnosis would you suggest and how might you confirm it?

- What other view should you obtain?

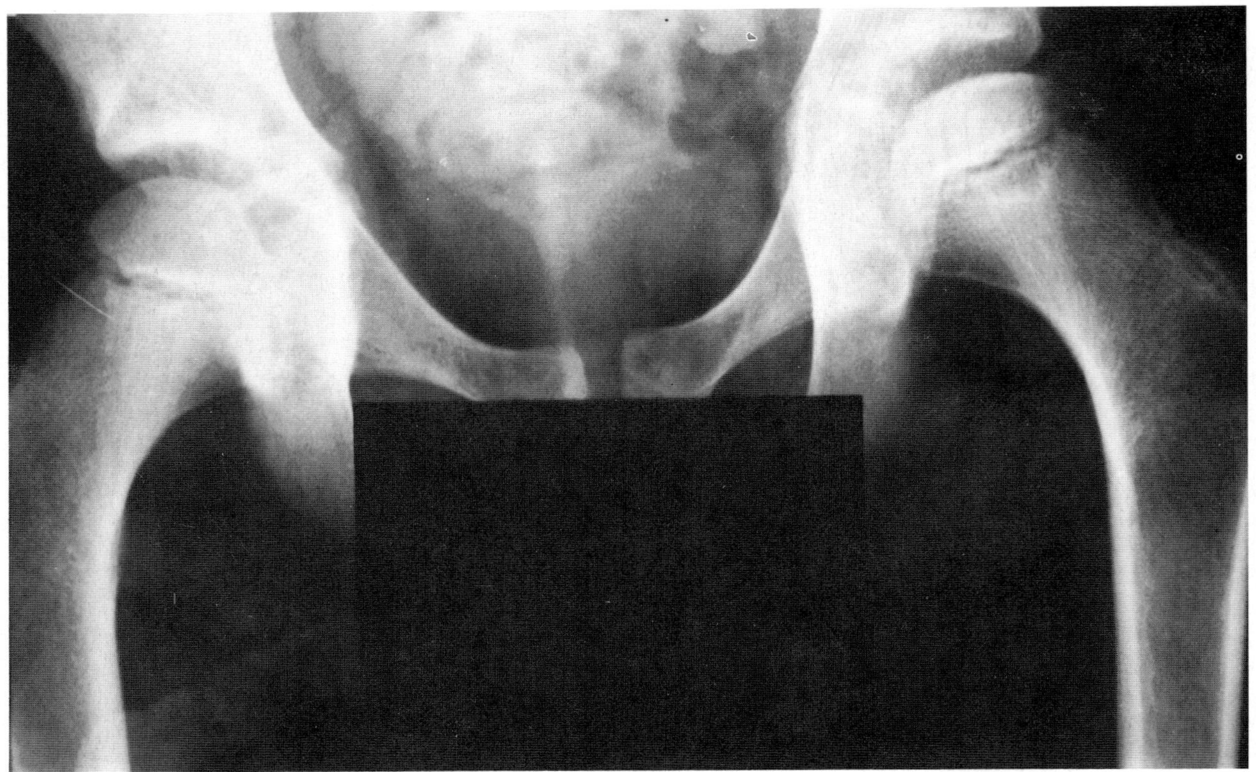

The initial film shows widening of the medial joint space of the left hip consistent with an effusion. This could be confirmed by ultrasonic examination.

Three months later the left femoral epiphysis shows flattening and irregularity. Fine sclerotic densities in the epiphysis confirm the presence of avascular necrosis which, in this case, is due to Perthes' disease.

Perthes' disease has a predilection for males and tends to occur between the ages of 4 and 12 years. Early in the disease, radiographs may be normal or show evidence of a joint effusion. Bone scintigraphy will often demonstrate an area of reduced or absent uptake due to avascular necrosis in the epiphysis before the typical radiographic changes develop. These include a small flattened femoral epiphysis, which may be laterally placed, and metaphyseal irregularity.

Necrosis tends to affect the anterolateral part of the epiphysis, an area better shown by the frog lateral (right) than the AP projection (above).

Perthes' disease is bilateral in up to ten per cent of patients, but this is rarely simultaneous. Other causes of avascular necrosis should always be considered, especially when the changes are bilateral and symmetrical.

Georg Clemens Perthes (1869-1927) was a surgeon in Leipzig and later Professor of Surgery in Tubingen. He described the disorder in 1910, the same year as Legg and Calvé, and so the disorder is often given the name of all three.

Reference

Catterall, A. (1971) The natural history of Perthes' disease. *J. Bone Joint Surg.*, 53-B, 37-53.

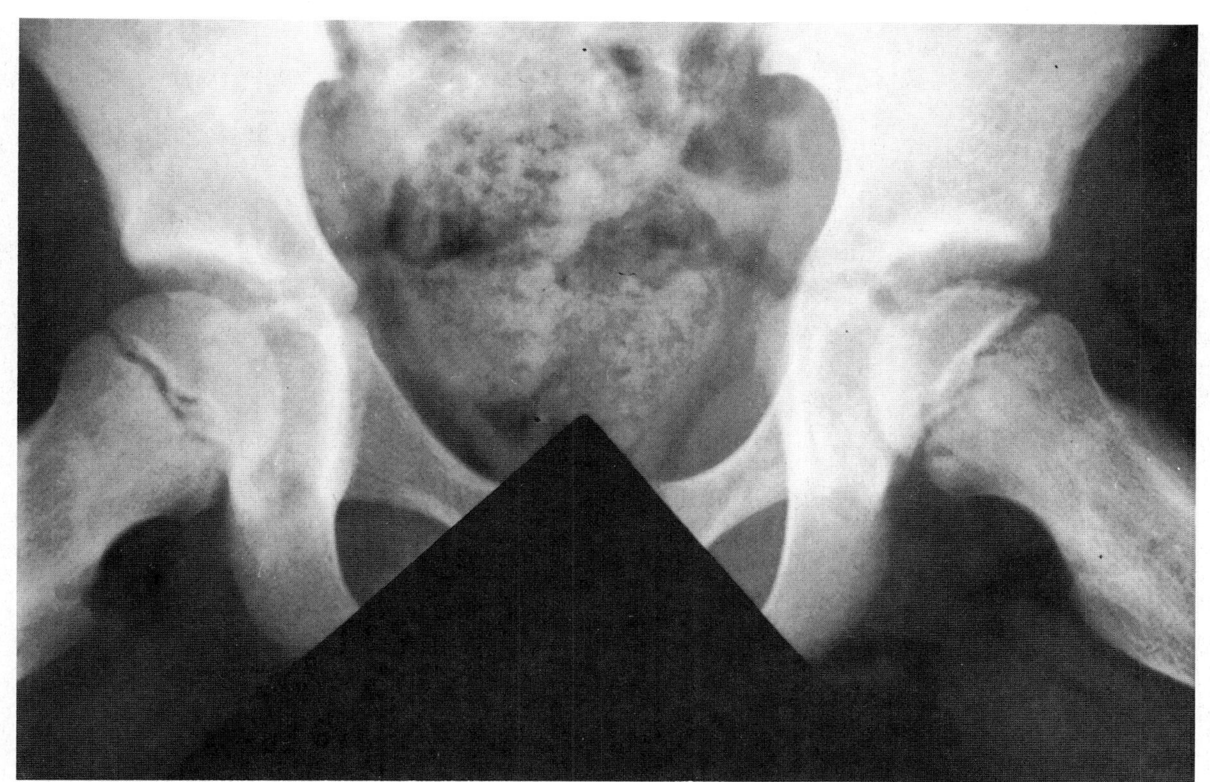

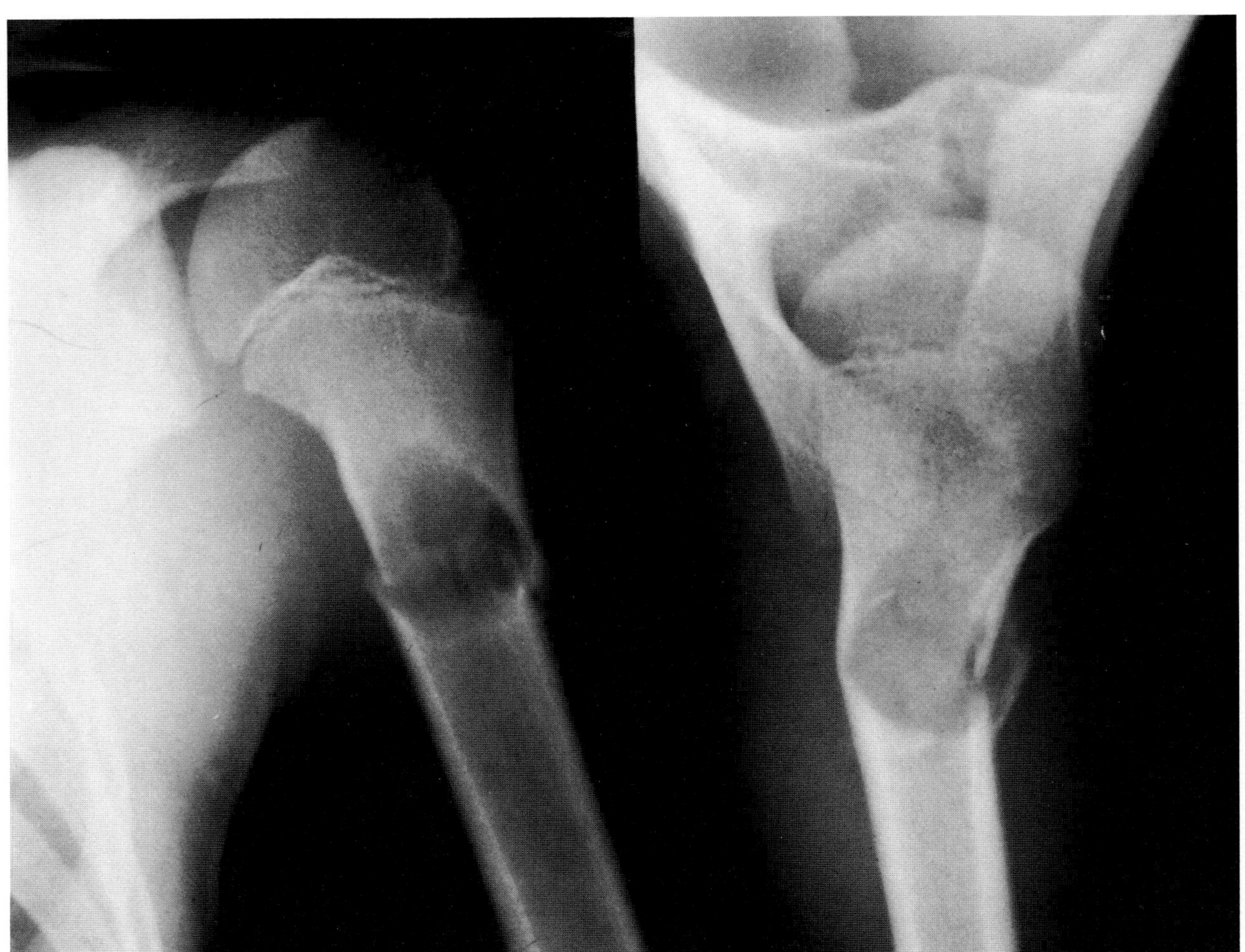

This 13-year-old boy was examined following a trivial injury.

- What is the diagnosis?
- How may such a lesion be managed?

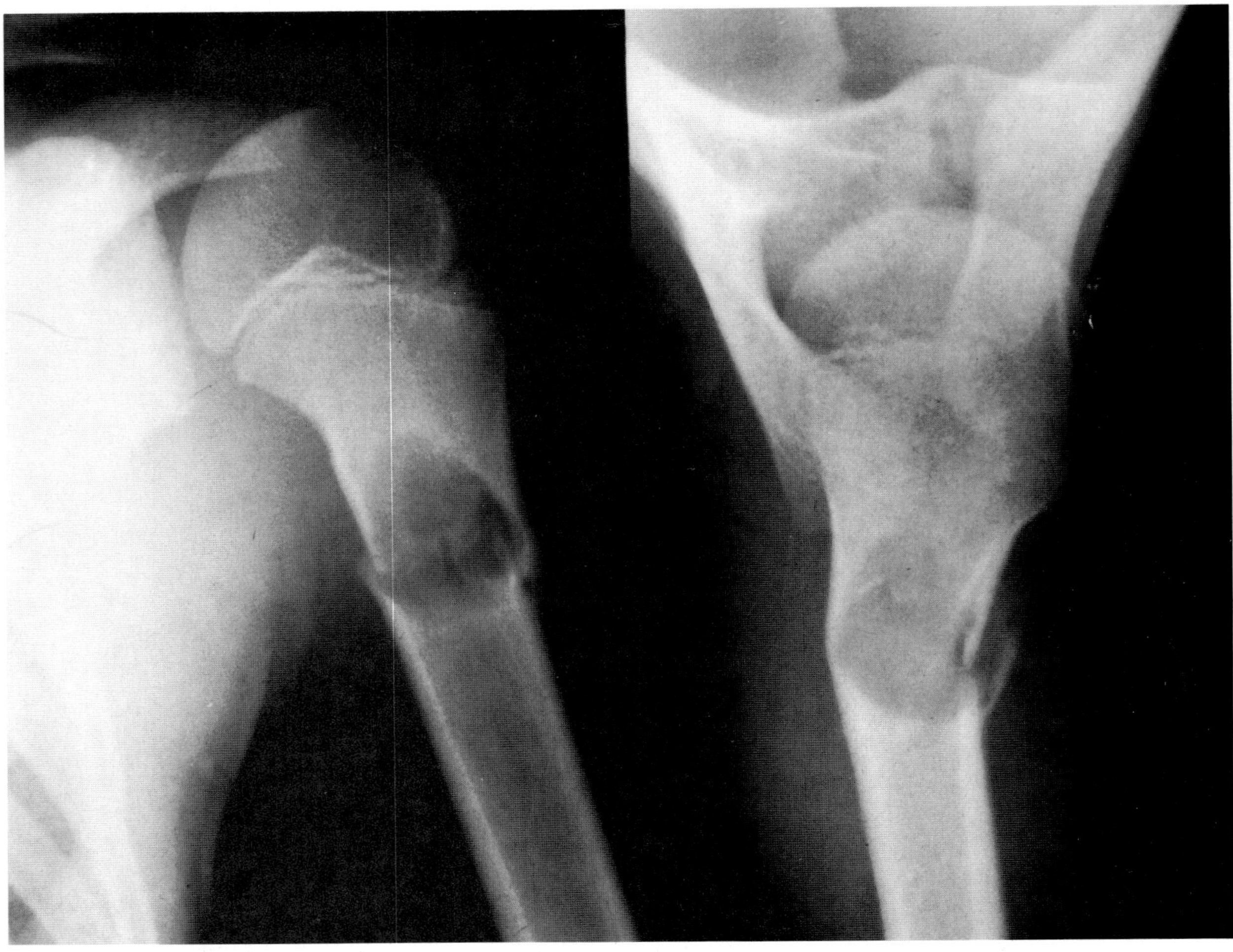

A pathological fracture has been sustained through a typical solitary bone cyst. These childhood lesions develop in the metaphysis and are well-defined, centrally located and usually unilocular. They may cause thinning and expansion of the cortex, and presentation with a fracture is common. Cysts in the proximal humerus and femur account for over 80 per cent of cases. Cysts may occur in the distal femur, proximal tibia and calcaneus in young adults.

Simple cysts are rarely symptomatic unless fractured, although a dull ache may be experienced. Following immobilisation, fractures usually heal but a part of the cyst may persist and enlarge. With growth, the cyst often migrates distally or may remain at the metaphysis. Orthodox treatment by curettage followed by packing with bone chips has been replaced recently in some centres by cyst puncture and injection of long-acting corticosteroids.

Fibrous dysplasia and aneurysmal bone cysts may cause diagnostic confusion although the latter are usually rapidly expansile and often eccentric.

References

Baker, D. M. (1970) Benign unicameral bone cysts. A study of 45 cases with long-term follow-up. *Clin. Orthop.*, 71, 140-151.

Fernbach, S. K. et al. (1981) Radiographic changes in unicameral bone cysts following direct injection of steroids. A report on 14 cases. *Radiology*, 140, 689-695.

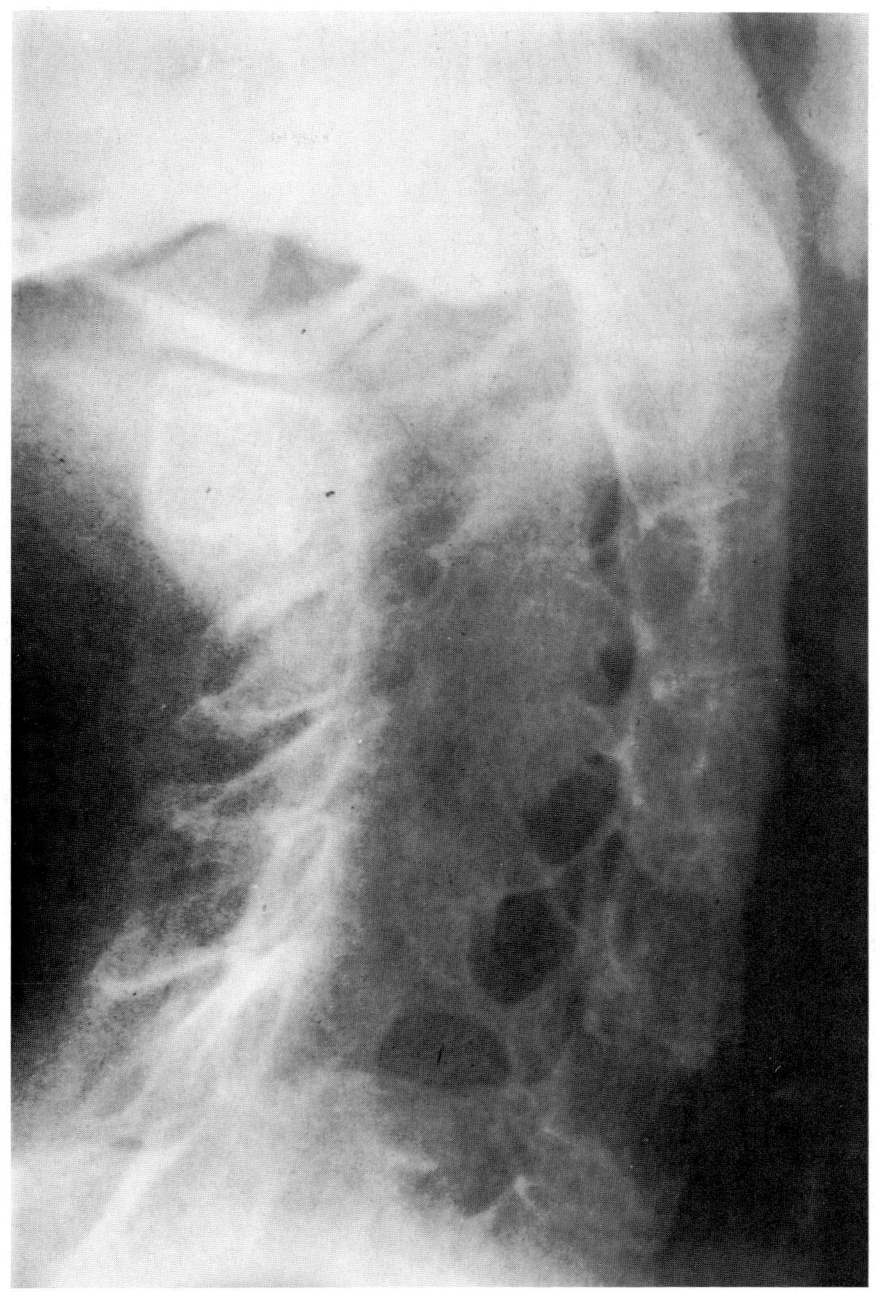

This woman aged 36 complained of neck stiffness.

- Describe the abnormalities in the cervical spine.

- What might be the cause?

A61

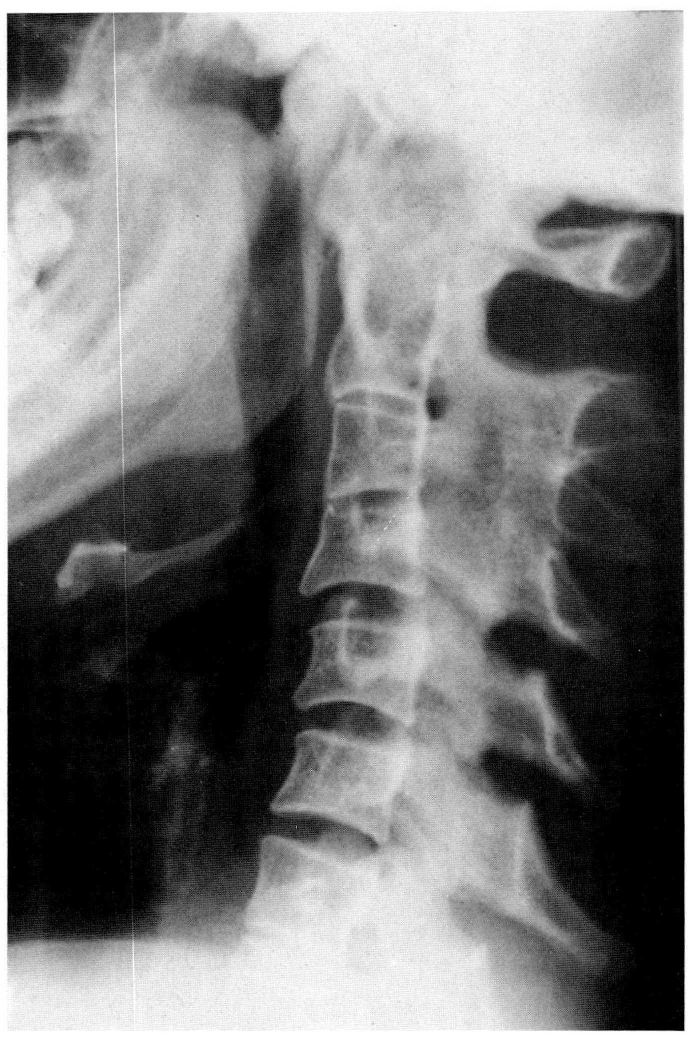

The lateral radiograph of the cervical spine shows ankylosis of the apophyseal joints, hypoplastic vertebral bodies and narrowed disc spaces between C2 and C4. The bodies of C1 and C2 are fused. These appearances may be observed following juvenile chronic arthritis and must be differentiated from localised congenital block vertebrae and the Klippel-Feil deformity, conditions where vertebral body height is maintained and fusion may also occur between the spinous processes.

The cervical spine is ultimately affected in two-thirds of those with juvenile chronic arthritis, predominantly at the C2/3 level. Inflammatory change and ankylosis in the apophyseal joints is followed by inhibition of growth in the contiguous vertebral bodies. The final deformity is more pronounced the younger the age of onset.

A second, less extensive example involving C2-4 is shown above.

Sir George Frederick Still (1868-1941) was paediatric physician at King's College Hospital and the first Professor of Paediatrics in Britain. He described the disorder in 1896 in his M.D. thesis while still a registrar.

Reference

Martel, W., Holt, J. F. and Cassidy, J. T. (1962) Roentgenologic manifestations of juvenile rheumatoid arthritis. *Amer. J. Roentgenol.*, 88, 400-423.

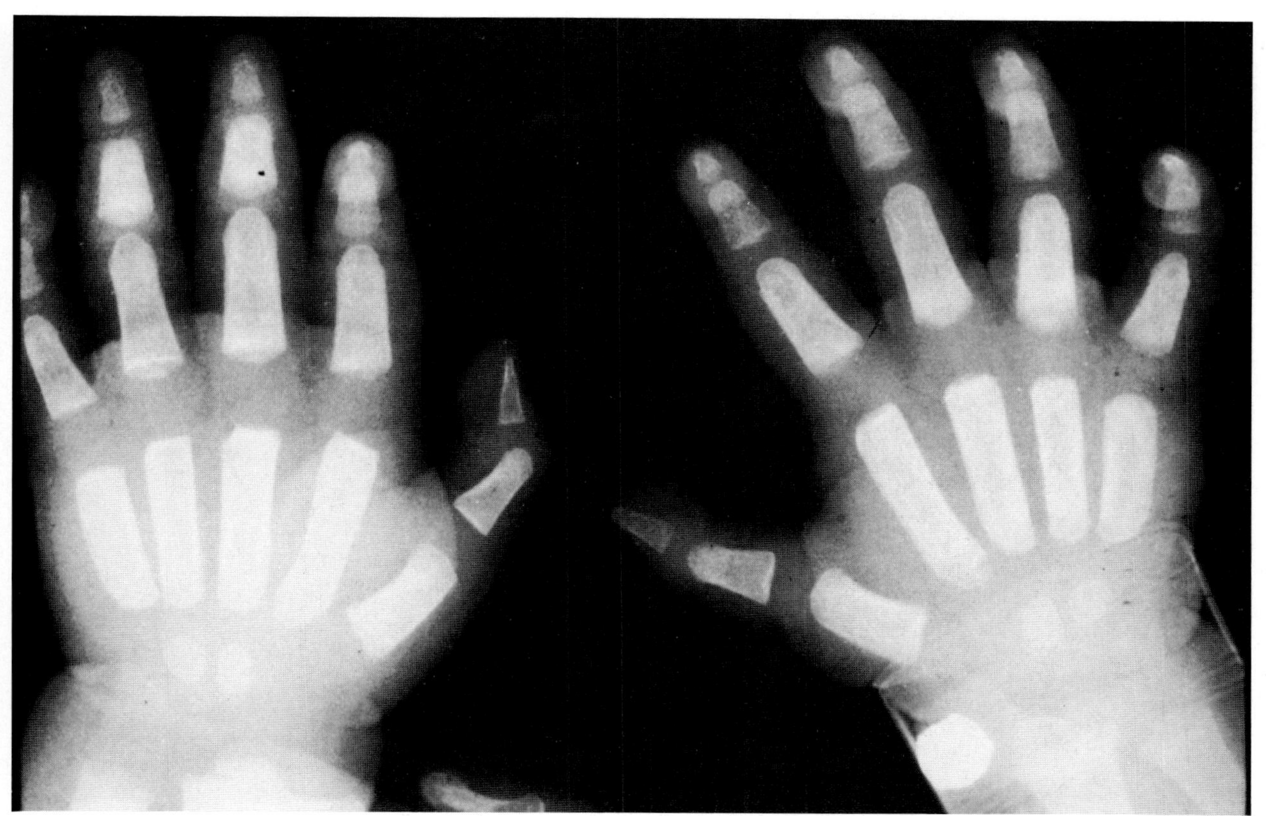

This 18-month-old black child presented with a
ten-day history of painful hands and feet.

- What diagnoses would you consider?

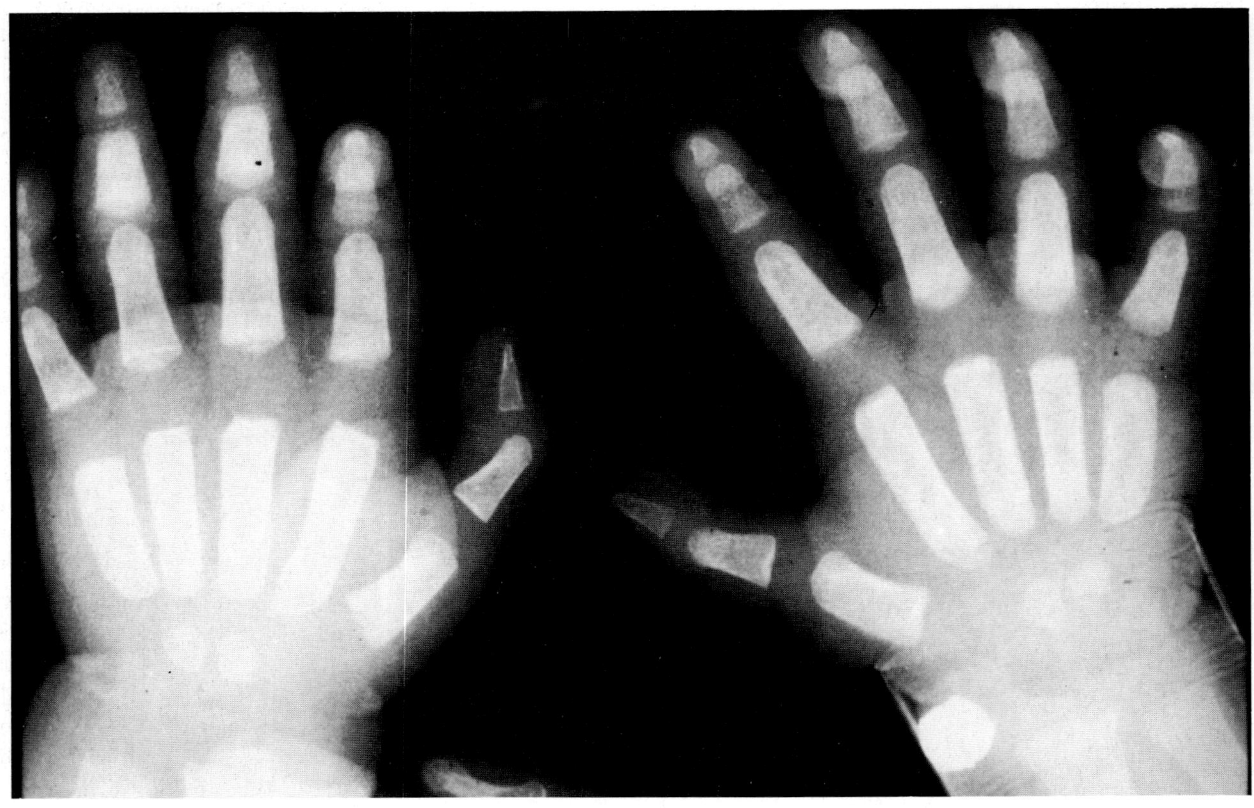

Patchy diaphyseal lucencies and the formation of periosteal new bone are evident in the metacarpals and phalanges, with generalised soft tissue swelling. Similar changes were present in the feet.

The differential diagnosis lies between sickle-cell dactylitis (the hand-foot syndrome) and/or osteomyelitis. In sickle-cell disease, osteonecrosis only affects the extremities between the ages of six months and two years, occurring in 20 per cent of such patients. The haemopoietic marrow in the hands and feet at this age appears particularly prone to circulatory stasis and infarction, particularly during vasoconstriction in the cold. Metaphyseal infarction can result in premature fusion and brachydactyly.

Patients with sickle-cell disease show an increased incidence of osteomyelitis as infarcted bone is particularly susceptible. Salmonella is a frequent pathogen, probably as a consequence of micro-infarction of the intestine leading to bacteraemia. Infarction and infection of bone cannot be reliably distinguished clinically or radiologically and all patients should initially receive antibiotics.

In this case, plasma electrophoresis confirmed the presence of sickle-cell disease and no evidence of infection was forthcoming.

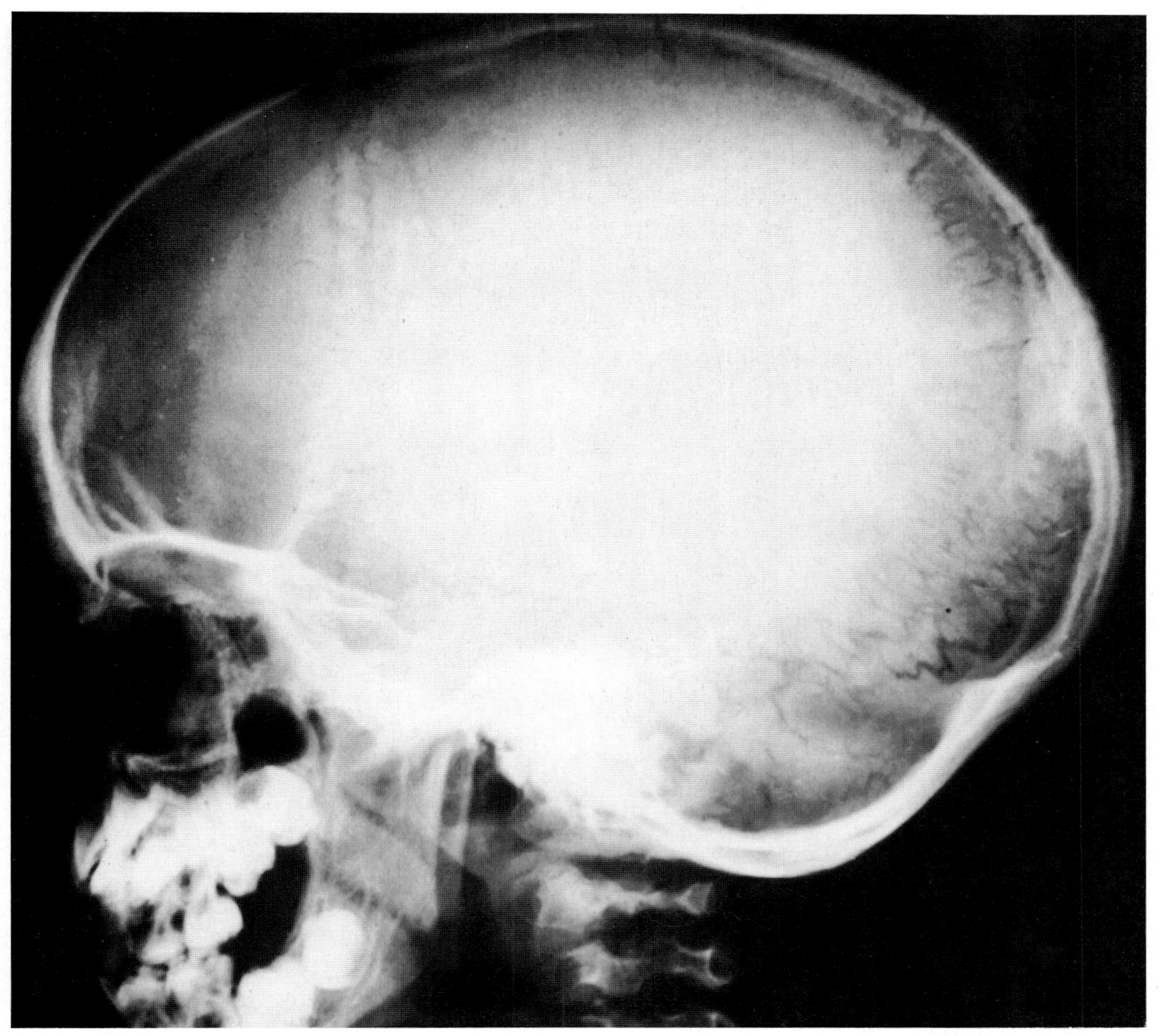

This skull radiograph was obtained following a head injury.

- What unusual feature is present?

- What differential diagnoses would you consider?

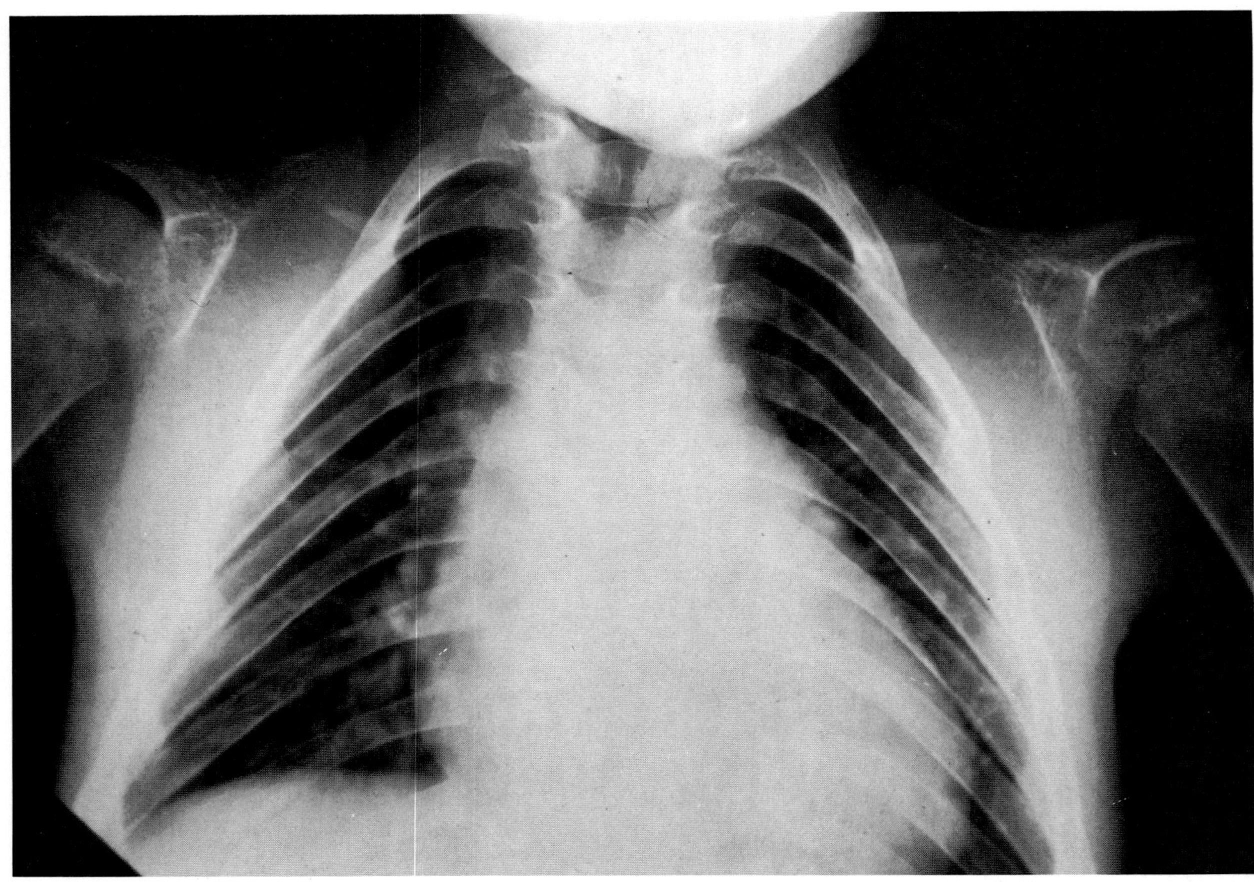

No fracture is evident but incidental multiple Wormian (sutural) bones are present. These occur in numerous conditions such as cleidocranial dysplasia, osteogenesis imperfecta, cretinism, Down's syndrome and hypophosphatasia.

A chest radiograph in this child revealed hypoplastic clavicles, consistent with cleidocranial dysplasia, a defective neural arch at C1, and cervical ribs.

Cleidocranial dysplasia usually has no major clinical significance; the clavicles may be absent or their lateral portions deficient to a variable degree. Inheritance is usually autosomal dominant in type. Other features include defects of cranial ossification, small facial bones, supernumerary teeth and incomplete ossification of the margins of the symphysis pubis.

Reference

Jarvis, L. J. and Keats, T. E. (1974) Cleidocranial dysostosis; a review of 40 cases. *Amer. J. Roentgenol.*, **121**, 5-16.

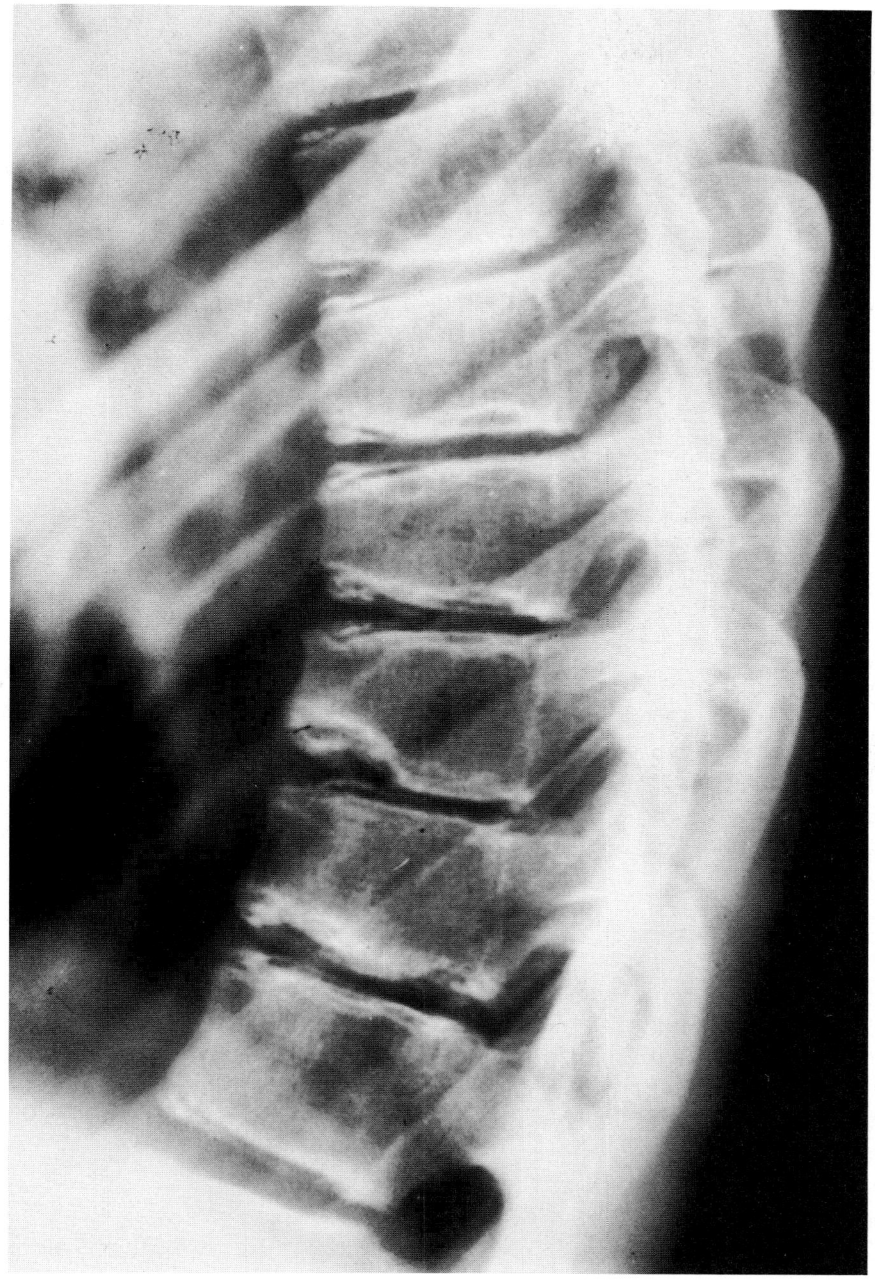

This adolescent complained of a rounded back deformity.

- What is the diagnosis and what are the characteristic radiographic changes in this condition?

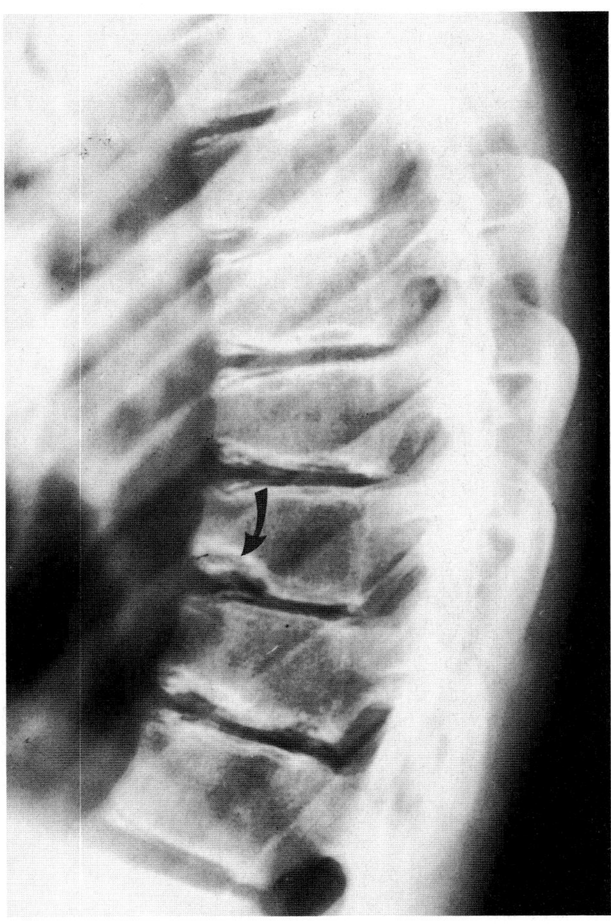

The appearances are characteristic of Scheuermann's disease. Irregularity of the end-plates is associated with intraosseous cartilaginous (Schmorl's) nodes (arrow), anterior wedging of the vertebral bodies, narrowing of the discs and a progressive kyphosis. The disorder presents in adolescence and affects the thoracic (75 per cent) or thoracolumbar (25 per cent) spine.

The aetiology is uncertain but probably related to stress-induced herniation of cartilage through constitutionally weak end-plates, with abnormal growth of the vertebral bodies.

Scheuermann's disease is self-limiting and does not progress after skeletal maturation. It may be complicated by thoracic disc herniation and anterior bony bridging.

The condition results from the normal stresses on the adolescent skeleton. Similar changes, although rarely widespread or at multiple levels, may occur as a result of athletic abuse of the vulnerable adolescent spine; activities such as gymnastics, trampolining, water-skiing and diving have all been implicated. Here again, the principal lesion is an intravertebral anterior discal herniation.

The differential diagnosis of kyphosis includes osteoporosis, trauma, infection and postural causes but the characteristic changes in Scheuermann's disease assist identification of this condition.

Holger Werfel Scheuermann (1877-1960) trained as both a radiologist and an orthopaedic surgeon in Denmark. The description of the disease in 1920 was in his doctoral thesis, which was rejected.

Reference

Bradford, D. S. (1977) Juvenile kyphosis. *Clin. Orthop.*, **128**, 45-55.

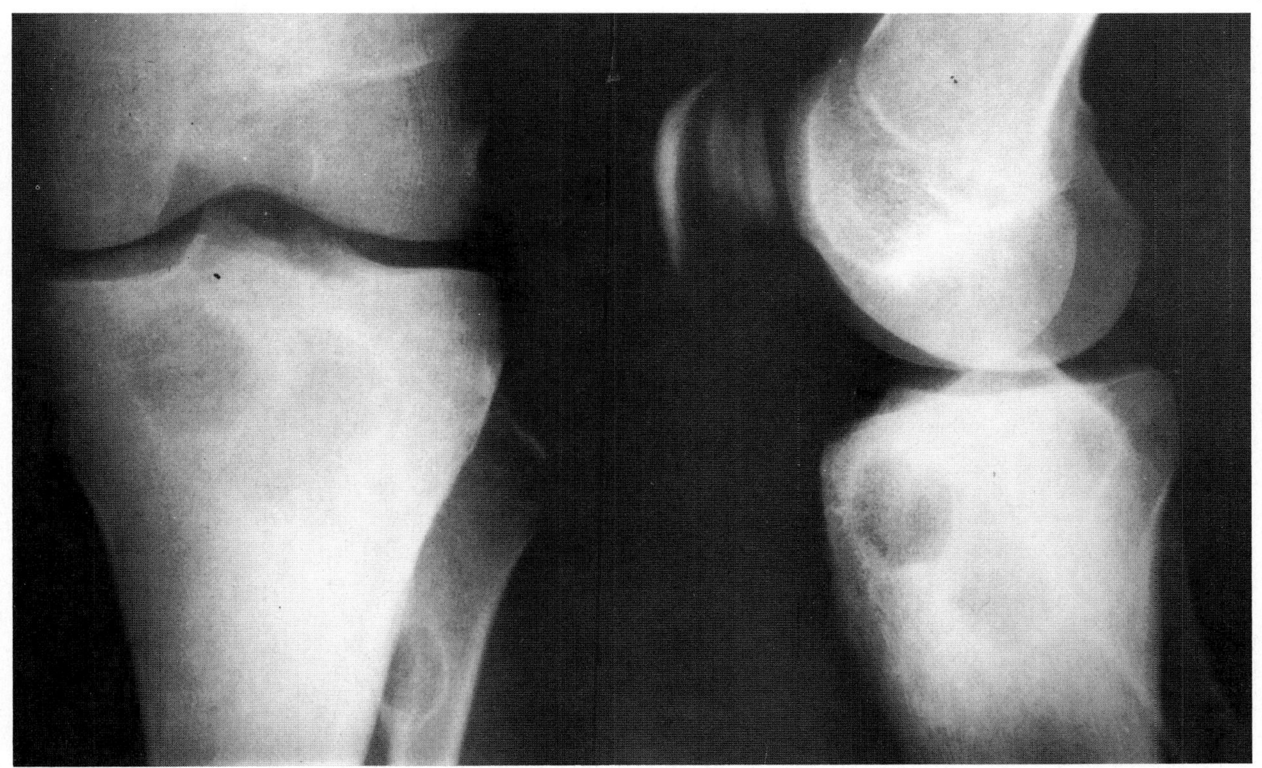

This 13-year-old girl presented with a six-month history of pain in the knee.

- Two lesions are shown; how do they differ in their radiological appearances?

- What is the likely aetiology of the tibial lesion?

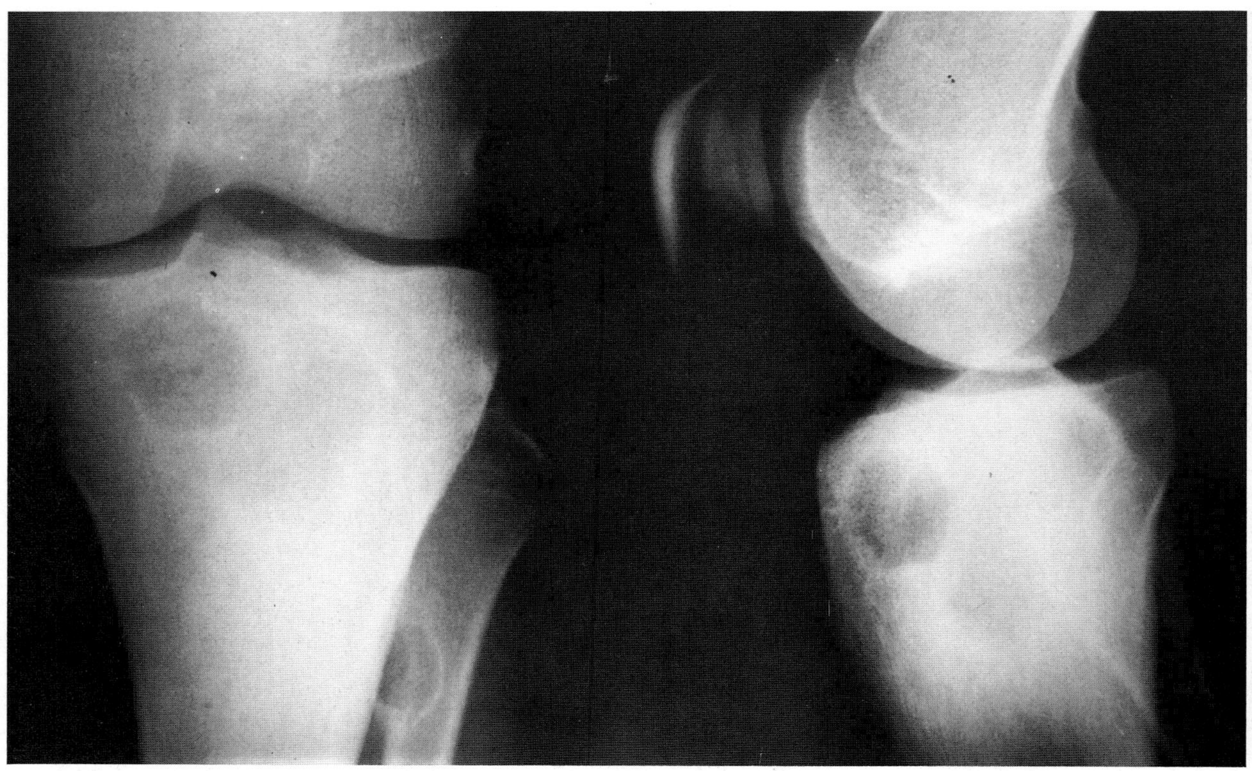

A multiloculated zone of medullary destruction with surrounding sclerosis is present in the proximal tibia. An organised periosteal reaction is demonstrated anteriorly on the lateral projection. These appearances are characteristic of a Brodie's abscess, where the infection is most commonly due to *Staphylococcus aureus*, as in this case.

Brodie's abscesses have a predilection for the ends of tubular bones and in particular the metaphyses in children. Pyogenic infections are, to some extent, confined by the growth plate; an associated septic arthritis is rare except when the metaphysis is intra-articular, e.g. in the hip joint.

Observe the incidental fibrous cortical defect in the fibula. This well-defined lucency has a fine sclerotic rim, and is eccentrically placed in the proximal part of the diaphysis. These benign lesions occur frequently in the growing child and most are found in the femur and tibia.

Sir Benjamin Brodie (1783-1862) was surgeon to St. George's Hospital and described the chronic abscess with no identifiable acute stage in 1832.

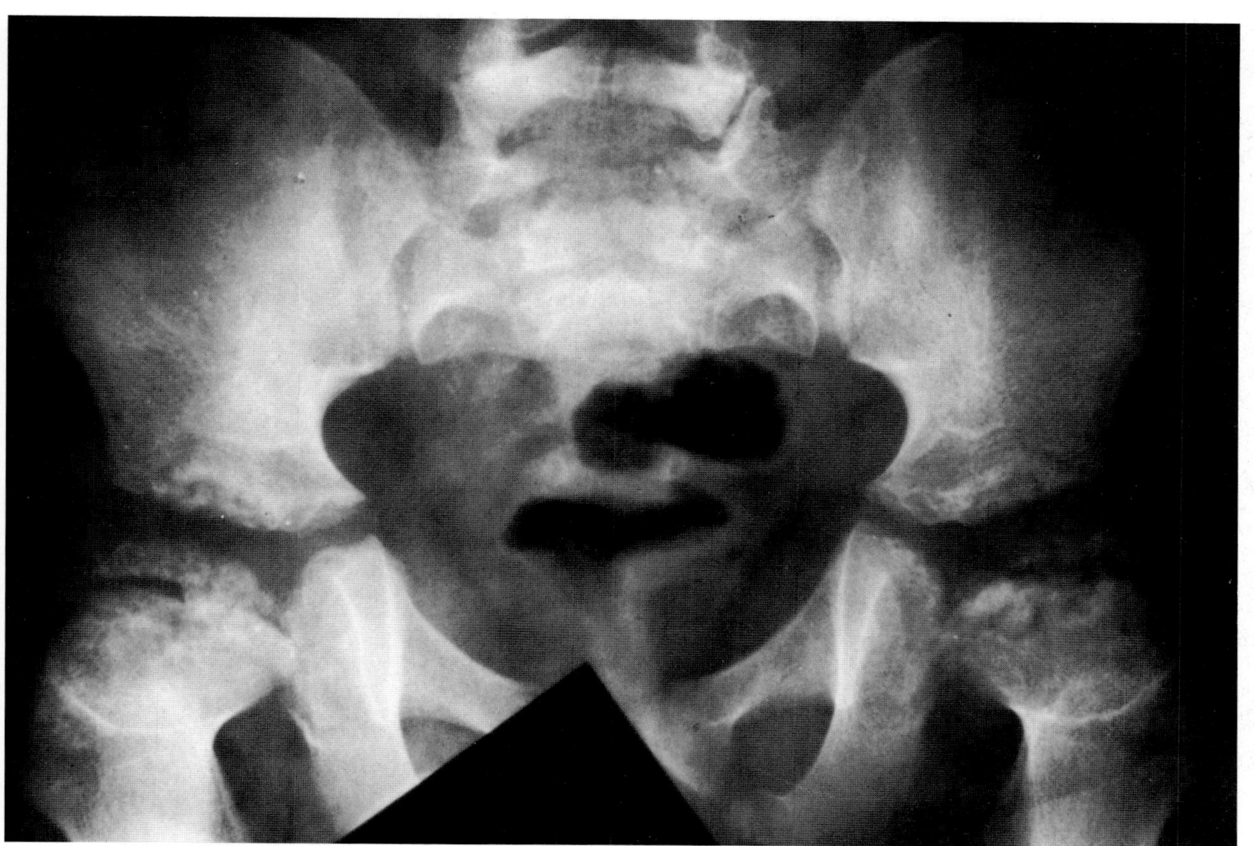

This 14-year-old boy presented for investigation of short stature.

- Describe the abnormalities on the radiograph and suggest possible diagnoses.

- What other conventional radiograph may be useful in the differential diagnosis?

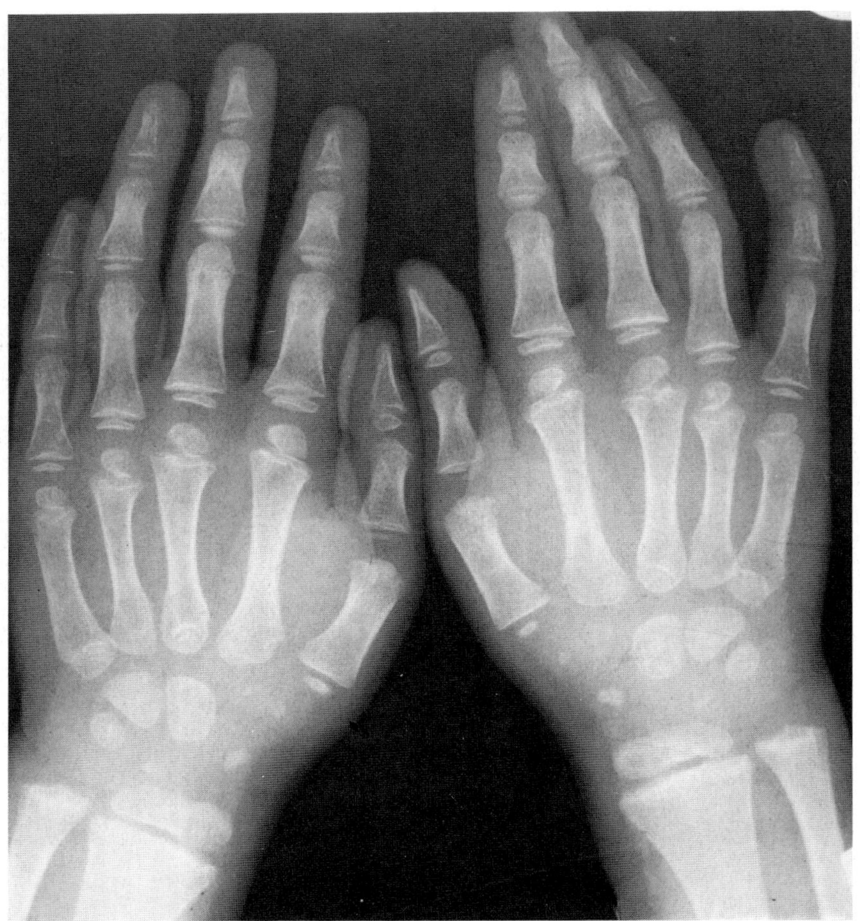

A view of the pelvis demonstrates the characteristic dysplastic fragmented femoral epiphyses and coxa vara seen in cretinism. The differential diagnosis might include bilateral Perthes' disease (which, however, is rarely symmetrical in onset or severity) and multiple epiphyseal dysplasia.

Assessment of the skeletal age from a radiograph of the hands is an important additional investigation. Here, skeletal maturation is severely retarded, with an estimated bone age of six years. Delayed development in a child with short stature may be due to severe constitutional disease, e.g. cretinism, rickets, hypopituitarism, hypogonadism, Turner's syndrome, mucopolysaccharidoses and other osteochondrodysplasias, and steroid therapy. This patient was clinically and biochemically hypothyroid and had none of the characteristic clinical or radiological features of the other disorders.

In hypothyroidism, skeletal blood flow and both the formation and resorption of bone are reduced, leading to a disturbance in modelling and delay in skeletal maturation.

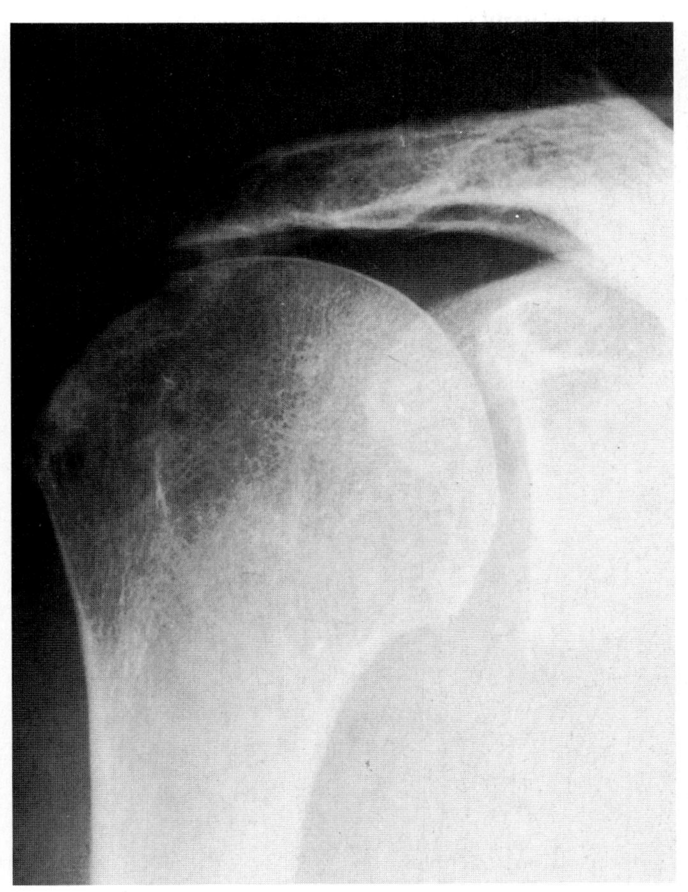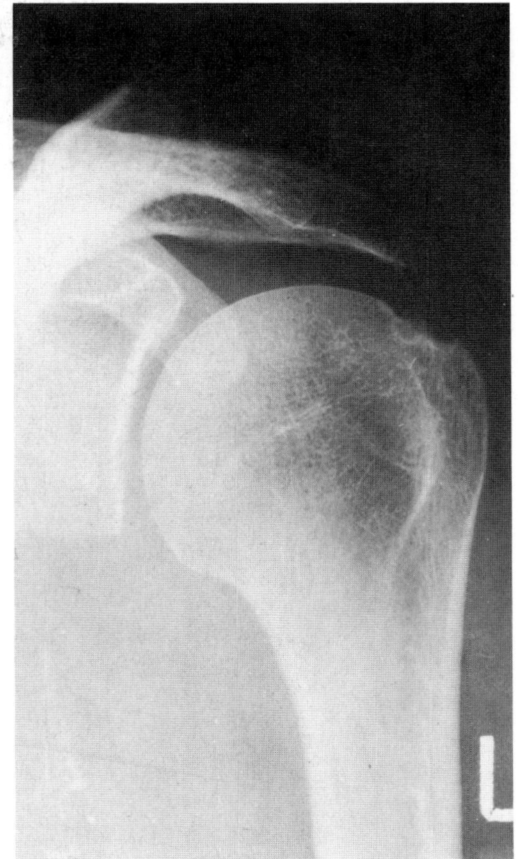

This middle-aged patient presented with chronic shoulder pain with limitation of abduction.

- Describe the radiological features.
- Can the diagnosis be made on these films?
- If not, what further investigation should be performed?

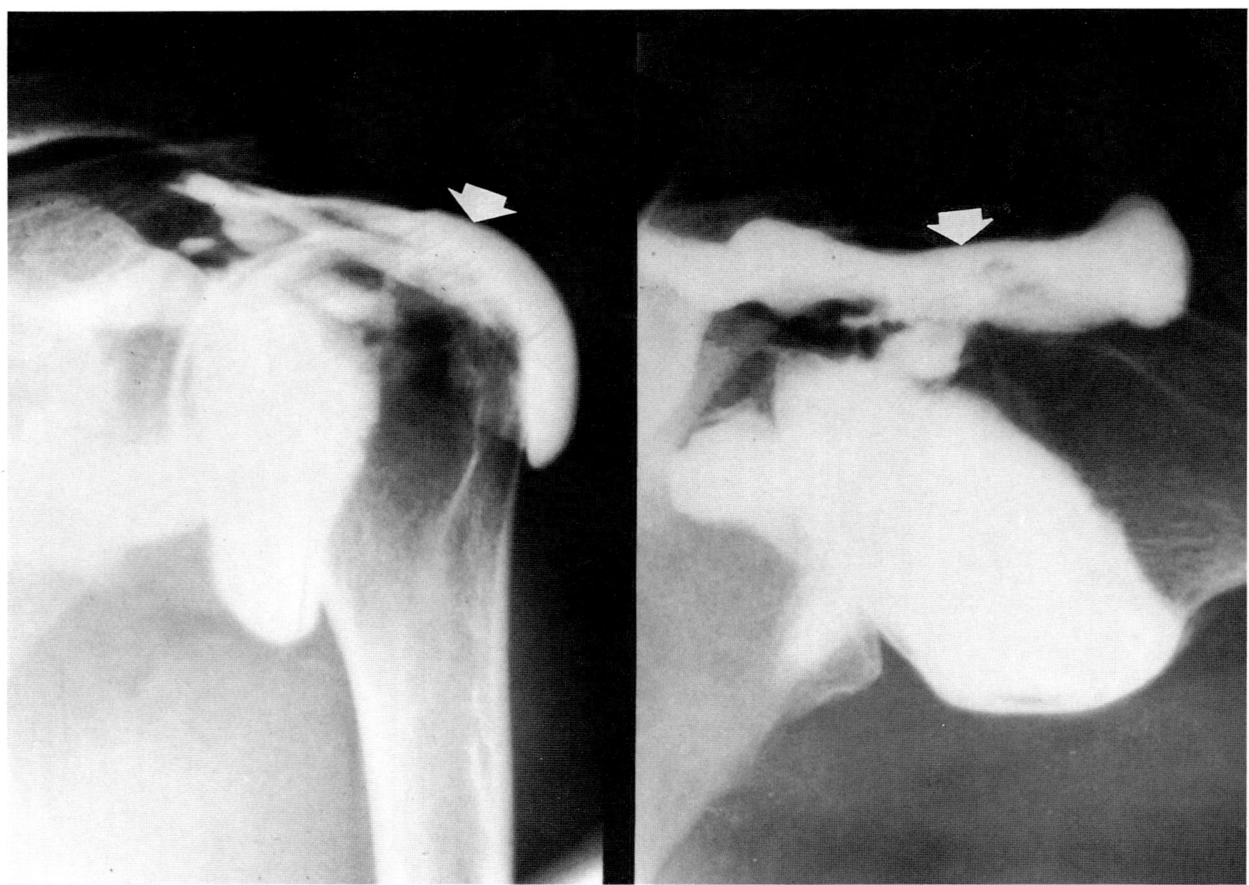

The AP view of the right shoulder shows narrowing of the acromiohumeral joint space, flattening and sclerosis of the humeral head at the site of insertion of the rotator cuff tendon and calcification within the tendon. These features indicate a chronic tear of the rotator cuff and no further investigation is required for diagnosis.

On the left, the acromiohumeral joint space is preserved, but cystic changes are present in the greater tuberosity and an abnormal concavity is shown by the inferior surface of the acromion. These appearances are suggestive of a previous injury to the rotator cuff, but a tear cannot be diagnosed without arthrography. In this examination contrast medium is shown to pass through a large rotator cuff tear and to fill the subacromial bursa (arrowed).

The muscles forming the rotator cuff comprise the supraspinatus, infraspinatus and teres minor muscles which arise from the posterior aspect of the scapula and are inserted into the greater tuberosity, and the subscapularis which inserts into the lesser tuberosity. The tendons fuse with each other and the capsule of the glenohumeral joint to form the rotator cuff tendinous expansion which lies between the humeral head and the acromion. It separates the glenohumeral joint from the subacromial bursa. Degenerative changes or trauma can result in a partial or complete tear and subsequent communication between the glenohumeral joint and the subacromial bursa. Tears due to attrition are particularly common in association with rheumatoid arthritis.

Reference

Kotzen, L. M. (1971) Roentgen diagnosis of rotator cuff tear. Report of 48 surgically-proven cases. *Amer. J. Roentgenol.*, **112**, 507-511.

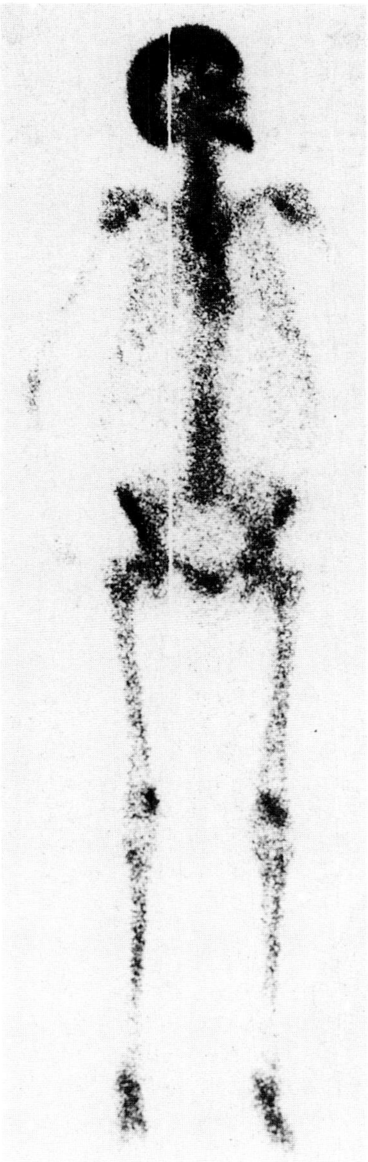

This patient was being treated for a chronic illness.

- What is abnormal in the radionuclide bone scan?

- What term is applied to the appearances shown?

- What disorder may this patient have?

A68

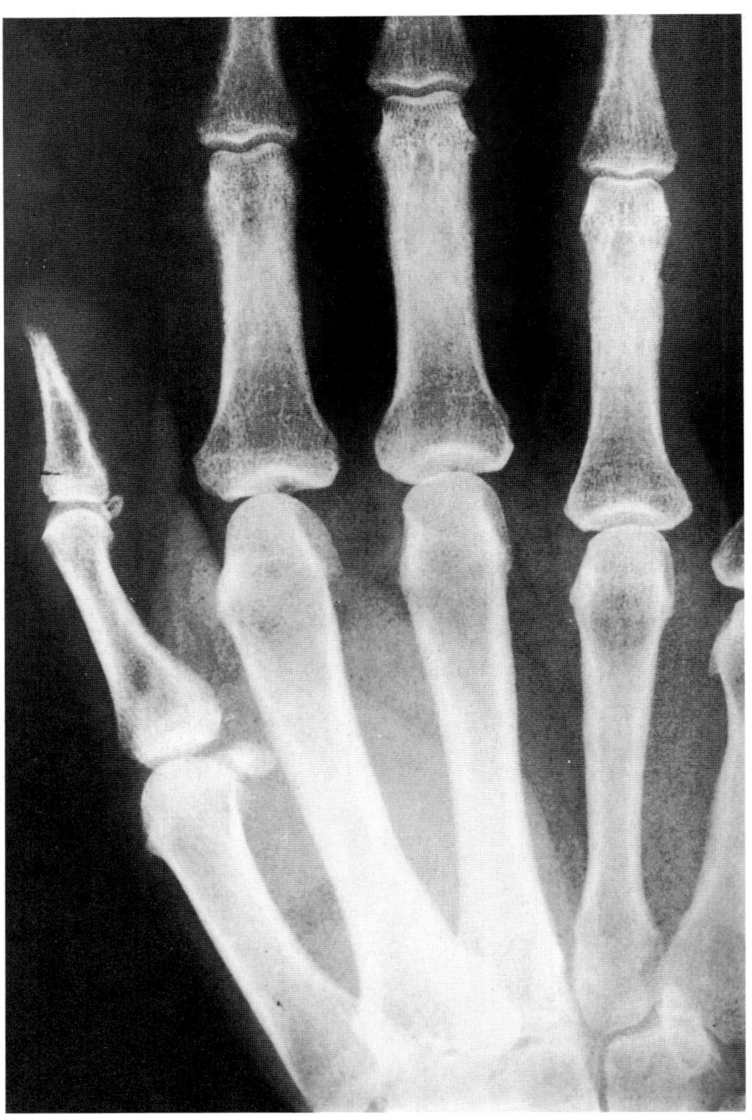

The ^{99m}Tc diphosphonate scan shows a genera-lised increase in skeletal isotope activity but no uptake in the kidneys or other soft tissues; this is often referred to as a 'superscan'. A generalised increase in bone activity is common to all conditions with increased bone turnover, such as osteomalacia, hyperparathyroidism, renal osteodystrophy, acromegaly, thyrotoxicosis and disseminated malignancy. The complete absence of renal activity is consistent with renal osteodystrophy where features of osteomalacia and hyperparathyroidism are combined; so much of the radionuclide is taken up by the bone that little if any is left for renal excretion. The patient had been in renal failure for several years, and the radiograph of his hand shows subperiosteal resorption along the radial aspects of the index and middle fingers, characteristic of hyperparathyroidism.

Reference

Rosenthall, L. and Keyes, M. (1975) Technetium-99m-pyrophosphate kinetics and imaging in metabolic bone disease. *J. Nucl. Med.*, **16**, 33-39.

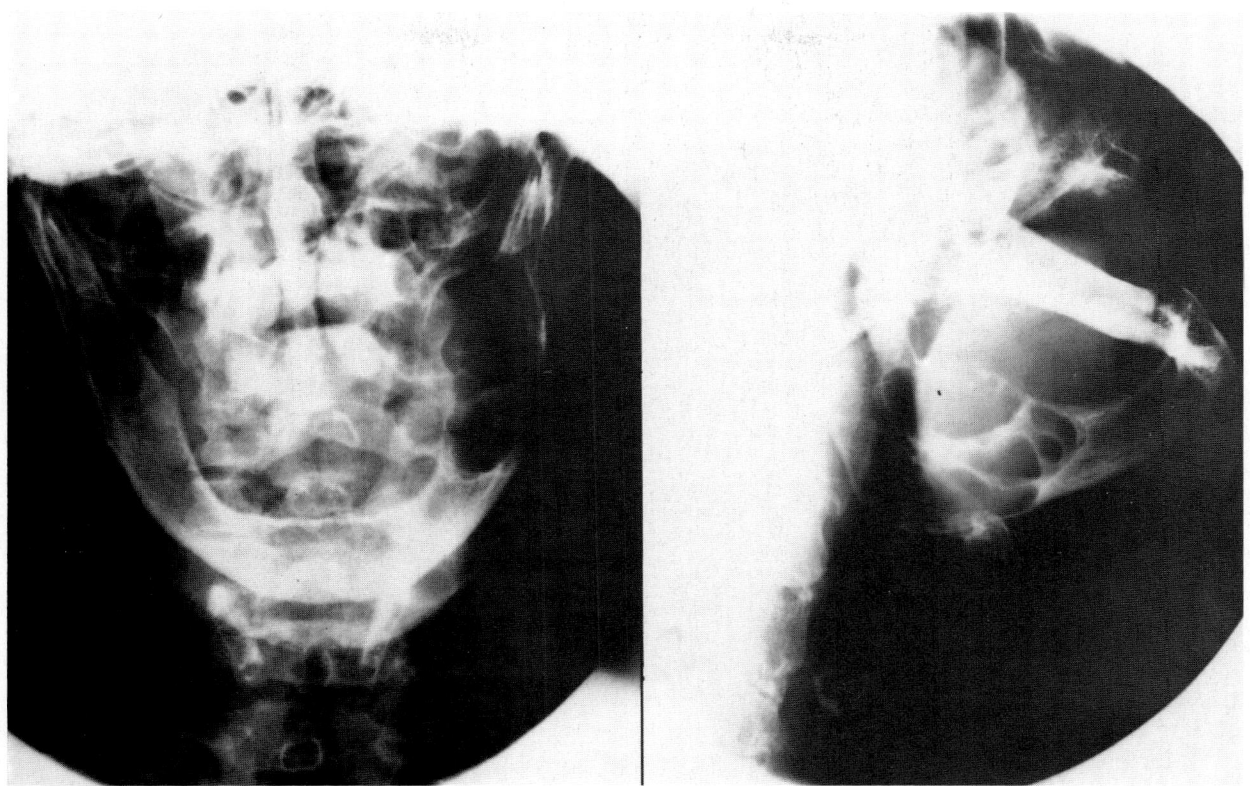

This middle-aged woman complained to her dentist of a painless lump inside her mouth.

- What is the diagnosis?
- Where else may such a lesion be found?

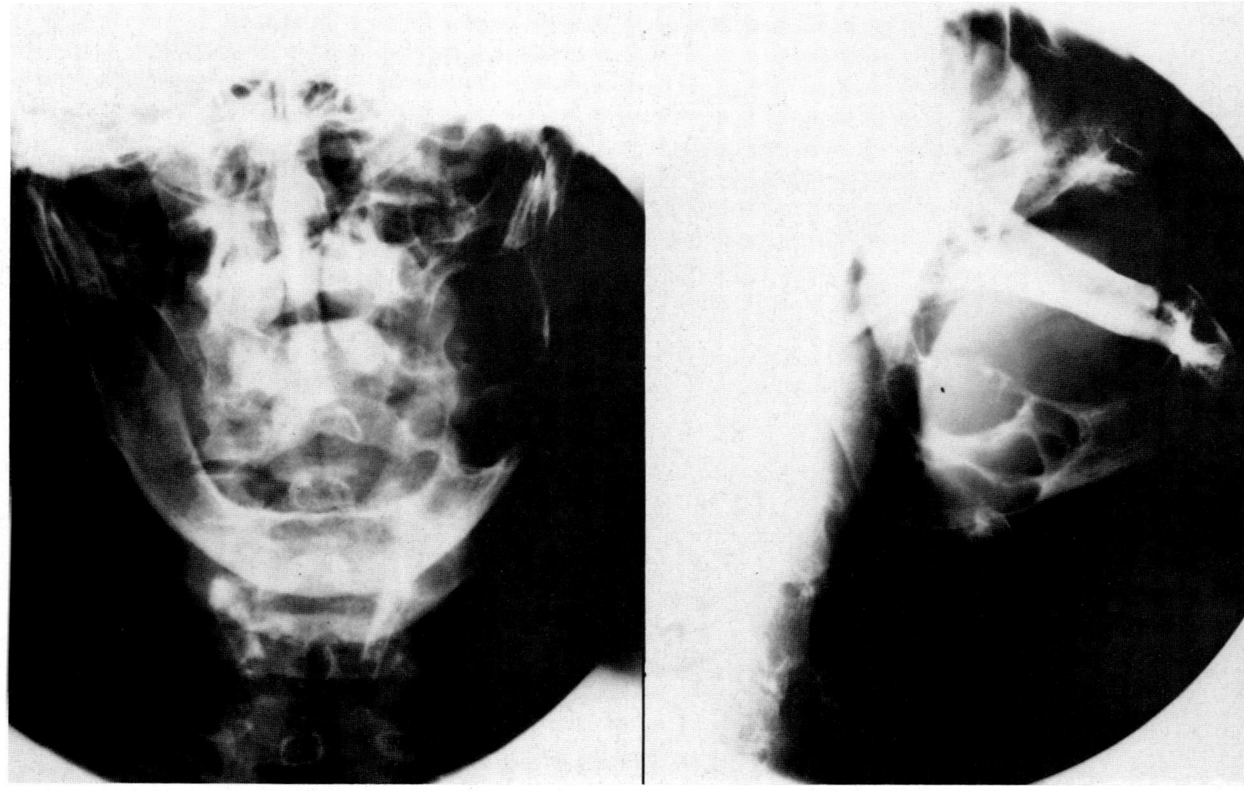

An expanded, multiloculated, lytic lesion occupies the left angle of the mandible. It is well-defined and has caused extreme thinning of the overlying cortex. The cortex may have been breached medially. This was an ameloblastoma, confirmed at biopsy. In this case there is no likely alternative radiological diagnosis, but other cystic lesions such as dental cysts, brown tumours and fibrous dysplasia can sometimes cause confusion.

Eighty per cent of ameloblastomas are found in the mandible, usually close to the angle, and 20 per cent affect the maxilla. They are epithelial in origin, have a peak incidence in the middle-aged and are locally invasive. Presentation is with a slowly enlarging mass which may be painful, particularly if complicated by a pathological fracture.

These lesions have in the past been termed adamantinomas, a name now reserved for lesions with similar histological features but affecting the long bones.

Reference

McIvor, J. (1974) The radiological features of ameloblastoma. *Clin. Radiol.*, **25**, 237-242.

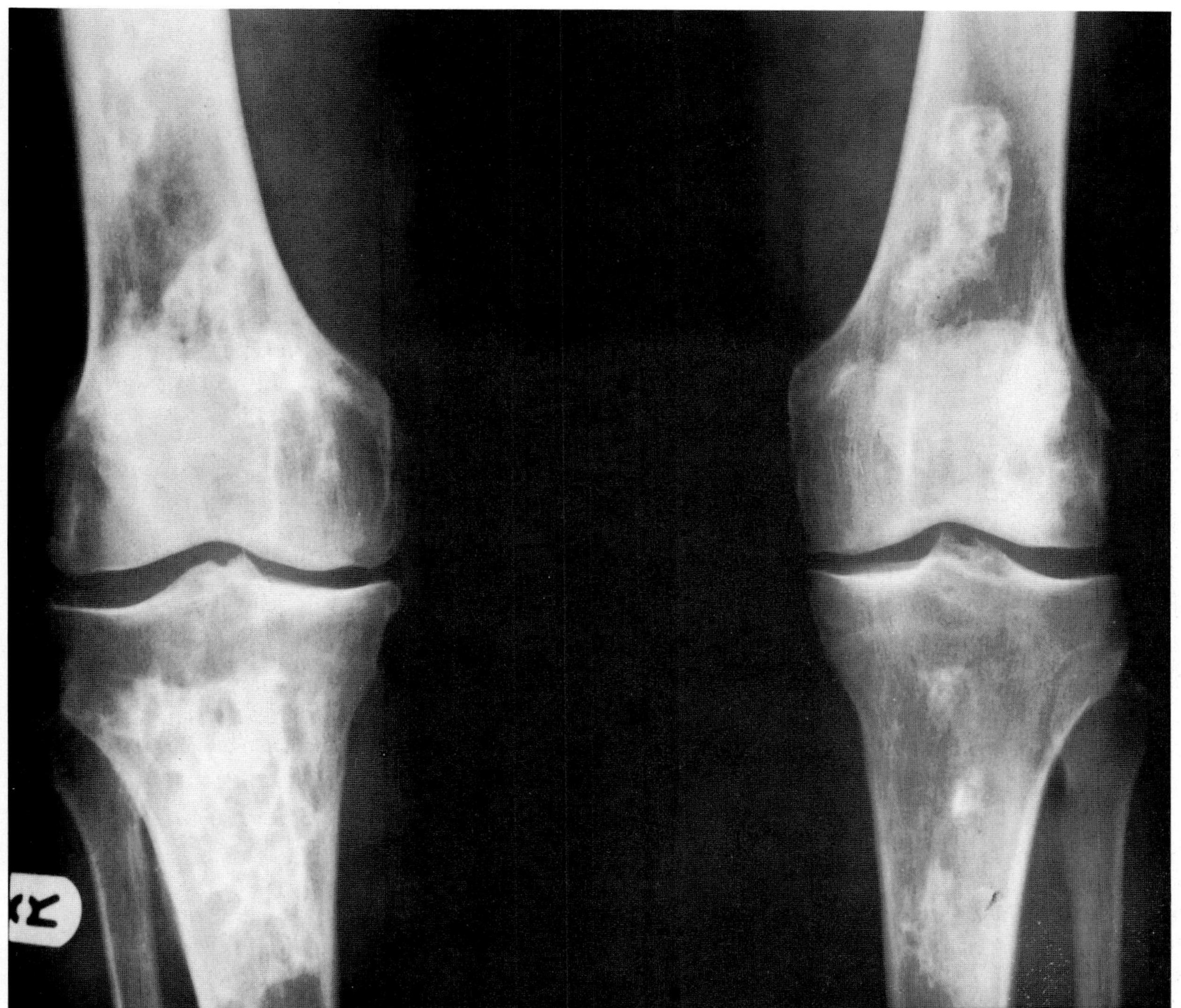

This radiograph was obtained during a routine occupational health examination. The patient was a 48-year-old man.

- What is the aetiology of the abnormalities?

- Suggest a differential diagnosis.

- What abnormality is likely at the hip joints?

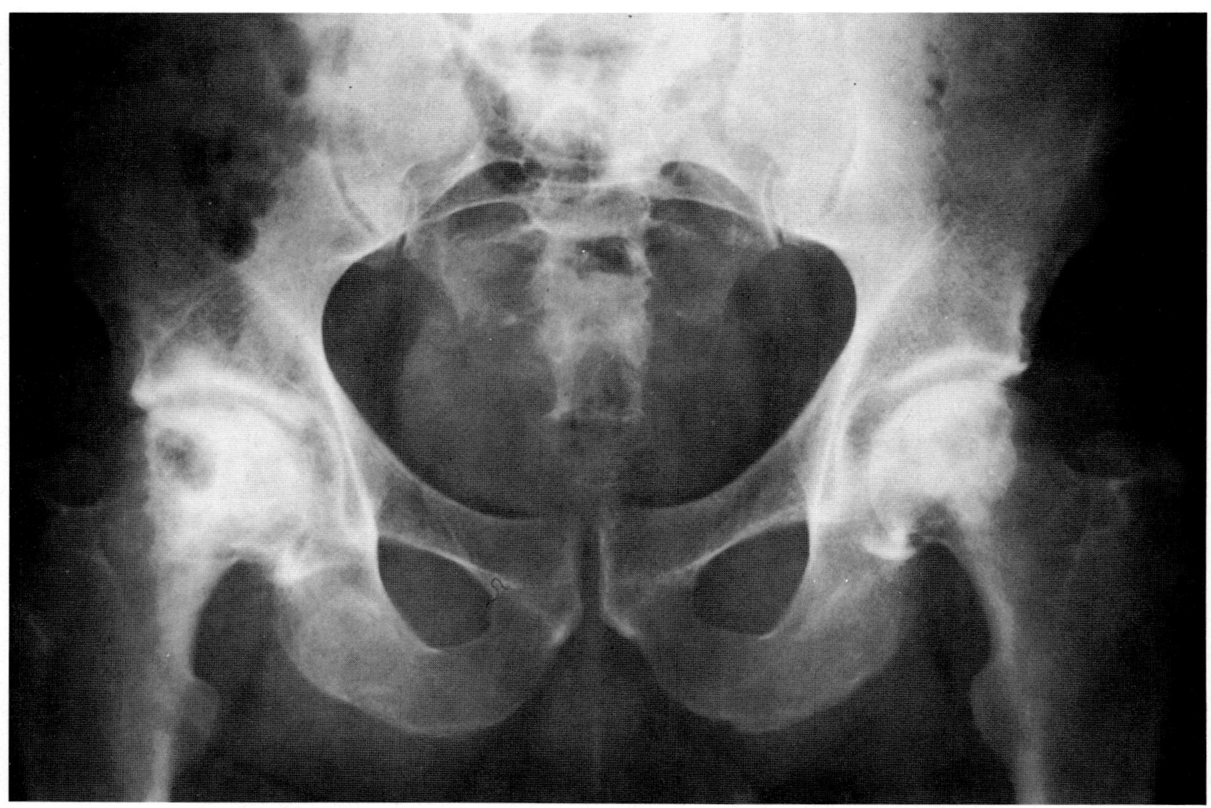

Irregular, but mainly well-defined densities are seen in the femora and tibiae, predominantly in the diaphyses. These are bone infarcts and their widespread distribution suggests a generalised cause, such as sickle-cell disease, Gaucher's disease, corticosteroid therapy or dysbaric osteonecrosis. The patient was working as a deep sea diver and had suffered an episode of decompression sickness one year prior to the examination.

Under hyperbaric conditions the blood is supersaturated with gases. If the subject is allowed to return to atmospheric pressure too rapidly, the gases come out of solution. Any oxygen or carbon dioxide is rapidly eliminated by respiration but nitrogen forms bubbles which act as emboli and obstruct small vessels, causing bony infarction.

The fatty bone marrow is particularly vulnerable to infarction as fat dissolves large amounts of nitrogen and there is an inadequate system of collaterals. The ends of the long bones are at risk because they are supplied by end-arteries.

If infarction is confined to the diaphyses of the long bones, the patient is often asymptomatic. Involvement of subchondral bone may cause pain in the affected joints and result in avascular necrosis which is typified by the 'snow-capping' shown in the femoral heads of this patient.

The incidence of decompression sickness in workers at risk varies with safety standards but is usually 10-20 per cent. The incidence is much higher in tunnel workers than in divers. Radiological changes of osteonecrosis may take 4-12 months to appear.

Reference

Heard, J. L. et al. (1978) Radiological findings in commercial divers. *Clin. Orthop.*, **130**, 129-138.

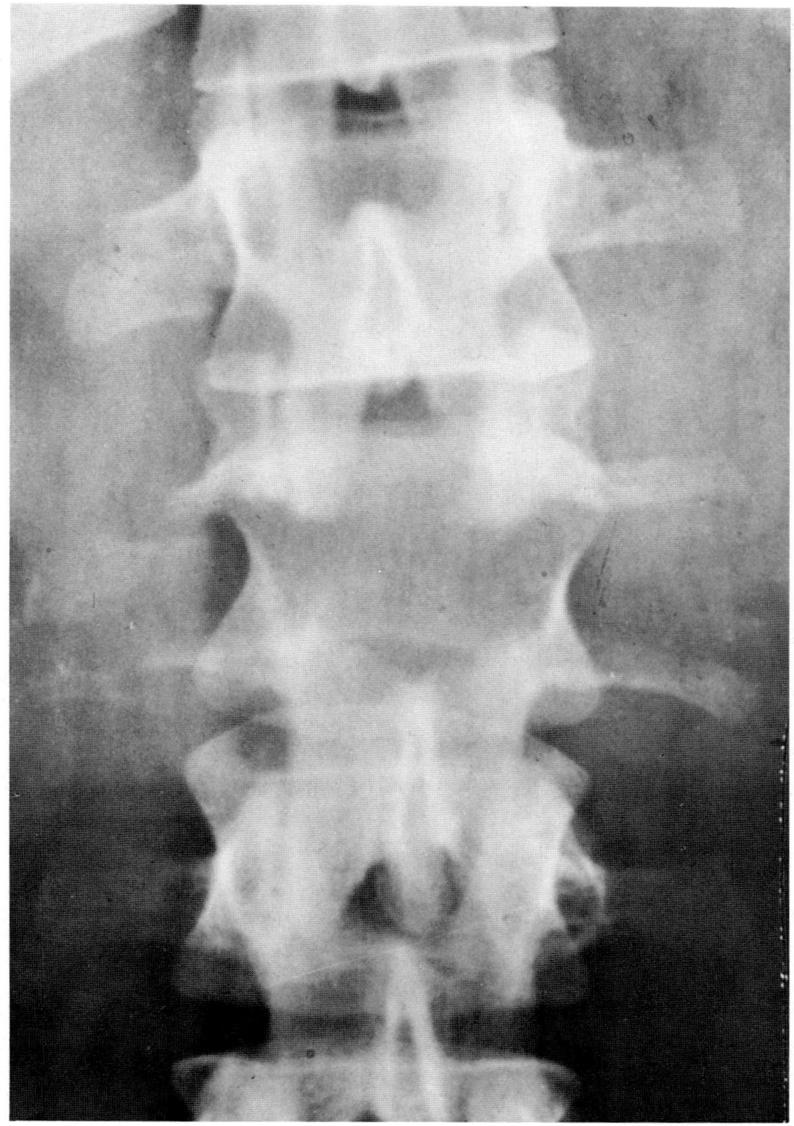

This man was a front seat passenger when involved in an RTA. He was wearing a seat belt at the time.

- What is the injury and how does it occur?

- What would you expect to see on the lateral view of the lumbar spine?

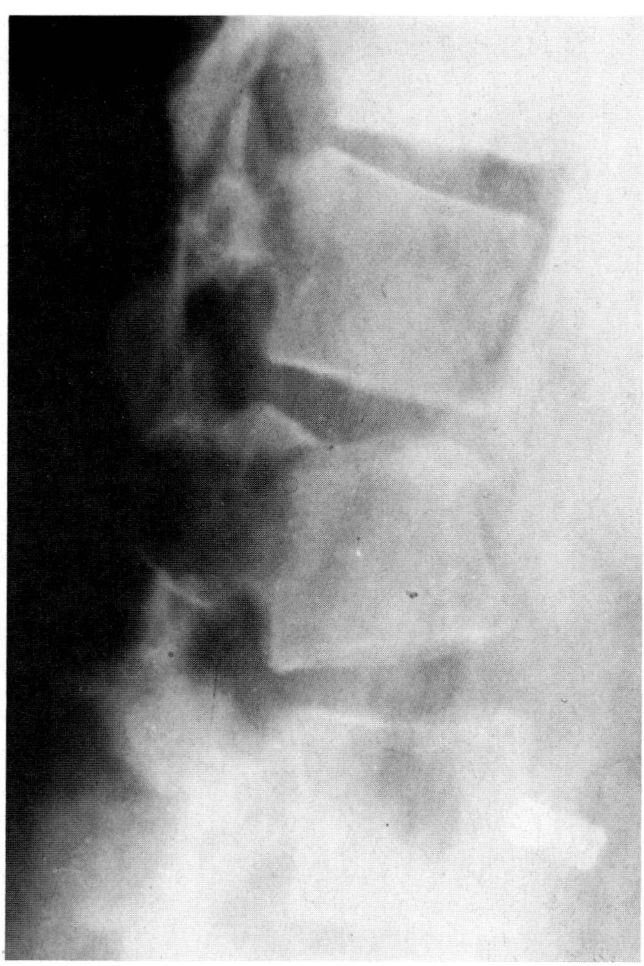

The AP view of the lumbar spine shows downward displacement of the spinous process of L2 and an apparent absence of the L2 pedicles. Fractures are present through the transverse processes of L1 and L2, which at L2 are essentially horizontal.

The appearances suggest a Chance (or lap-strap) fracture, an injury which occurs when the body is forced into flexion over a lap seat belt or other object acting as a fulcrum. The hyperflexion may result either in rupture of the posterior ligaments, transverse fractures of the posterior bony elements, transverse processes and vertebral body, or a combination of these injuries. It is the separation of the posterior elements which gives the apparently empty appearance to the vertebral body on the AP view. The diagnosis was confirmed in this patient by the lateral view, which shows the transverse fracture through the pedicles and vertebral body of L2.

Chance fractures are often associated with soft tissue injuries, which include rupture of the anterior abdominal wall muscles, tears in the relatively fixed second and third parts of the duodenum and elsewhere in the small bowel, mesenteric tears and spinal cord injuries.

C. Q. Chance was consultant radiologist to the Derbyshire Royal Infirmary when he described the radiological appearances of the fracture in 1948.

References

Dehner, T. R. (1971) Seatbelt injuries of the spine and abdomen. *Amer. J. Roentgenol.*, **111**, 833-843.

Rogers, L. F. (1971) The roentgenographic appearance of transverse or Chance fractures of the spine; the seat belt fracture. *Amer. J. Roentgenol.*, **111**, 844-849.

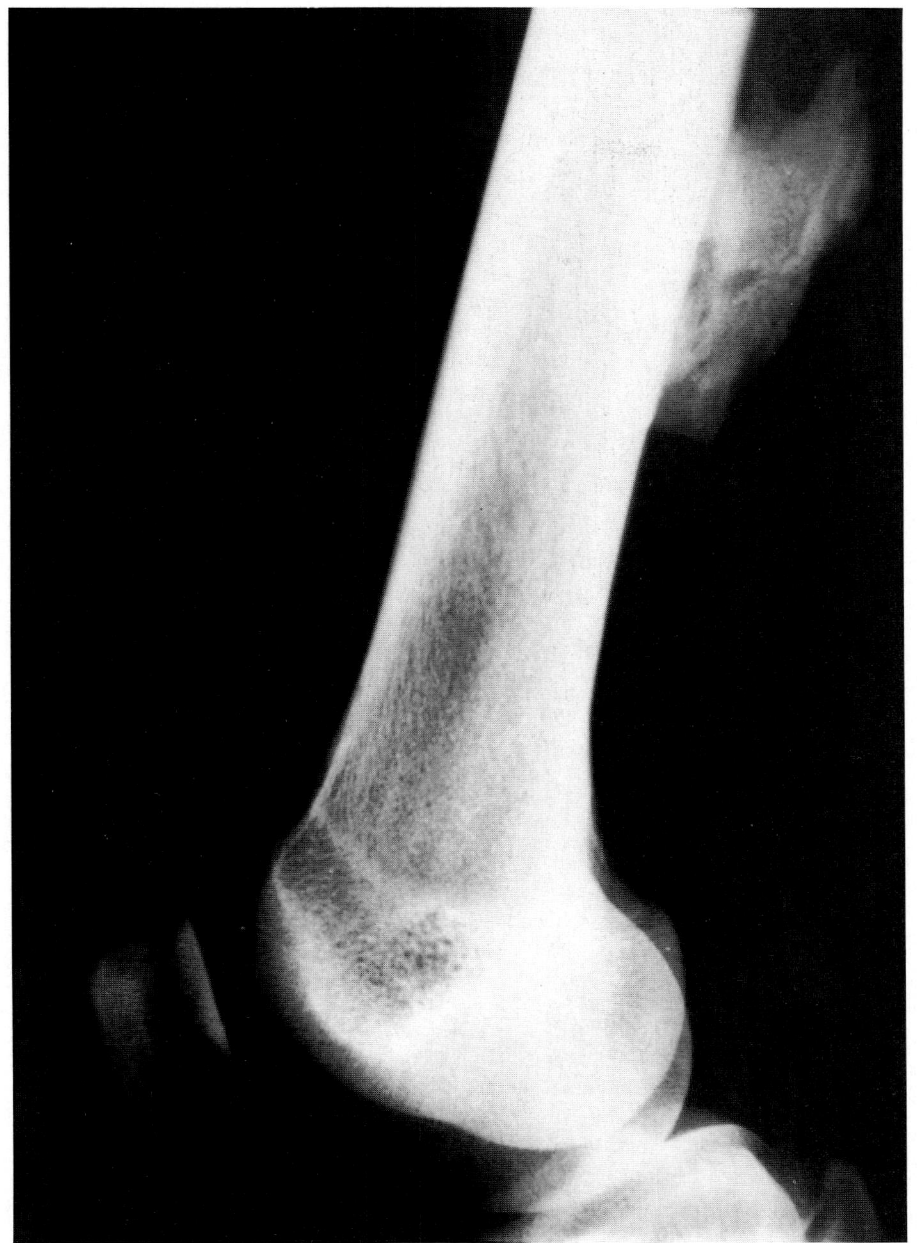

This 25-year-old man complained of swelling and discomfort in the left thigh.

- What is the differential diagnosis?

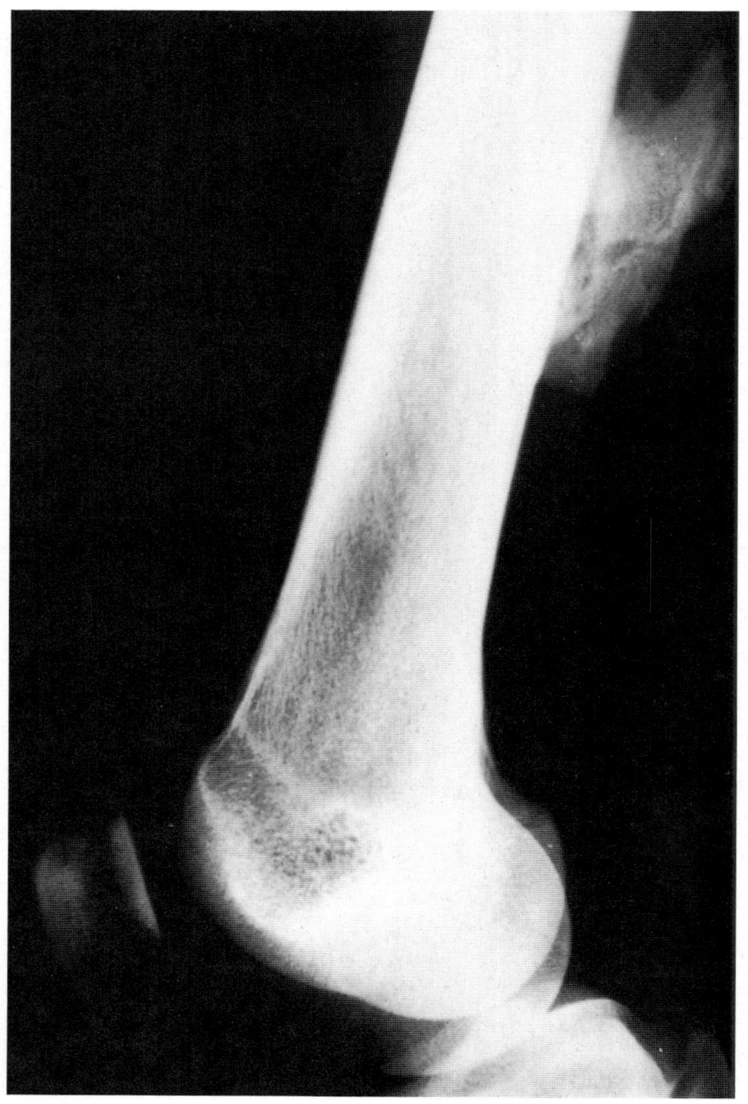

A clearly defined bony excrescence arises from the posterior aspect of the femoral shaft.

The differential diagnosis lies between an osteochondroma and an exostosis due to post-traumatic myositis ossificans. Radiological evidence of a cartilage cap would not be expected, but continuity of the medulla and the cortical contour between the femur and the lesion would help to support the former. A parosteal osteosarcoma is an unlikely diagnosis as such tumours have irregular, lobular margins and relatively dense centres.

Myositis ossificans follows injury to the soft tissues sufficient to give either a soft tissue or subperiosteal haematoma and is unrelated to fracture of the underlying bone. It is particularly common in the thigh and this patient had sustained an injury there while playing football three years earlier. He had developed a large haematoma and subsequently a bony lump which proved, at operation, to be an ossified subperiosteal haematoma. Ossification begins within weeks of injury, and patients may present at this stage with a tender lump which then gets smaller. Diagnosis is easier if the ossification is clearly separated from the underlying bone, but continuity with the associated periosteal reaction often occurs.

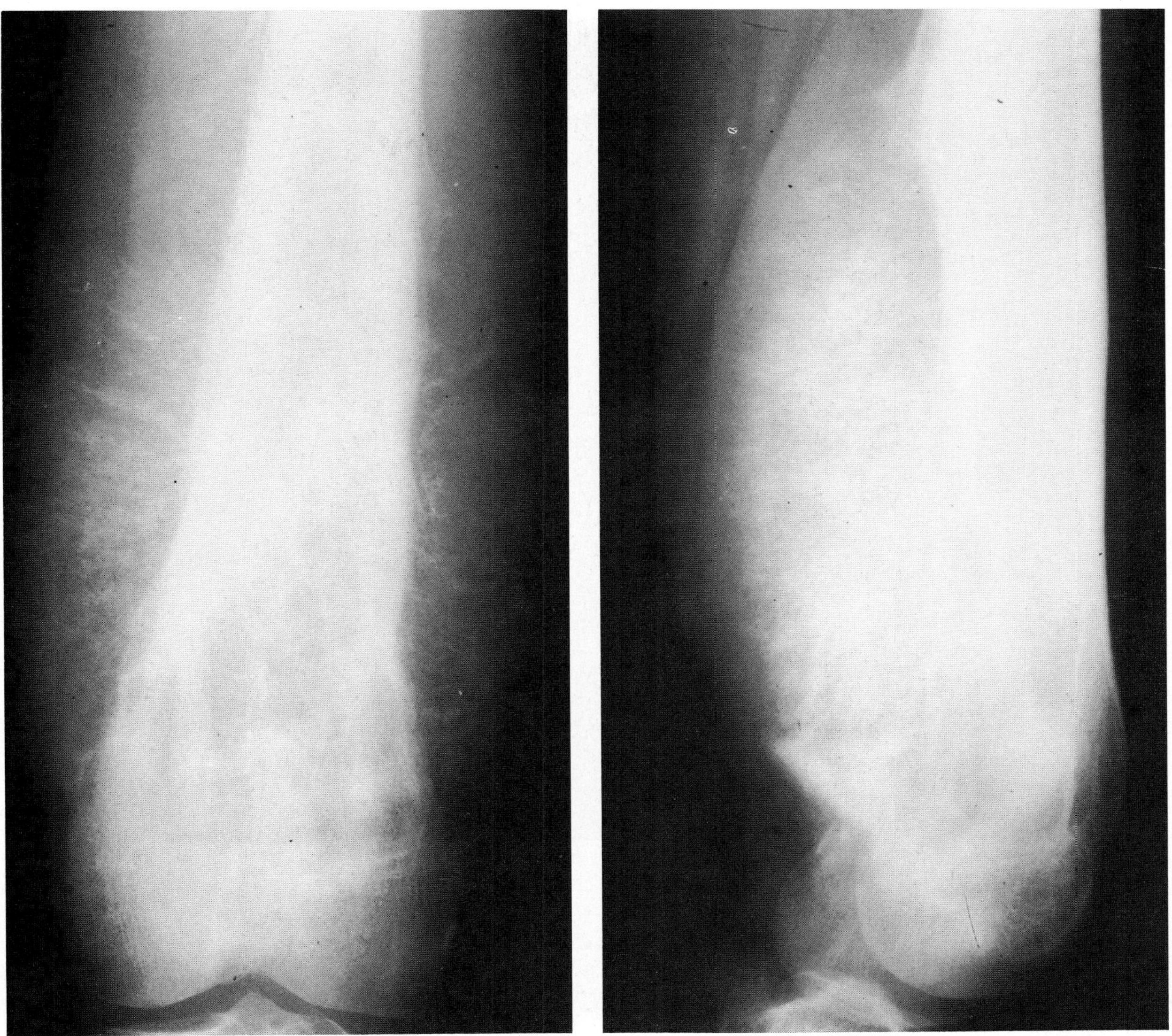

This 17-year-old boy had complained of pain
and swelling above his knee for one year.

- Describe the appearances.
- What is the most likely diagnosis?

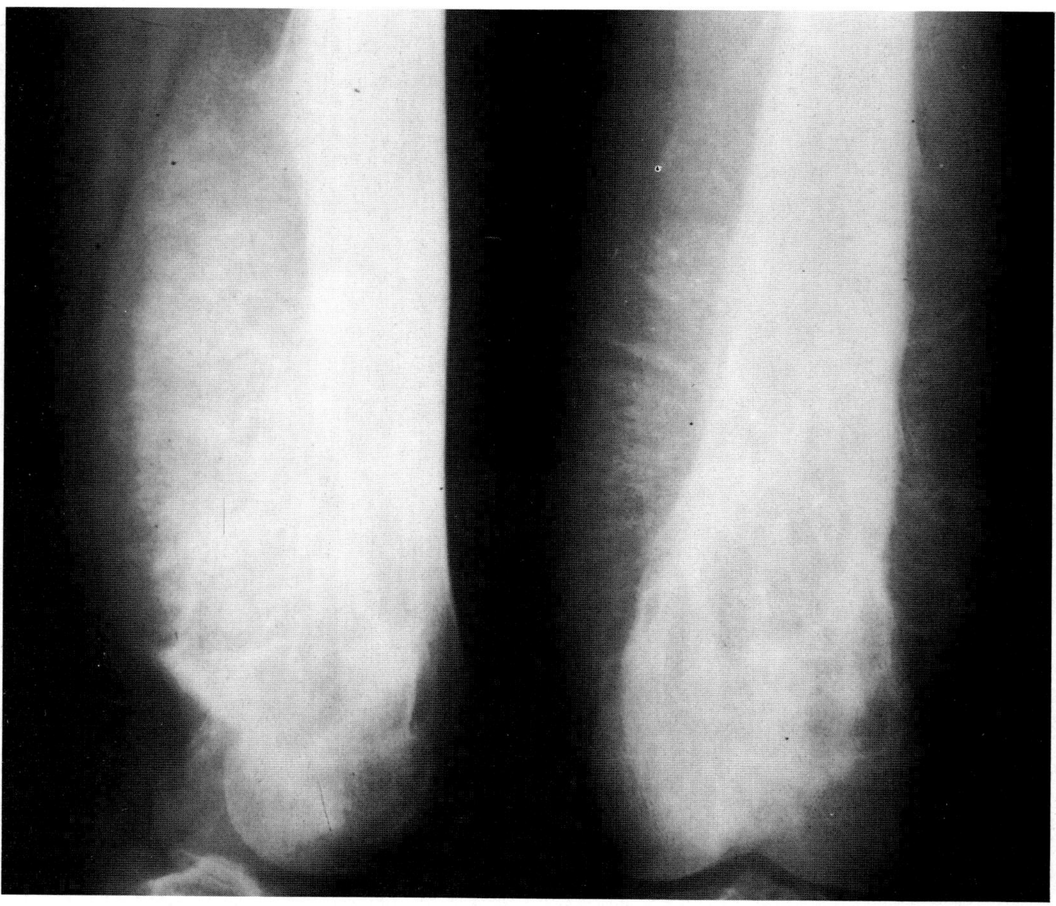

An ill-defined region of cortico-medullary destruction is present at the distal end of the femur. It shows a wide zone of transition and a well-defined mass extending into the soft tissues. Spicules of bone arranged in a radiating or 'sunburst' pattern lie within the mass and the periosteum is elevated at its superior and inferior margins to form reactive or Codman's triangles.

The radiological features indicate an aggressive malignant lesion. The most likely cause is an osteosarcoma, but because of the serious implications of the diagnosis, biopsy is necessary. This patient's lesion had originally been treated as fibrous dysplasia following the report of a biopsy at an earlier stage of the disease. A second biopsy was correctly interpreted histologically as an osteosarcoma.

It should be remembered that sunburst bony spiculation is not pathognomonic of an osteosarcoma. In this condition it is due to perpendicular growth of reactive and tumour bone from the periosteum, but a similar pattern of reactive bone may sometimes be seen in Ewing's sarcoma, haemangioma, meningioma, osteomyelitis and other conditions.

Reference

Dahlin, D. C. and Coventry, M. B. (1967) Osteogenic sarcoma: a study of 600 cases. *J. Bone Joint Surg.*, **49-A**, 101-110.

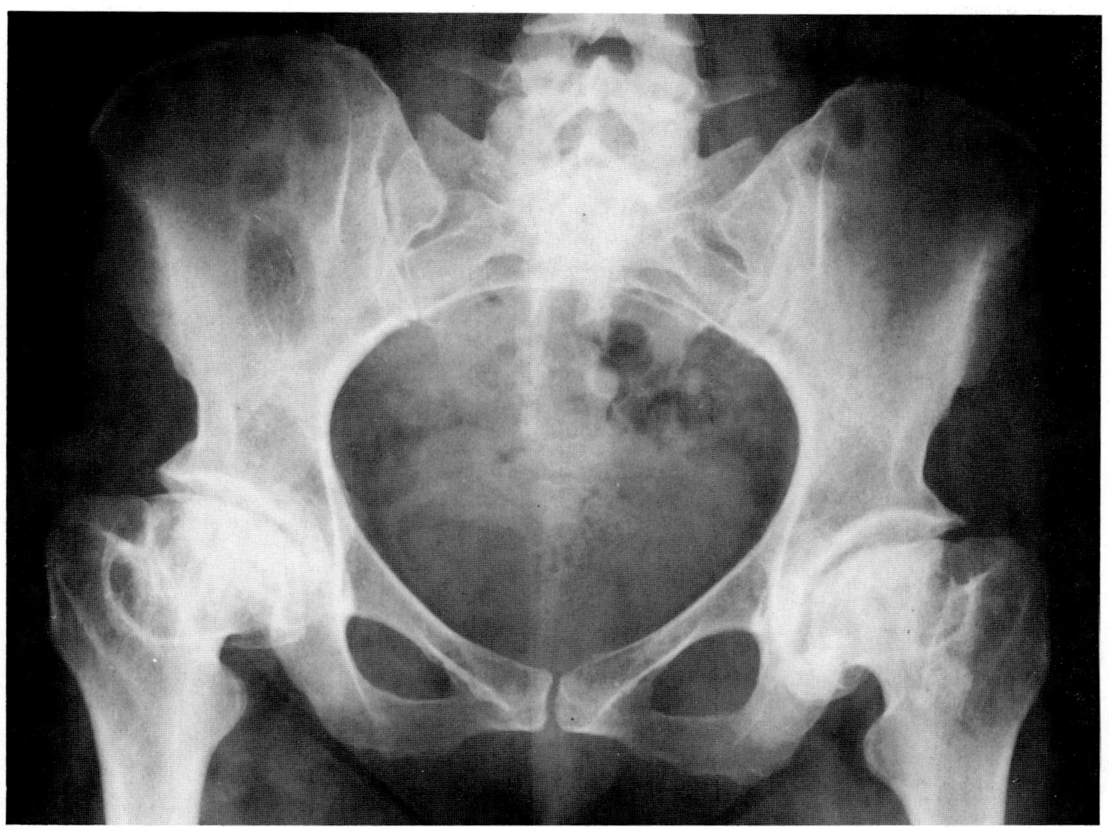

This 35-year-old woman presented with painful hips.

- What further radiographs should be obtained in order to confirm the diagnosis?

- How tall is the patient likely to be?

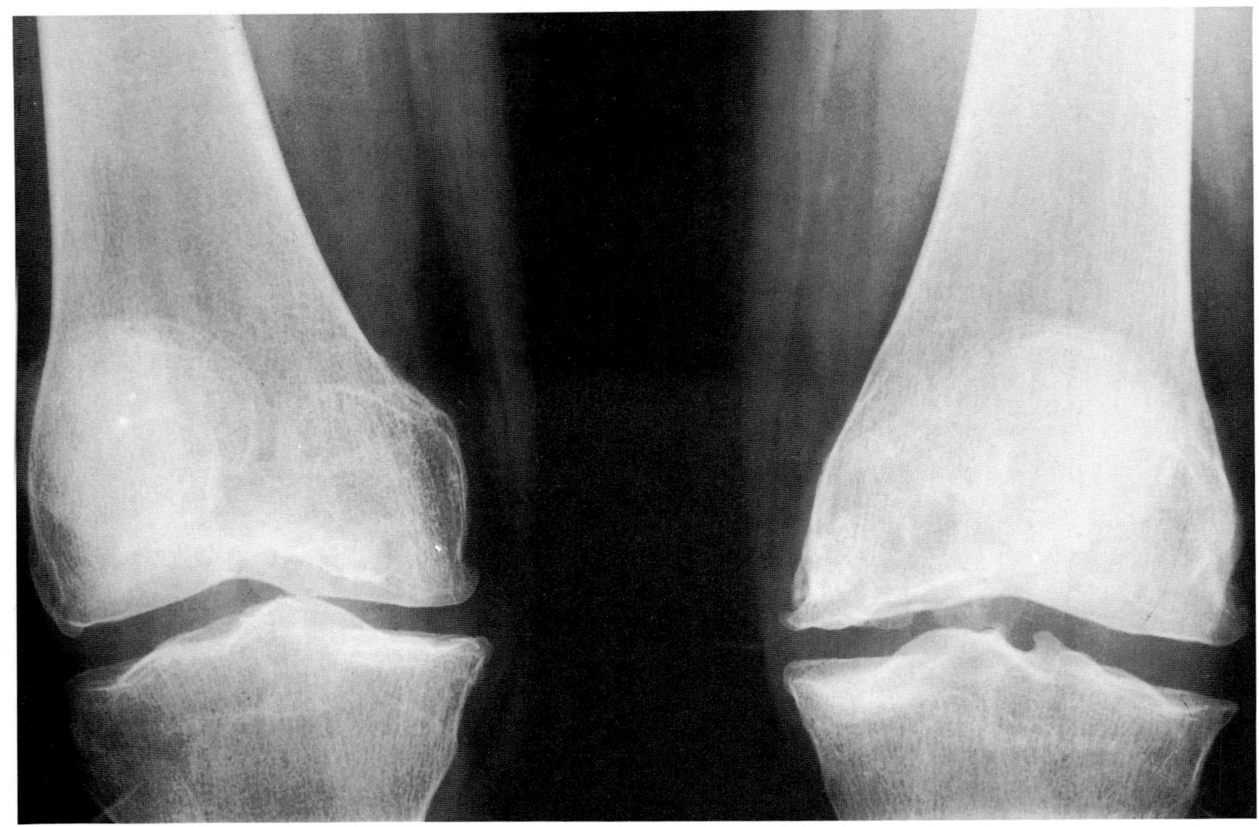

Both hips are abnormal. The acetabula are shallow and the femoral heads are flattened with irregular articular surfaces and secondary degenerative articular changes. Mild coxa vara is present.

The femoral abnormalities alone would be consistent with the long term sequelae of conditions such as Perthes' disease and slipped epiphyses but the associated symmetrical acetabular dysplasia is more likely to suggest an epiphyseal dysplasia. Radiographs of other joints and the spine were obtained. A radiograph of the knees (above) also shows bilateral defects of modelling of the articular surfaces and early degenerative change.

Epiphyseal dysplasias are divided into two main groups: spondyloepiphyseal dysplasia, where there is always a severe platyspondyly, and multiple epiphyseal dysplasia, which shows little or no spinal involvement, as in this case.

Multiple epiphyseal dysplasia is of autosomal dominant inheritance and manifests itself from the age of one to two years. Patients are of normal or moderately short stature, with normal proportions and, depending on the location and severity of the disorder, may walk with a waddling gait. In children, the secondary ossification centres are slow to develop and fragmented, and there may be radiological confusion with hypothyroidism. Early degenerative change is common.

Reference

Spranger, J. W., Langer, L. O. and Wiedemann, H.-R. (1974) *Bone Dysplasias: An Atlas of Constitutional Disorders of Skeletal Development*. W. B. Saunders, Philadelphia.

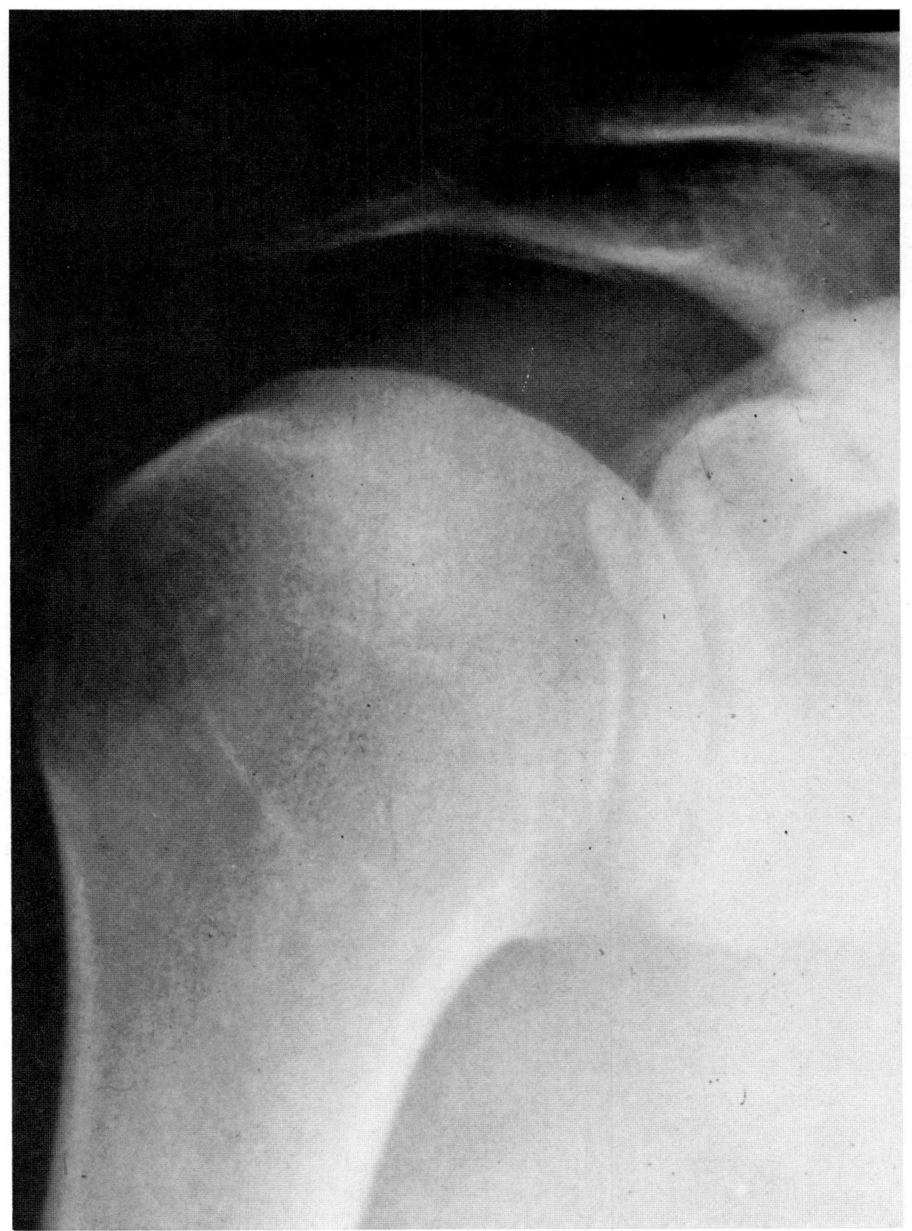

This patient sustained an injury during a fall.

- Can you make the diagnosis from this view?
- How would you confirm it?

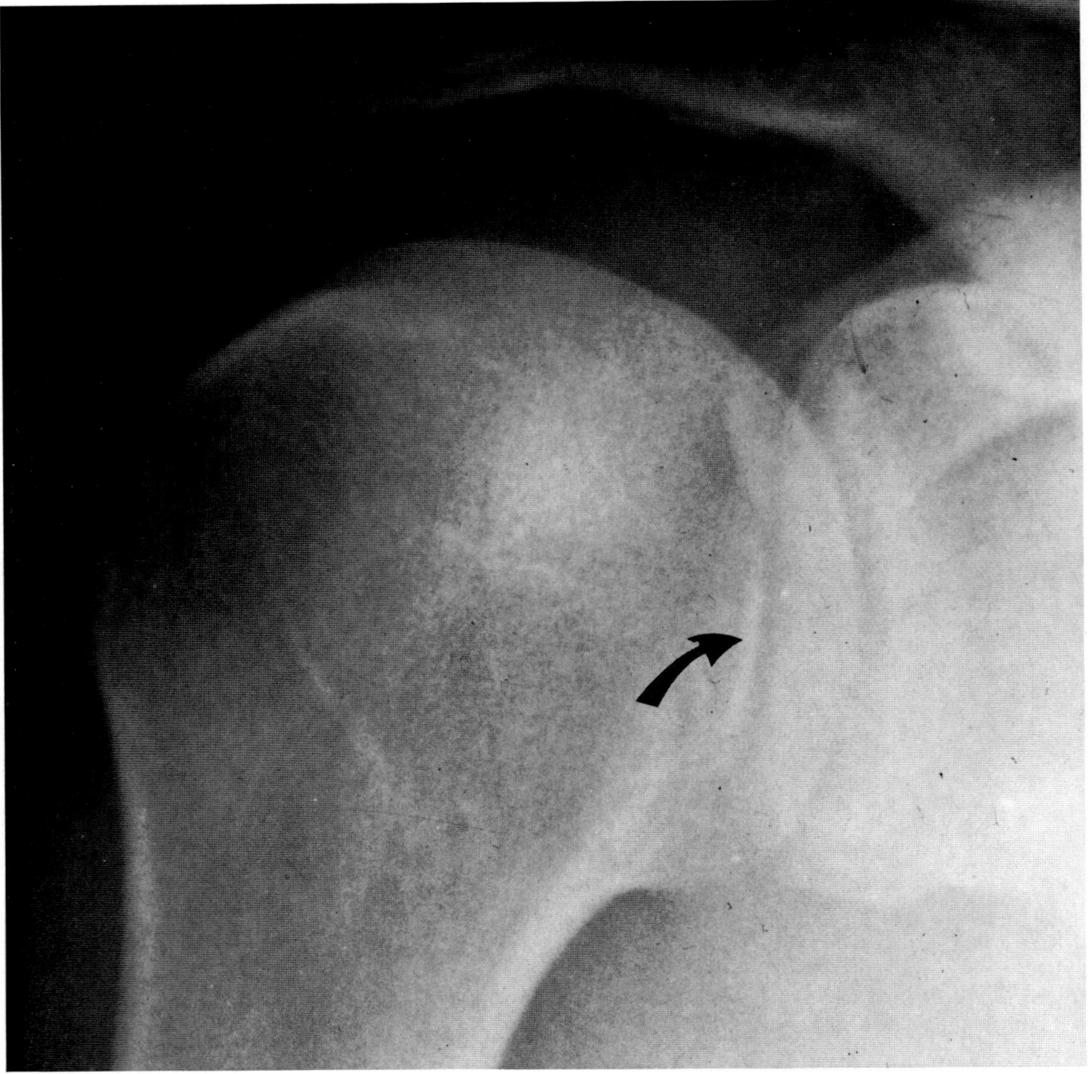

The AP projection of the shoulder shows a lack of congruity at the glenohumeral joint and the humeral head overlaps the profile of the glenoid. The humeral head appears abnormally rounded as it is held in internal rotation. These features indicate posterior dislocation, and the small cortical line running parallel to the medial articular surface of the humeral head (arrowed—see above) enables a definitive diagnosis to be made. This is a trough line and represents the margin of the notch-like impaction fracture which occurs during posterior dislocation at the glenohumeral joint. The unreduced dislocation was demonstrated, and the impaction fracture seen in profile, on the axial view on page 173.

Only 2-4 per cent of shoulder dislocations are posterior and as many as 50 per cent will be missed if an axial or scapula Y projection is not obtained.

The commonest cause is the muscular unco-ordination of an epileptic fit, as in this patient.

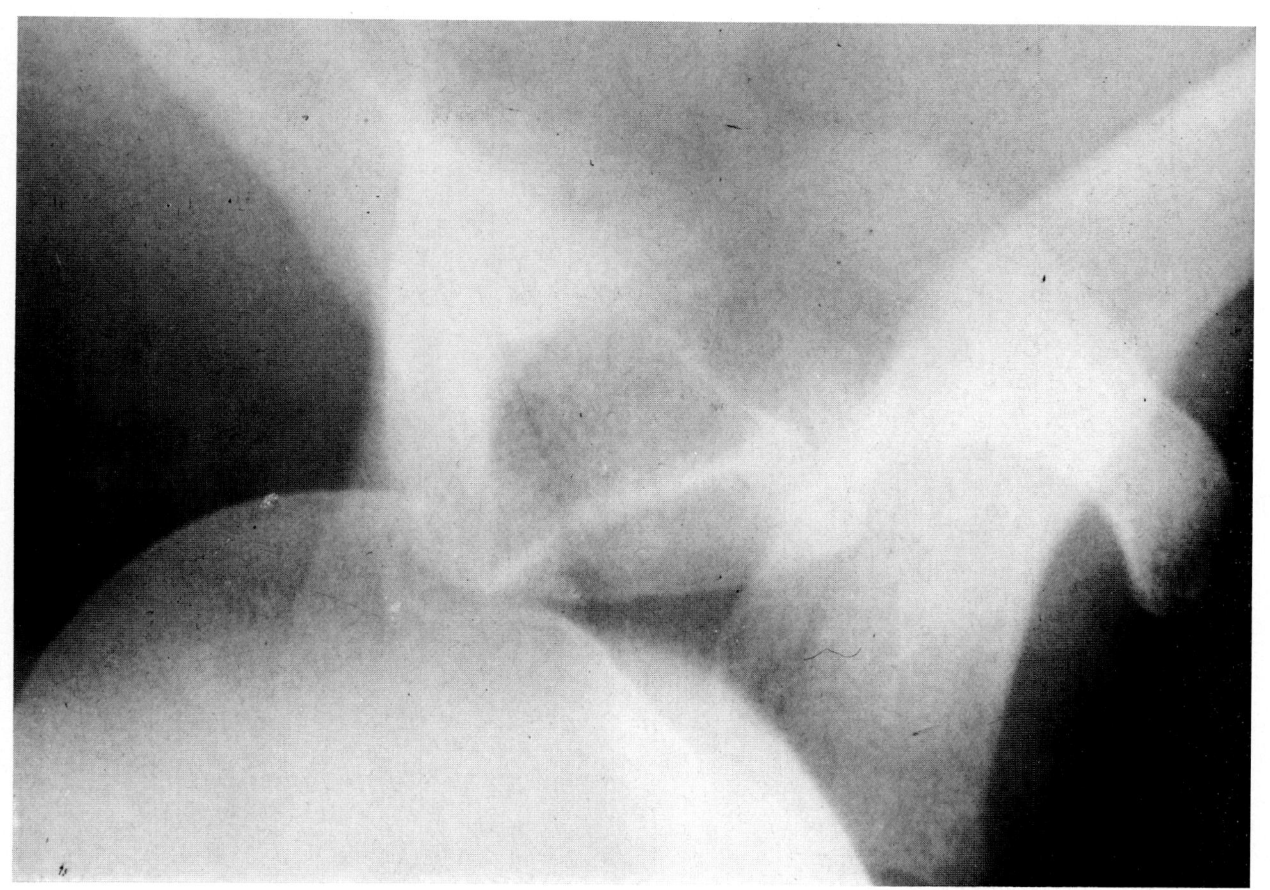

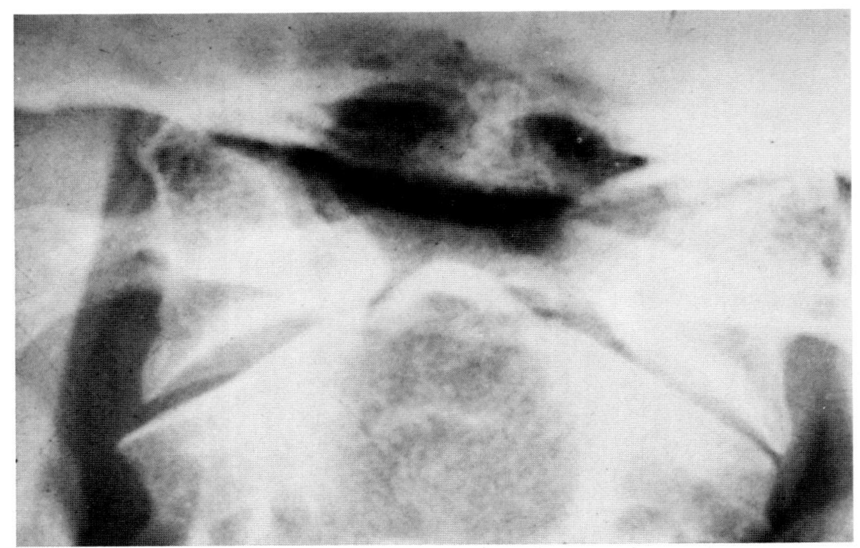

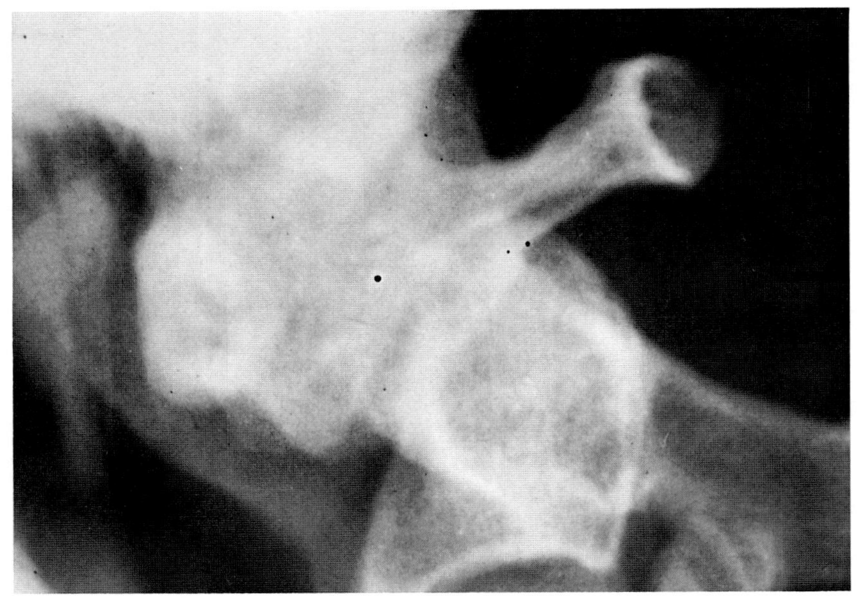

This 63-year-old man presented with increasing weakness in his right arm following a fall two years before.

- What do the radiographs show?
- What further view should be obtained?

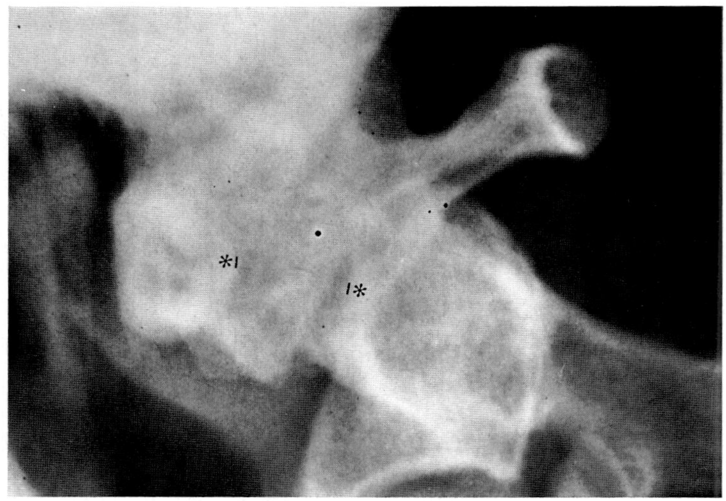

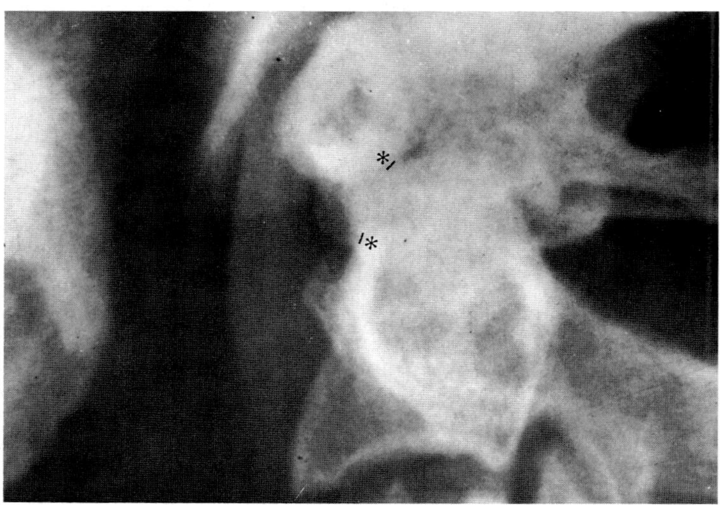

The AP and lateral views of the upper cervical spine shows a wide separation between the odontoid peg and the atlas with sclerosis of the well-defined superior margin of the axis. The appearances are not specific and possible causes include an old non-united odontoid fracture, hypoplasia of the odontoid or an os odontoideum. The patient's symptoms had followed a fall flat on his back; no radiographs were obtained at the time but it is assumed that he sustained a fracture which had not subsequently united.

It is important to recognise odontoid abnormalities as they are often associated with atlanto-axial instability. Instability may be evaluated with flexion views, as shown above in this patient. The markers show the excessive amount of movement permitted at this inter-vertebral level. The injury may only cause neck ache, but the nerve root compression in this patient is not uncommon and trivial injuries have the potential for causing severe cord compression.

Reference

McRae, D. L. (1960) The significance of abnormalities of the cervical spine. *Amer. J. Roentgenol.*, 84, 1-9.

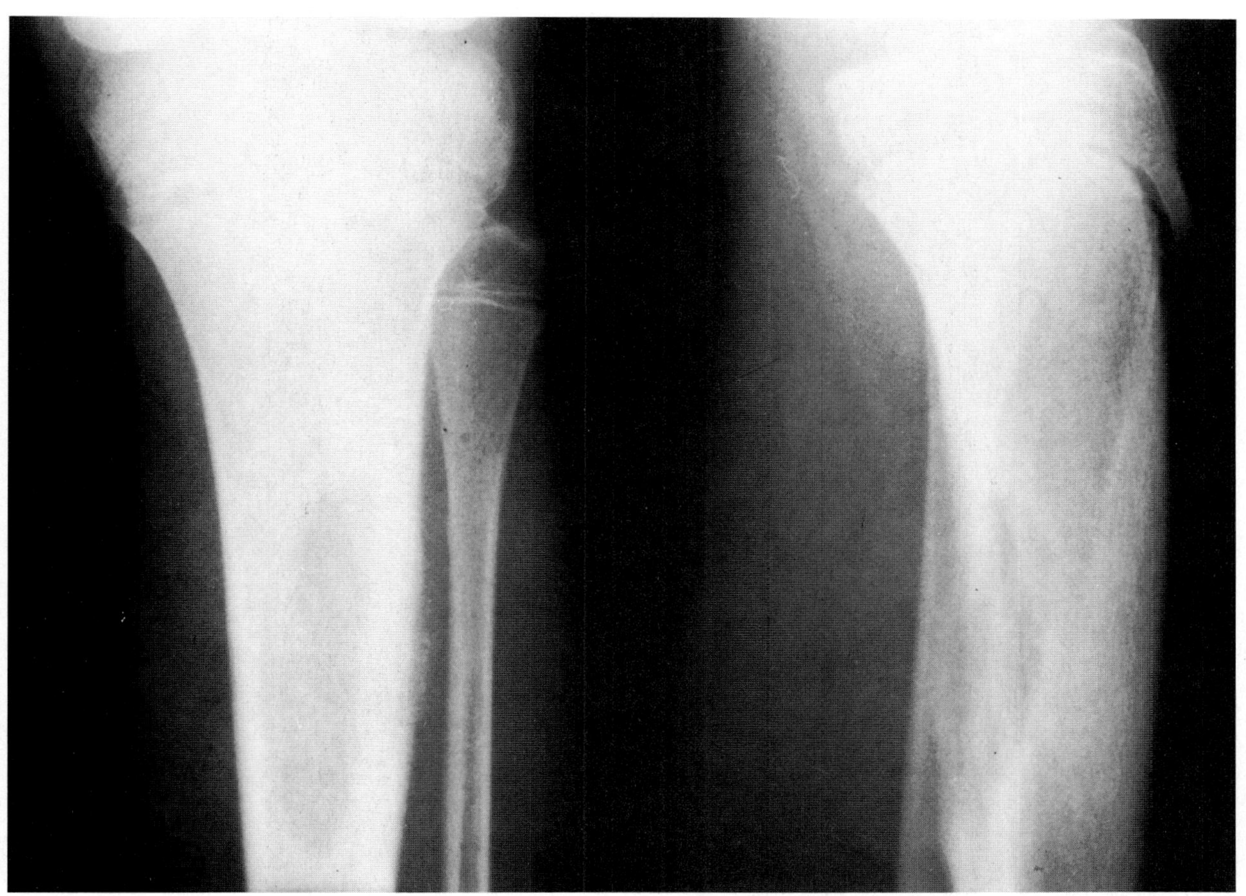

This 6-year-old boy complained of a painful swelling over the left tibia. On examination he had a fever and a raised WBC.

- Give three possible differential diagnoses.

- How might you establish the correct diagnosis?

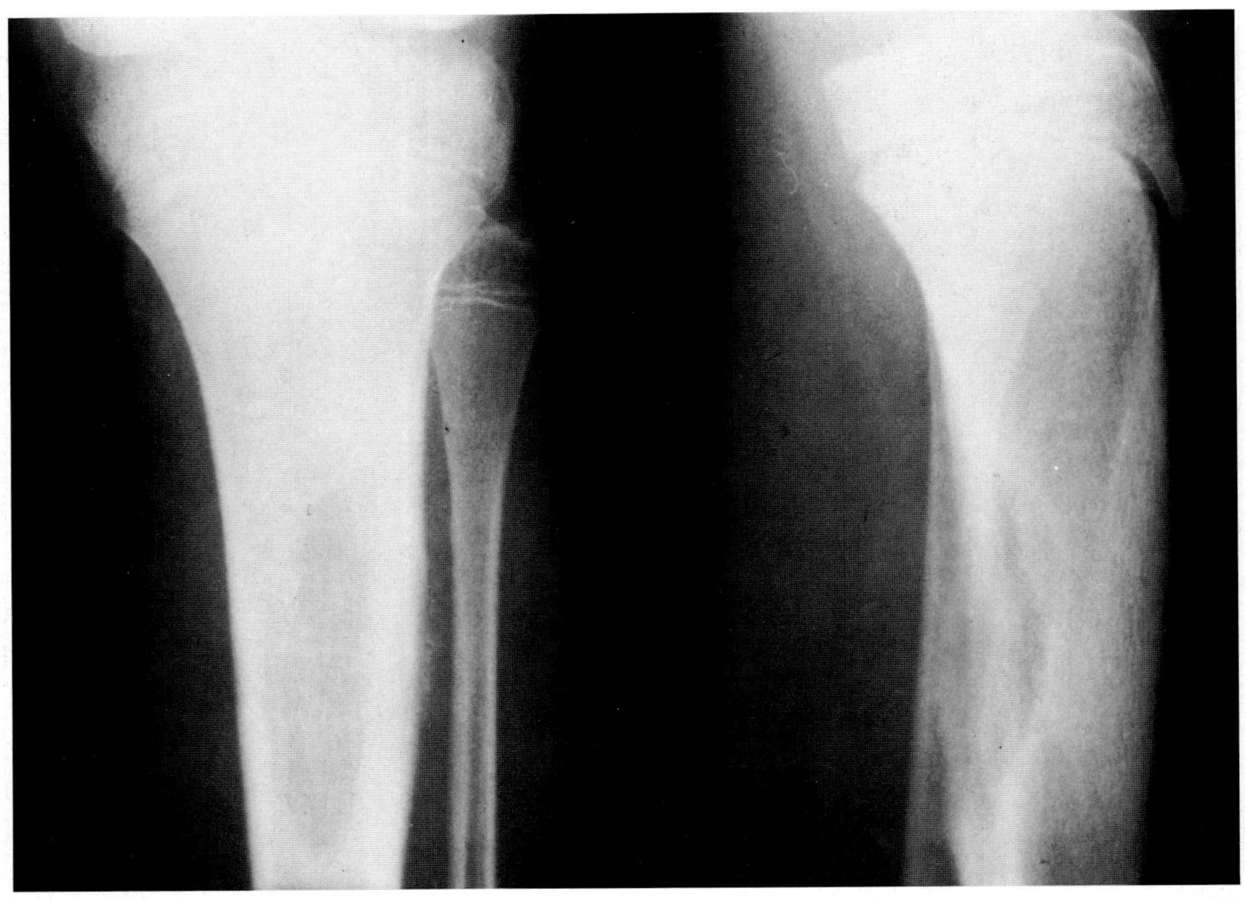

An area of medullary destruction is associated with cortical destruction and a periosteal reaction in the proximal part of the tibial diaphysis. At this age the differential diagnosis based on the clinical and radiological findings lies between an eosinophil granuloma, Ewing's sarcoma and osteomyelitis. If bone scintigraphy demonstrates a second lesion or shows a localised increase in uptake a diagnosis of Ewing's sarcoma is unlikely. CT scanning in Ewing's sarcoma commonly shows extension of the tumour into the soft tissues. In the present case a diagnosis could only be established by biopsy with histological examination. The patient had a biopsy-proven eosinophil granuloma.

Fifty to seventy five per cent of eosinophil granulomas are solitary and the sites most frequently affected are the skull, mandible, spine, ribs and long bones. The radiological appearances vary with site and those seen in this patient are typical of long bone involvement.

Reference

Nugert, C. et al. (1983) Eosinophil granuloma of bone: diagnosis and management. *Skeletal Radiol.*, 10 227-235.

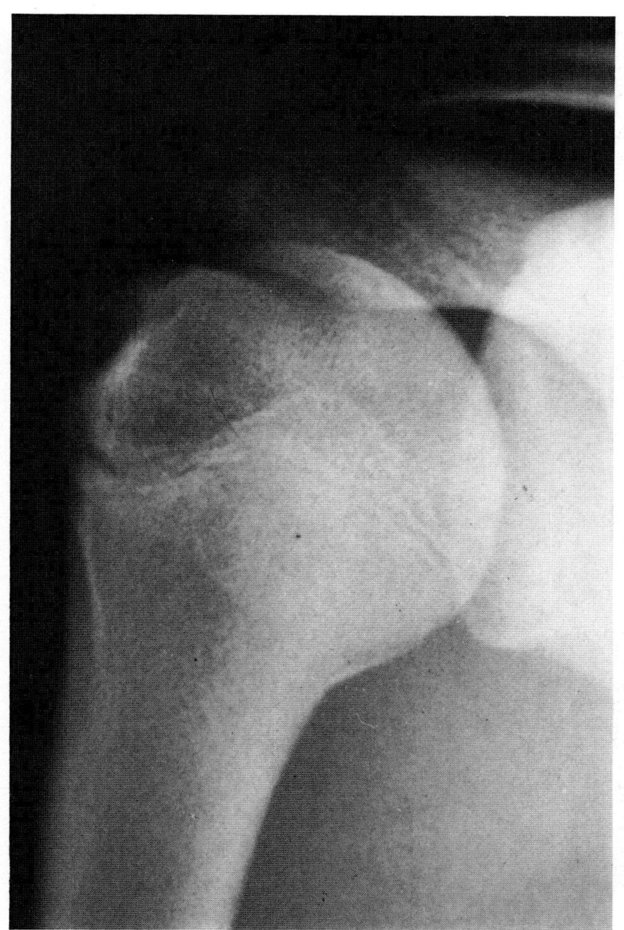 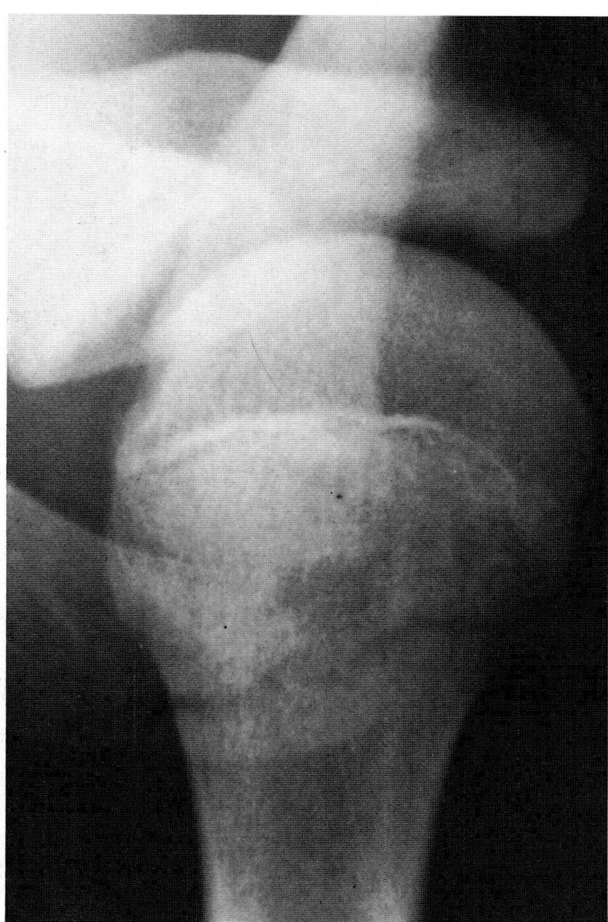

This adolescent boy's right shoulder dislocated
readily with certain simple active movements.

- What do the films show?
- What is the aetiology?

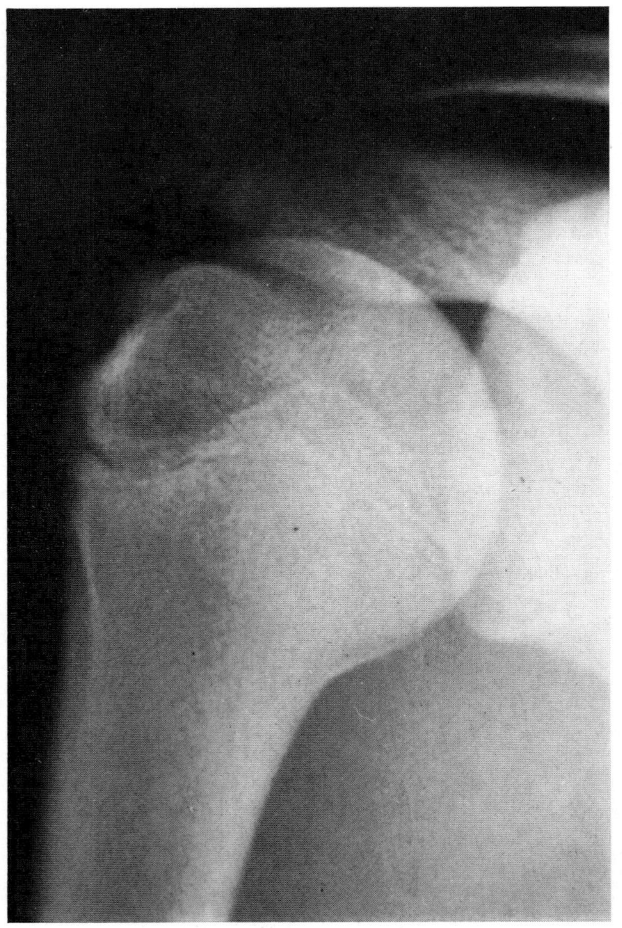
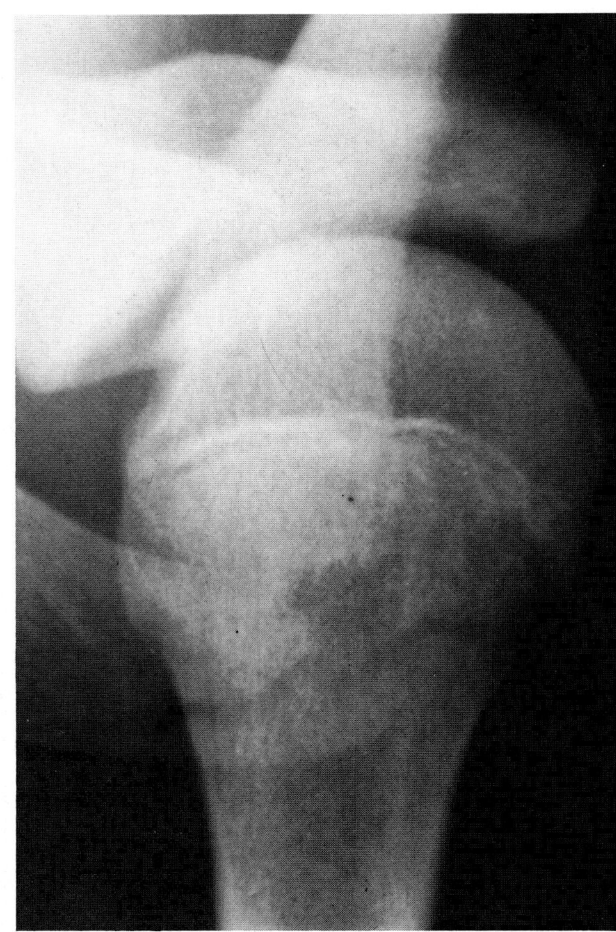

The AP and axial views of the right shoulder show a small cortical notch on the posterolateral aspect of the humeral head. This is known by various terms, including hatchet defect, Hill-Sachs lesion and Broca lesion, and indicates the presence of recurrent anterior dislocation at the glenohumeral joint. Its occurrence was recognised long before the discovery of X-rays.

It results from a compression fracture of the humeral head produced by impaction of the head on the anterior edge of the glenoid and may be produced by a single episode of anterior dislocation. An alternative, but less common result of anterior dislocation is a fracture of the osteocartilaginous rim of the glenoid (the Bankart lesion). The reported incidence of the Broca defect following anterior dislocation varies between 27 and 100 per cent. The wide variation is probably related to the ability to demonstrate it radiologically. The defect is often not visible on the AP and axial films and radiographs with the shoulder in 60° internal rotation, or in the Stryker projection, may be necessary for its demonstration.

References

Pavlov, H. and Freiberger, R. H. (1978) Fractures and dislocations about the shoulder. *Seminars in Roentgenol.*, **13**, 185-196.
Stoker, D. J. (1982) The radiology of the humeral defect in anterior dislocation of the shoulder—a comparative study. In: *Shoulder Surgery*. Editors, Bayley, I. and Kessel, L. Springer Verlag, Berlin, Heidelberg.

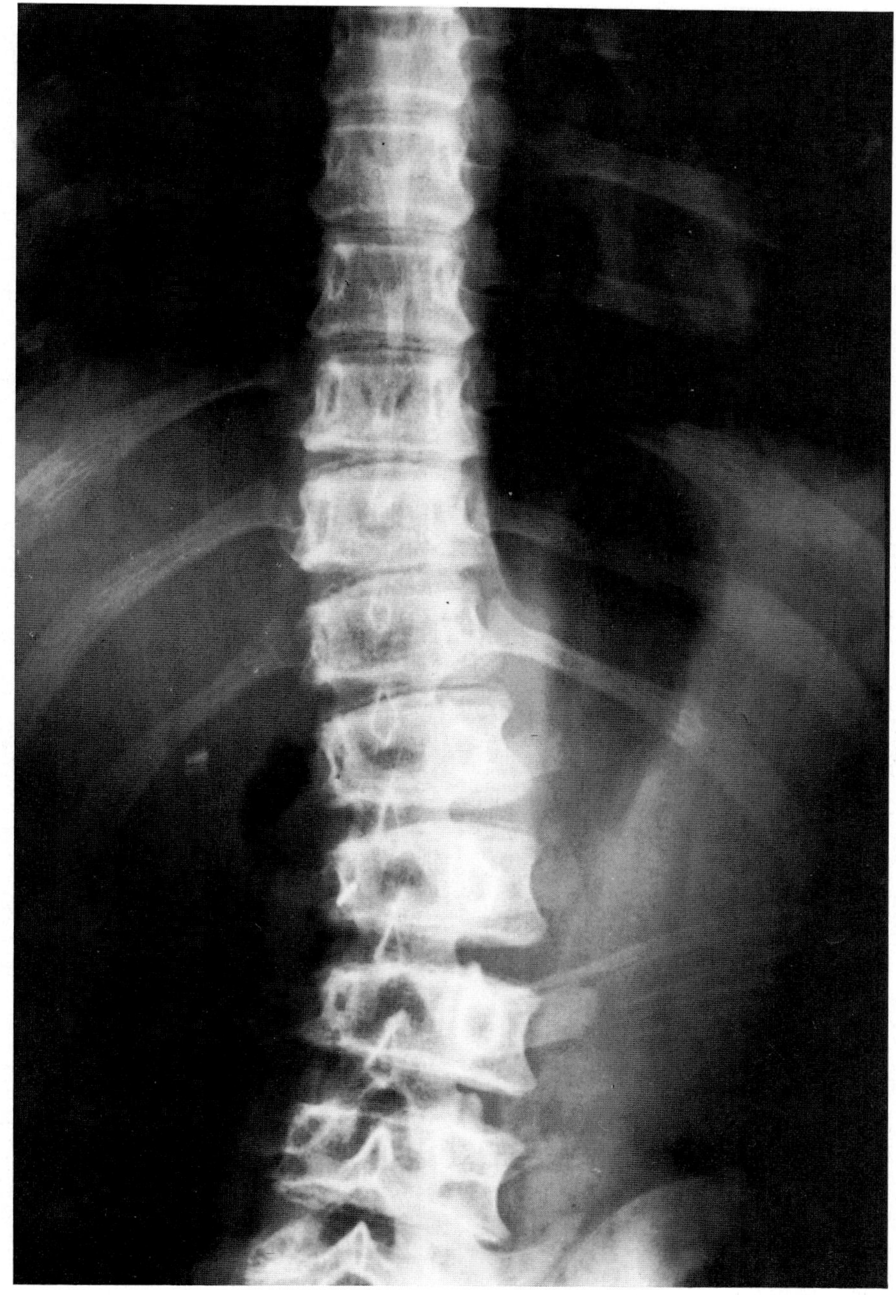

This 30-year-old woman had been treated for a
serious illness in early childhood.

- What was the nature of the illness?
- What complications might have occurred?

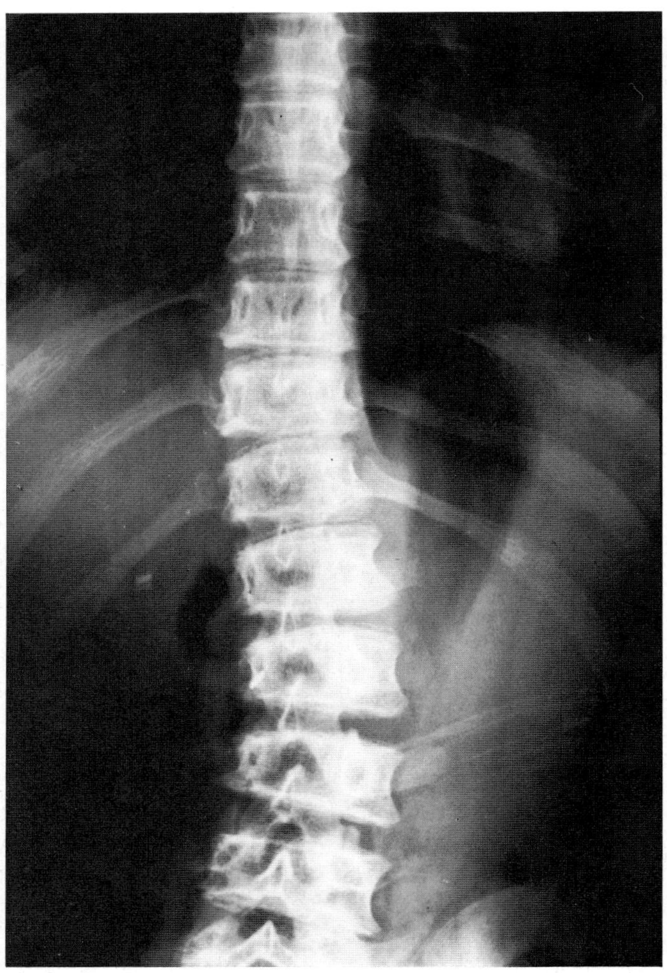

A lumbar scoliosis, convex to the left, is associated with a relative reduction in size of the vertebral bodies and a relative increase in height of the disc spaces on the right side. The right-hand pedicles between L1 and L3 are also small. Surgical clips are projected over L2 and to the right of L1.

The patient had been irradiated for a nephroblastoma (Wilms' tumour) of the right kidney at two years of age and the field had included the right side of the spine, causing unilateral retardation of growth. Current treatment plans include the whole of the vertebral body in the field, although even this technique cannot reliably prevent a mild scoliosis. The iliac crest and femoral head are excluded from the field. Radiological changes usually occur at least one year after treatment and are age and dose dependent: a scoliosis is more likely if the patient is under two years of age and receives a dose of >20 Gy. An increase in the scoliosis often occurs during the pubertal growth spurt and there may be an associated kyphosis. Long term complications include exostoses within the irradiated field (up to 20 per cent) and post-irradiation sarcomas.

References

Riseborough, E. T., Grabial, S. L., Burton, R. and Jaffe, N. (1976) Skeletal alterations following irradiation for Wilms' tumour with particular reference to scoliosis and kyphosis. *J. Bone Joint Surg.*, **58-A**, 526-536.

Rutherford, H. and Dodd, G. D. (1974) Complications of radiation therapy: growing bone. *Semin. in Roentgenol.*, **9**, 15-27.

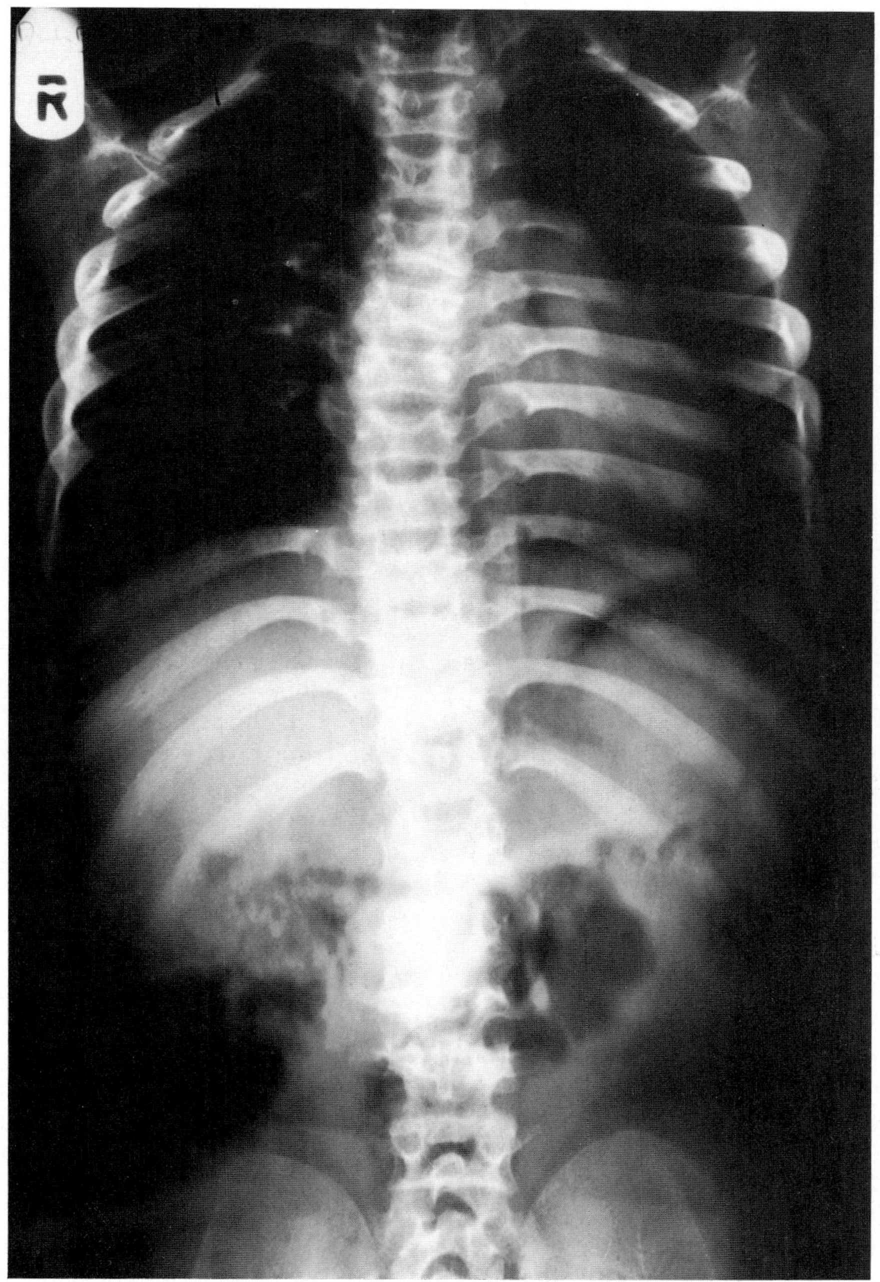

This 10-year-old child complained of a back deformity.

- What is the diagnosis?
- What features would you expect to see on the lateral view of the lumbar spine?

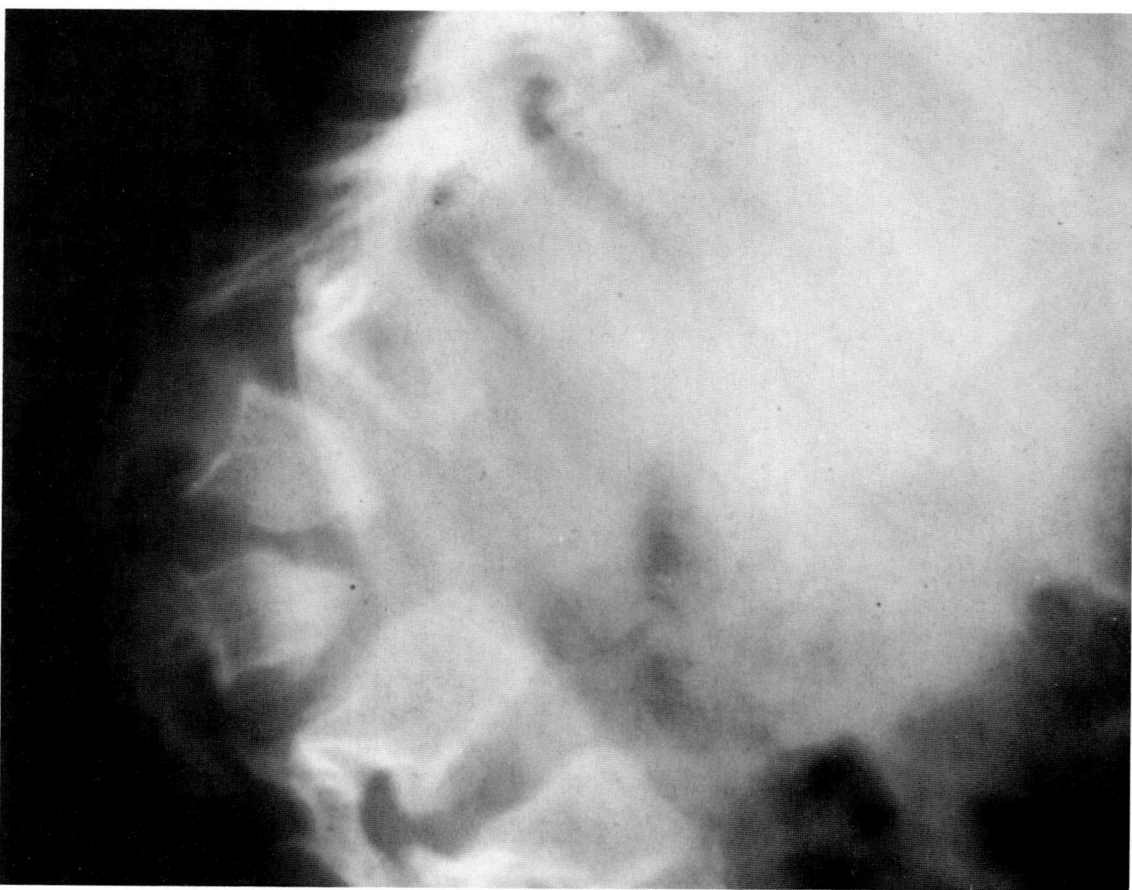

The AP view of the trunk shows a mild thoracic scoliosis, apparent overlap of the lower thoracic vertebrae suggestive of a localised kyphosis and an abnormal narrowing of the interpediculate distance in the lower lumbar spine. The last feature is diagnostic of achondroplasia.

Other characteristic radiological features are present in the lateral view. An angular kyphosis in the thoracolumbar region is associated with vertebral bodies which have a beak-like anterior projection, the so-called 'bullet' vertebral deformity. The lumbar lordosis is exaggerated and the disc to body height ratio is increased from the normal 1:3 to 1:2. Posterior scalloping of the bodies is present and the AP diameter of the neural canal is reduced due to the short pedicles.

Achondroplasia is an autosomal dominant condition recognisable at birth by the rhizomelic dwarfism. Spontaneous mutation is common.

The thoracolumbar kyphosis and abnormally-shaped vertebral bodies are common to several congenital conditions such as Hurler's syndrome, Down's syndrome and cretinism, and may be related to hypotonia. The interpediculate distance normally shows a progressive increase towards L5; in achondroplasia, inadequate development of the neural arches causes a progressive narrowing. In some other developmental syndromes, the interpediculate distance may simply fail to increase from L1 to L5. Spinal stenosis is not uncommon in achondroplastic adults and severe neurological impairment can result from a simple disc protrusion.

Reference

Swischuk, L. E. (1970) The beaked, notched or hooked vertebra. Its significance in infants and young children. *Radiology*, **95**, 661-664.

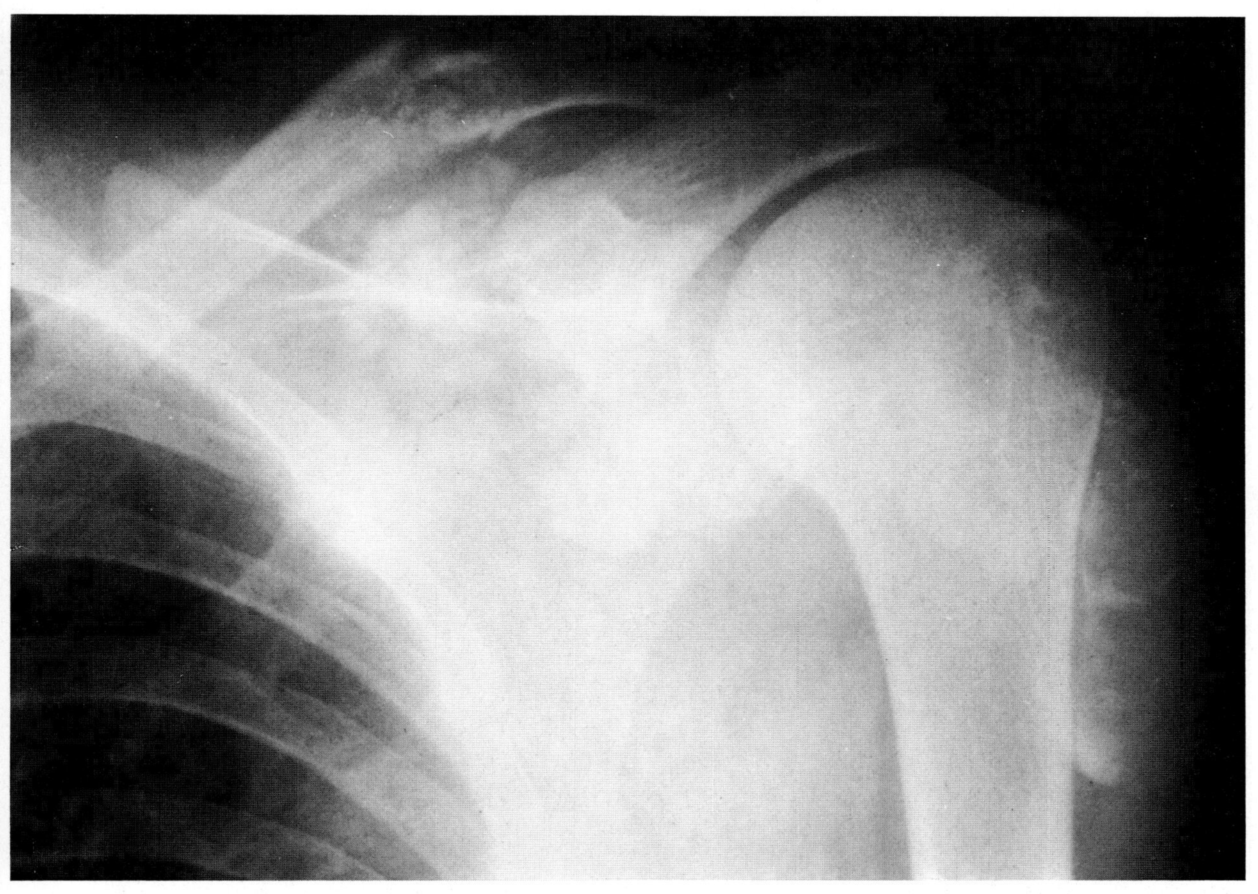

This middle-aged woman complained of a painful shoulder.

- Describe the features.

- What treatment had the patient been receiving?

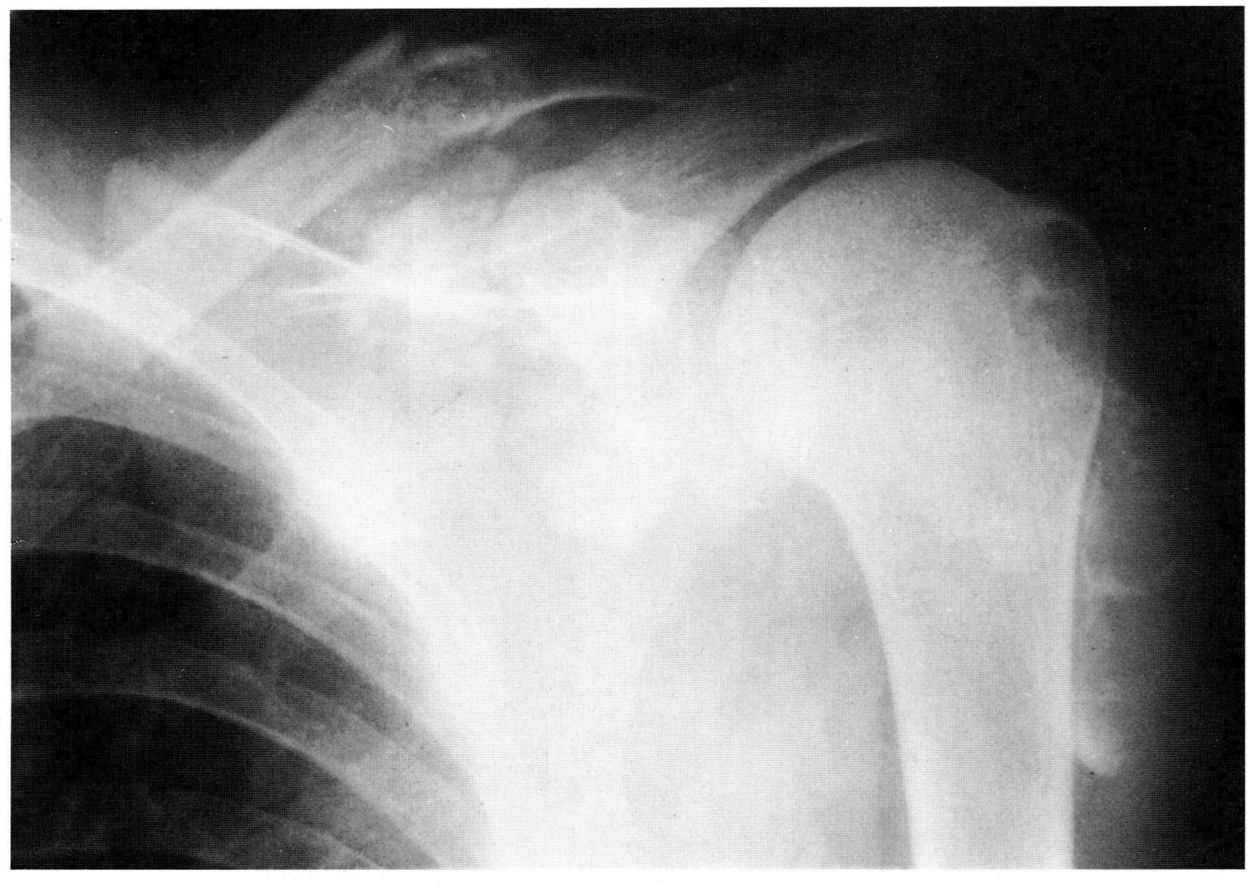

Amorphous areas of calcification are seen around the left shoulder. A fracture involves the distal third of the clavicle and the lateral end of the clavicle is eroded. This combination is typical of renal osteodystrophy and is due mainly to the secondary hyperparathyroidism. The patient had been receiving haemodialysis for chronic renal failure for several years.

The radiological findings in renal osteodystrophy are variable and include osteoporosis, osteomalacia, secondary hyperparathyroidism and osteosclerosis. In addition, aluminium hydroxide, given as a phosphate binder during long term haemodialysis, has been reported to be associated with osteomalacia, periosteal reaction and an increased incidence of fractures.

The soft tissue calcification is also a feature of secondary hyperparathyroidism and may produce tumoural masses. It may involve more than one joint and is often symmetrical. Periarticular calcification is also seen in other conditions such as hypoparathyroidism, sarcoidosis and hypervitaminosis D.

Reference

Chambers, S. E. et al. (1985) Periosteal new bone in patients on intermittent haemodialysis: an early indicator of aluminium-induced osteomalacia? *Clin. Radiol.*, 36, 163-168.

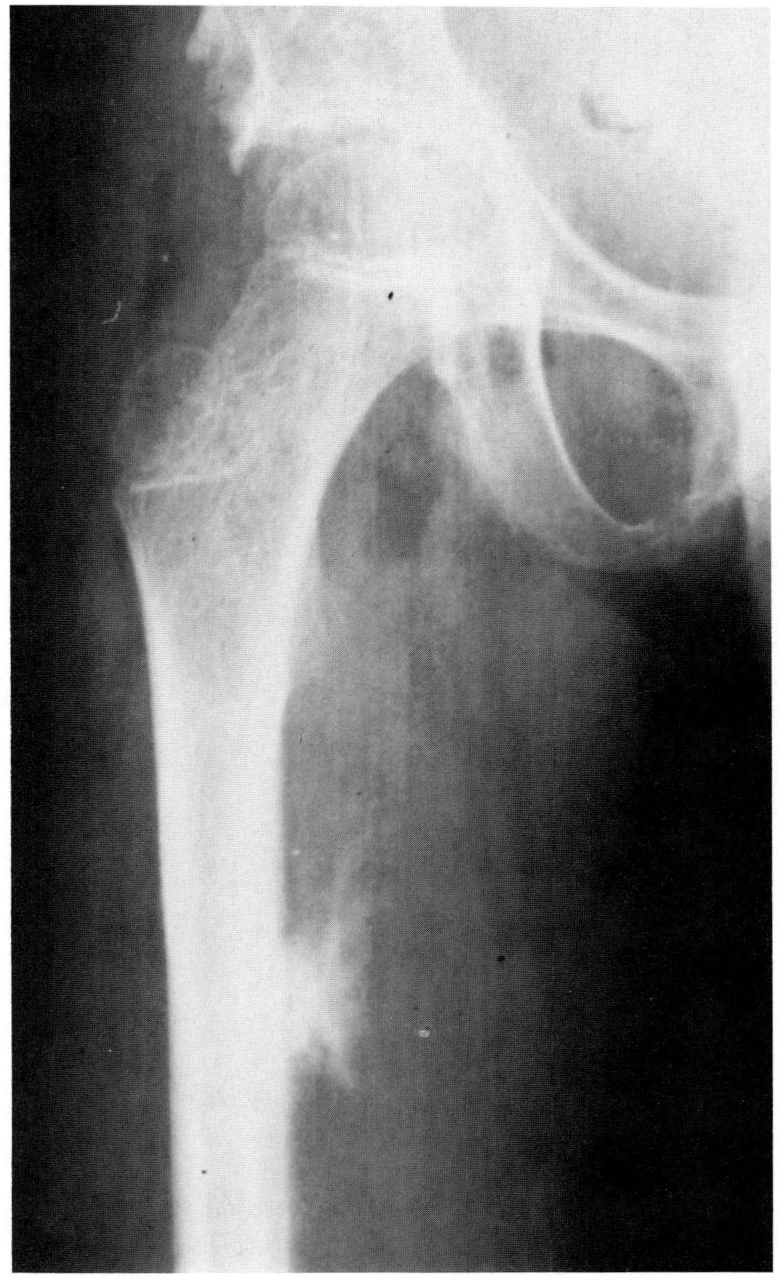

This 6-year-old girl complained of a painful thigh. There was no history of trauma.

- What is the diagnosis?

- How do you account for the appearances?

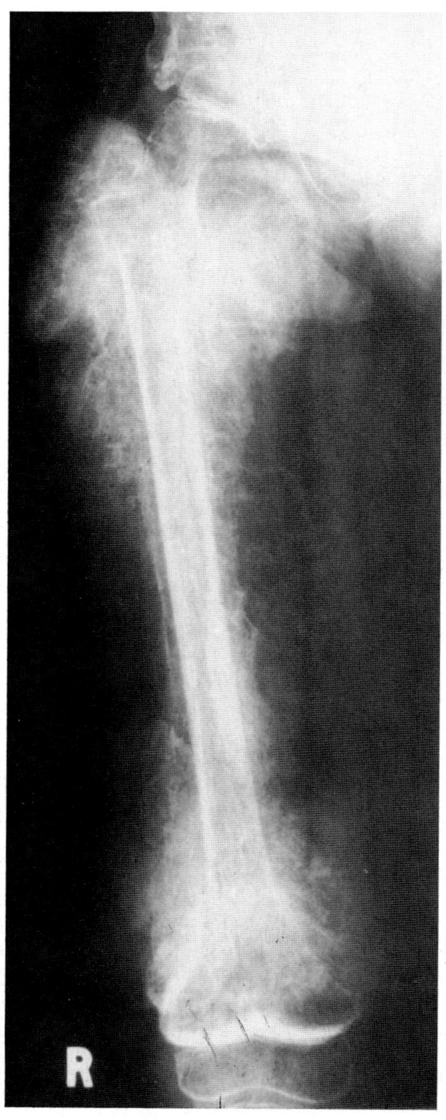

The initial film shows a generalised reduction in bone density and coarse bony trabeculation consistent with osteoporosis. A large amount of callus is present adjacent to the medial aspect of the femoral shaft, but with no identifiable femoral fracture. The combination of generalised osteopenia and exuberant callus is characteristic of osteogenesis imperfecta, a disorder that had been diagnosed in this child in infancy. Long-term administration of corticosteroids might simulate this appearance.

The radiograph above was taken six months later; the callus is more extensive and a fracture is now visible in the proximal femoral shaft. The mild protrusio acetabuli shown on both films is secondary to the osteopenic state.

In osteogenesis imperfecta the long bones usually show a typical gracile appearance in childhood when the condition is of genetically dominant inheritance.

Reference

Bauze, L. J., Smith, R. and Francis, M. J. O. (1975) A new look at osteogenesis imperfecta. *J. Bone Joint Surg.*, 57-B, 2-12.

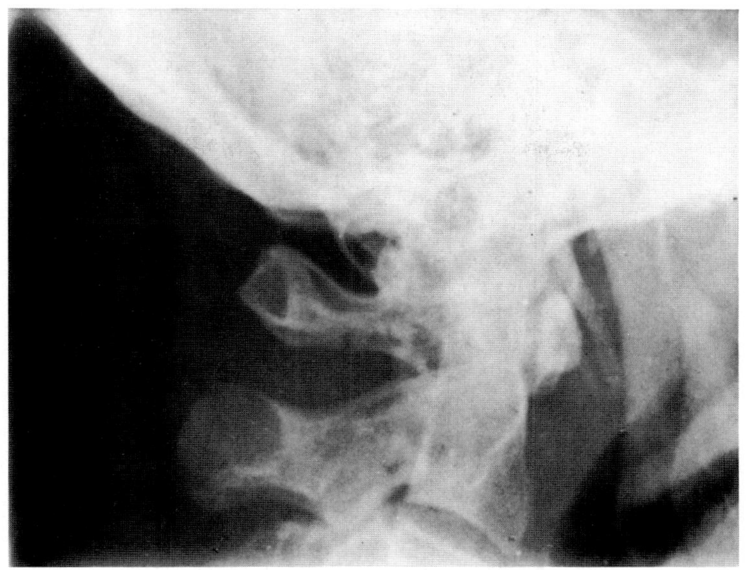

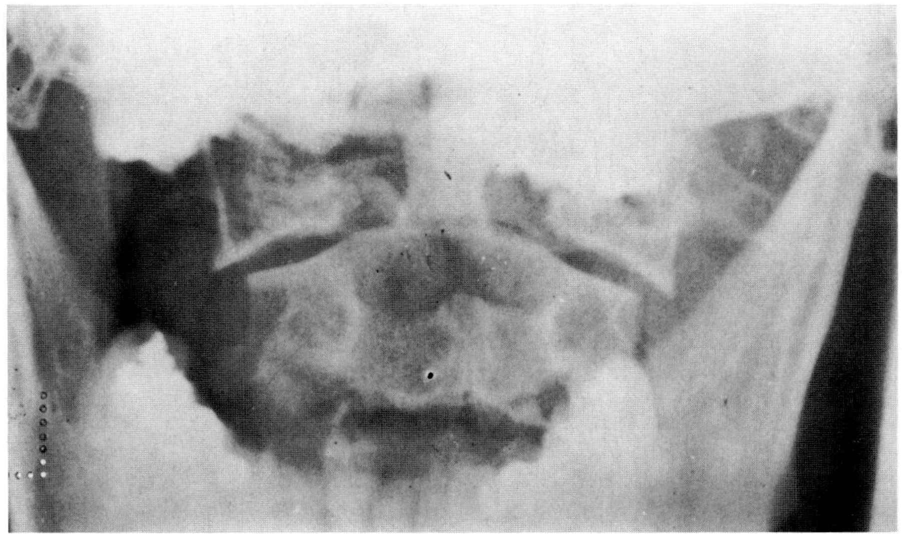

This young man dived into a partly filled swimming pool while under the influence of alcohol.

- What is the injury?

- What other techniques may be useful in evaluating this type of fracture?

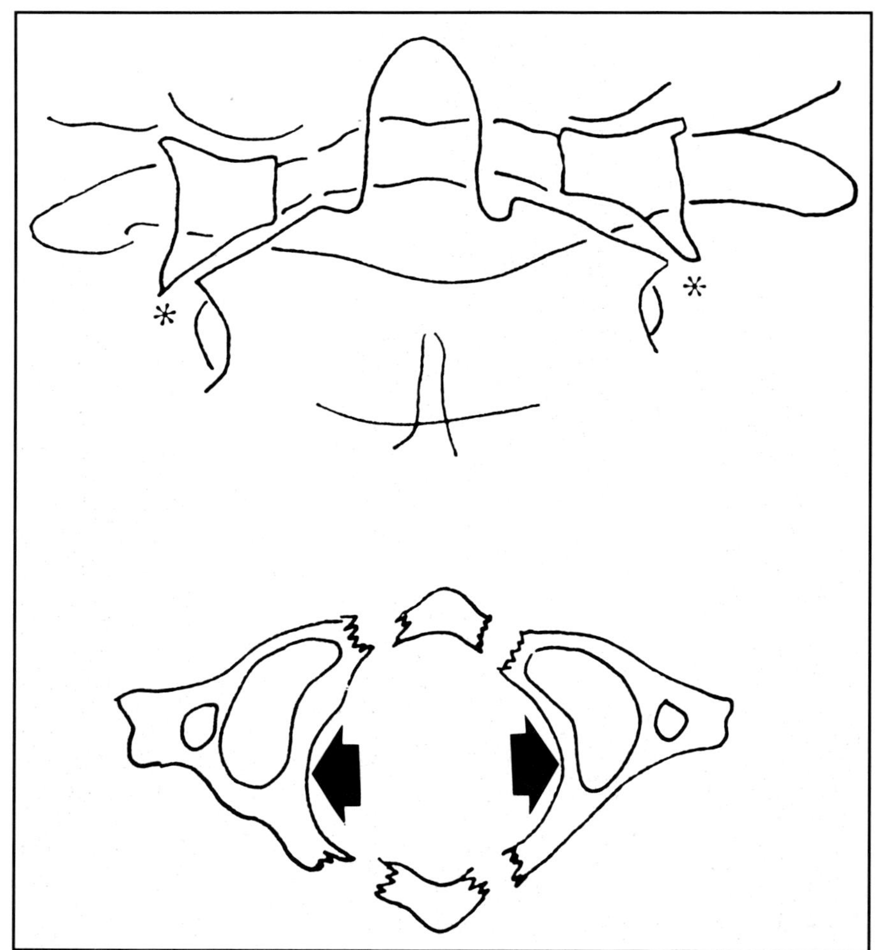

The AP open mouth view of C1/2 shows the lateral masses of C1 displaced outwards beyond the lateral margins of the superior articular facets of C2. The lateral projection shows a fracture through the posterior arch of C1. These are the appearances of a Jefferson (burst) fracture where the bony ring, formed by the anterior and posterior arches of C1, has been fractured at more than one site. It is caused by downward pressure of the occipital condyles on the atlas, which may be due to a heavy blow on the head, or a fall by the subject from a height on to the head, as in this case. Although it is an unstable fracture, the fragments usually do not encroach on the spinal canal and neurological impairment is unusual.

The fracture is usually shown on an AP open mouth view but plain tomography or CT sometimes may be necessary. The injury is differentiated from rotation by the fact that *both* lateral masses of the atlas lie more laterally than those of the axis.

Sir Geoffrey Jefferson (1886-1961), consultant neurosurgeon to the Manchester Royal Infirmary, described four cases with this fracture in 1919-1920 and reviewed the earlier literature.

Reference

Harris, J. H. Jr. (1978) *The Radiology of Acute Cervical Trauma.* Williams & Wilkins, Baltimore.

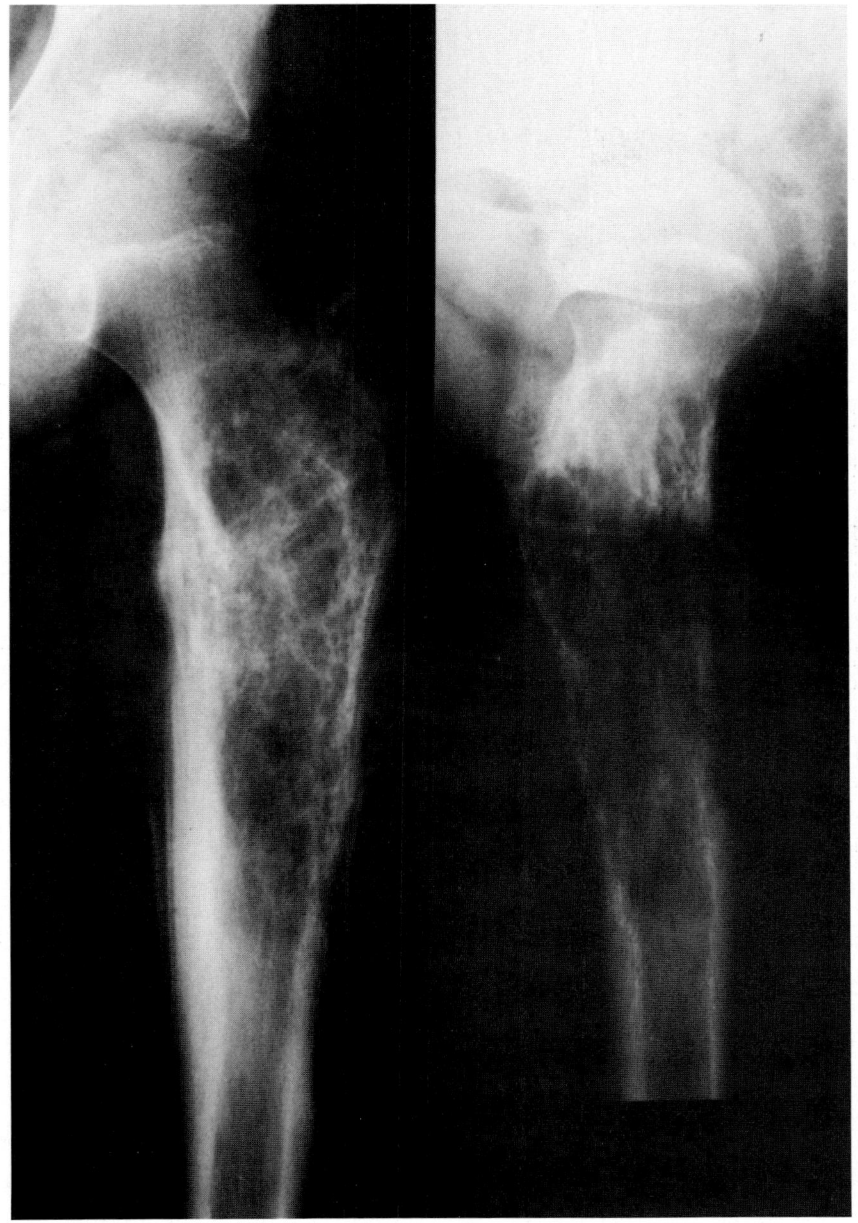

This 12-year-old boy presented with a two-month history of pain and swelling in his left thigh.

- Describe the appearances.

- What diagnoses would you consider?

- What other investigations are indicated?

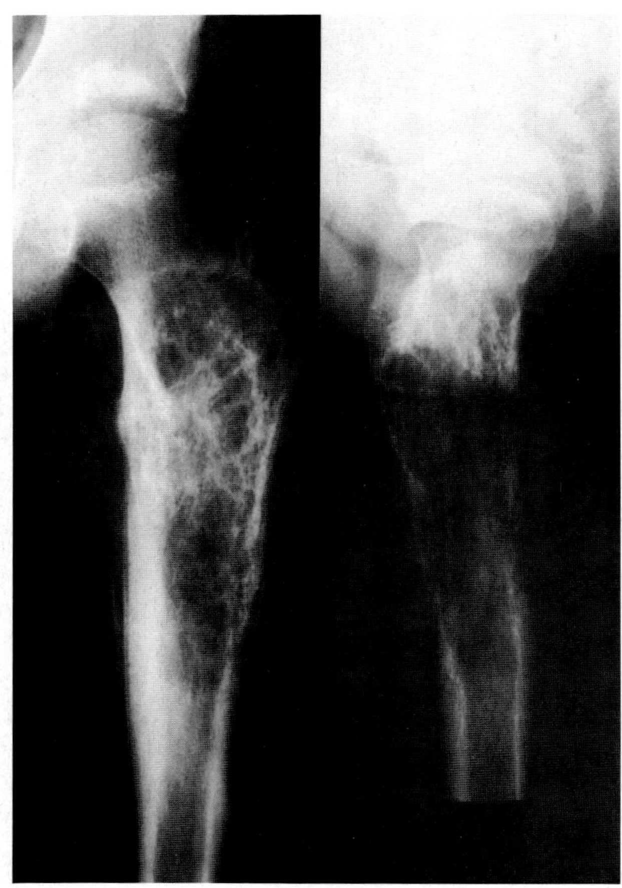

The AP and lateral views of the proximal half of the femur show an extensive and permeative region of medullary and cortical destruction in the diaphysis, associated with a lamellated ('onion skin') periosteal reaction.

The radiological findings are consistent with a malignant process and at this age especially, a Ewing's sarcoma. Although often described as the hallmark of this tumour, the classical 'onion skin' appearance is present only in a minority of cases. The differential diagnoses to consider with a diaphyseal lesion of this type include neuroblastoma in a younger child, non-Hodgkin's lymphoma and leukaemia. A radionuclide scan is required to exclude multiple lesions and CT of the thorax to demonstrate any pulmonary metastases.

Ewing's sarcoma has a peak incidence in the 5-15 age group and is rare beyond the third decade. It occurs most commonly in the diaphyseal and diametaphyseal regions of the long bones, and in the pelvis, vertebrae and ribs.

Although the initial response to radiotherapy is often dramatic, most of the neoplasms will recur, with metastatic spread to skeletal and extraskeletal sites. Modern therapy therefore is aimed at eradication of micrometastases by systemic chemotherapy. In appropriate cases, the primary tumour may be excised following an initial course of chemotherapy.

James Ewing (1866-1943) was the first Professor of Pathology at Cornell University. He described the tumour that now bears his name as 'diffuse endothelioma of bone' in 1920.

Reference

Vohra, V. G. (1967) Roentgen manifestations in Ewing's sarcoma: a study of 156 cases. *Cancer*, 20, 727-733.

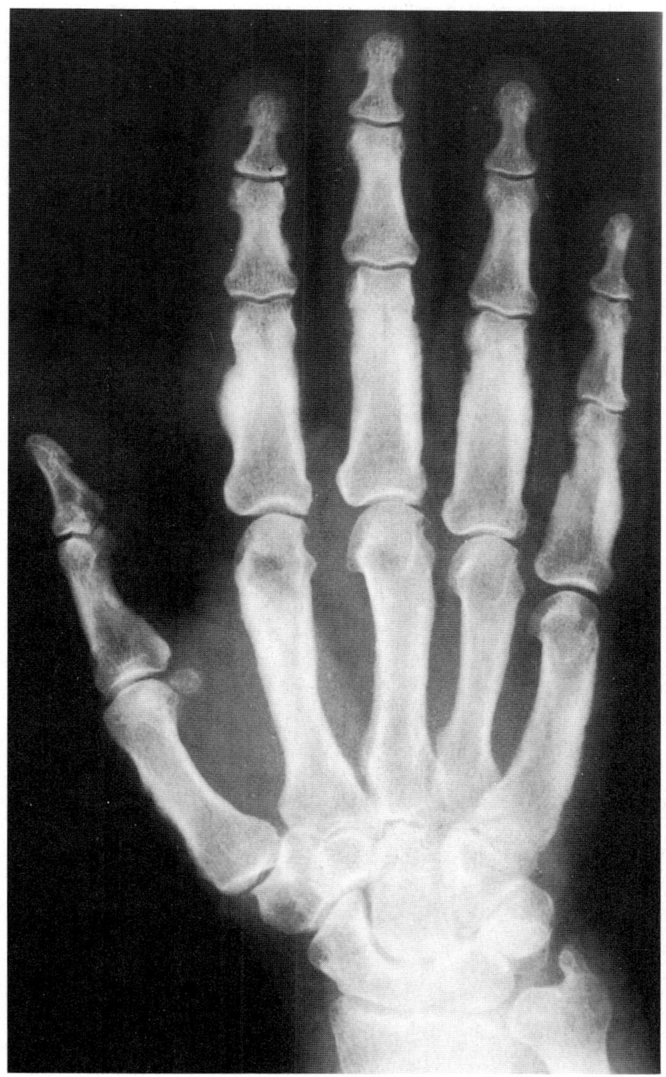

This middle-aged woman presented with swollen fingers.

- What abnormalities are shown in this radiograph?

- What is the diagnosis?

- What are the typical clinical findings in this condition?

- What is the differential diagnosis?

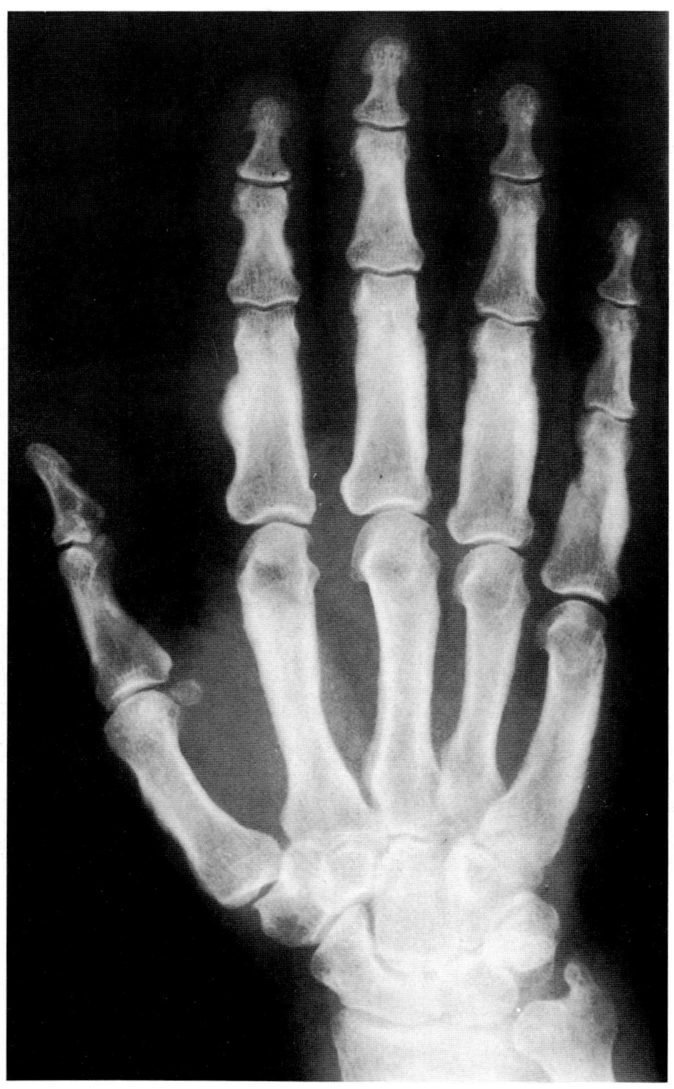

Formation of periosteal new bone has occurred on the diaphyses of the proximal phalanges and, to a lesser degree, in the metacarpals and middle phalanges. The distribution is consistent with a diagnosis of thyroid acropachy, although the new bone has a less feathery margin than usual. These features present, as on this occasion, several years after treatment for hyperthyroidism when the patient is either euthyroid or hypothyroid. Such treatment is usually surgical, but the condition can follow the administration of radioiodine or even antithyroid drugs. The typical clinical findings are soft tissue swelling, exophthalmos and pretibial myxoedema.

The differential diagnosis includes hypertrophic osteoarthropathy and pachydermoperiostosis, both of which predominantly involve the distal shafts of the bones of the forearm. Pachydermoperiostosis is associated with a typical facies and hyperhidrosis. Venous stasis or infective periostitis should only be considered as causes in the presence of relevant clinical findings.

Reference

Moule, B., Grant, M. C., Boyle, I. T. and May, H. (1970) Thyroid acropachy. *Clin. Radiol.*, **21**, 329-333.

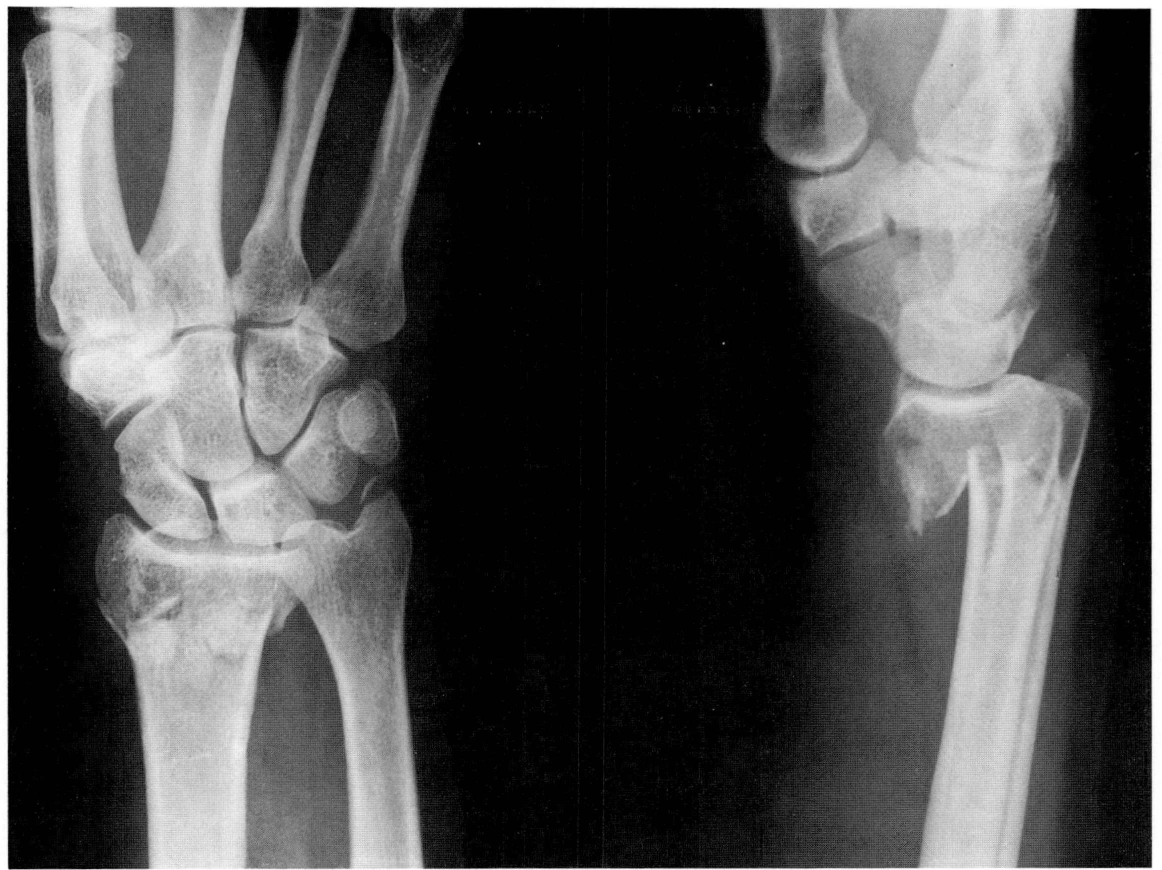

This man fell over while playing basketball. He came to the Casualty Department with a painful wrist.

- What is the diagnosis?

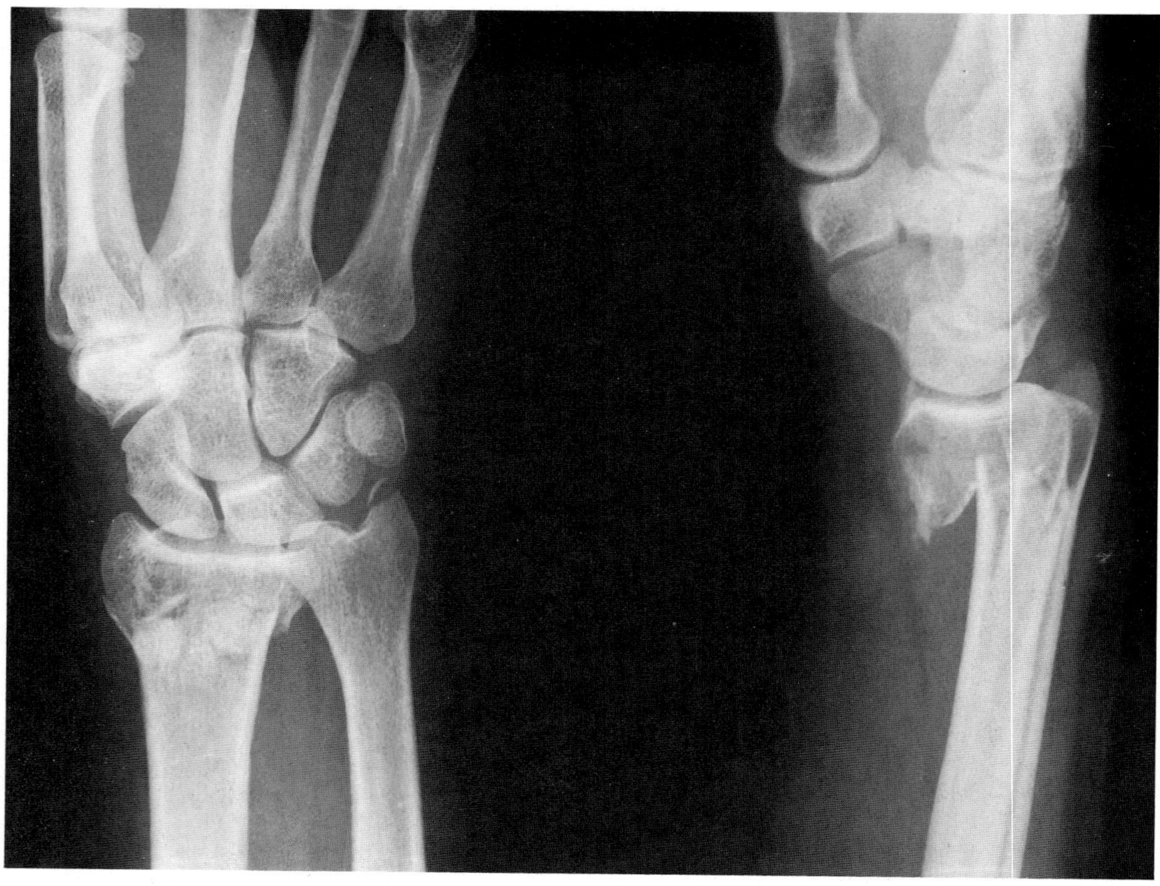

The PA projection of the right wrist shows a transverse fracture through the distal radius. In the lateral projection, the fracture is shown to be oblique with volar and proximal displacement of the distal fragment. Dislocation at the radio-ulnar joint and avulsion of the ulnar styloid have also occurred. This is a Smith's fracture (sometimes called a reversed Colles' fracture), an injury caused by a fall either on to the dorsiflexed wrist or on to the back of the hand.

It is important to distinguish between Smith's and Colles' fractures. They look similar in the PA projection and may only be diagnosed by the direction in which the distal fragment is displaced in the lateral view (see Question 10). If a Smith's fracture is erroneously treated as a Colles' fracture, the deformity will be increased, leading to malunion and subsequent weakness, pain and limitation of movement at the wrist.

Robert William Smith (1807-1873) succeeded Abraham Colles as Professor of Surgery at Trinity College, Dublin. He described the fracture in 1847.

Reference

Woodyard, J. E. (1969) A review of Smith's fractures. *J. Bone Joint Surg.*, **51-B**, 324-329.

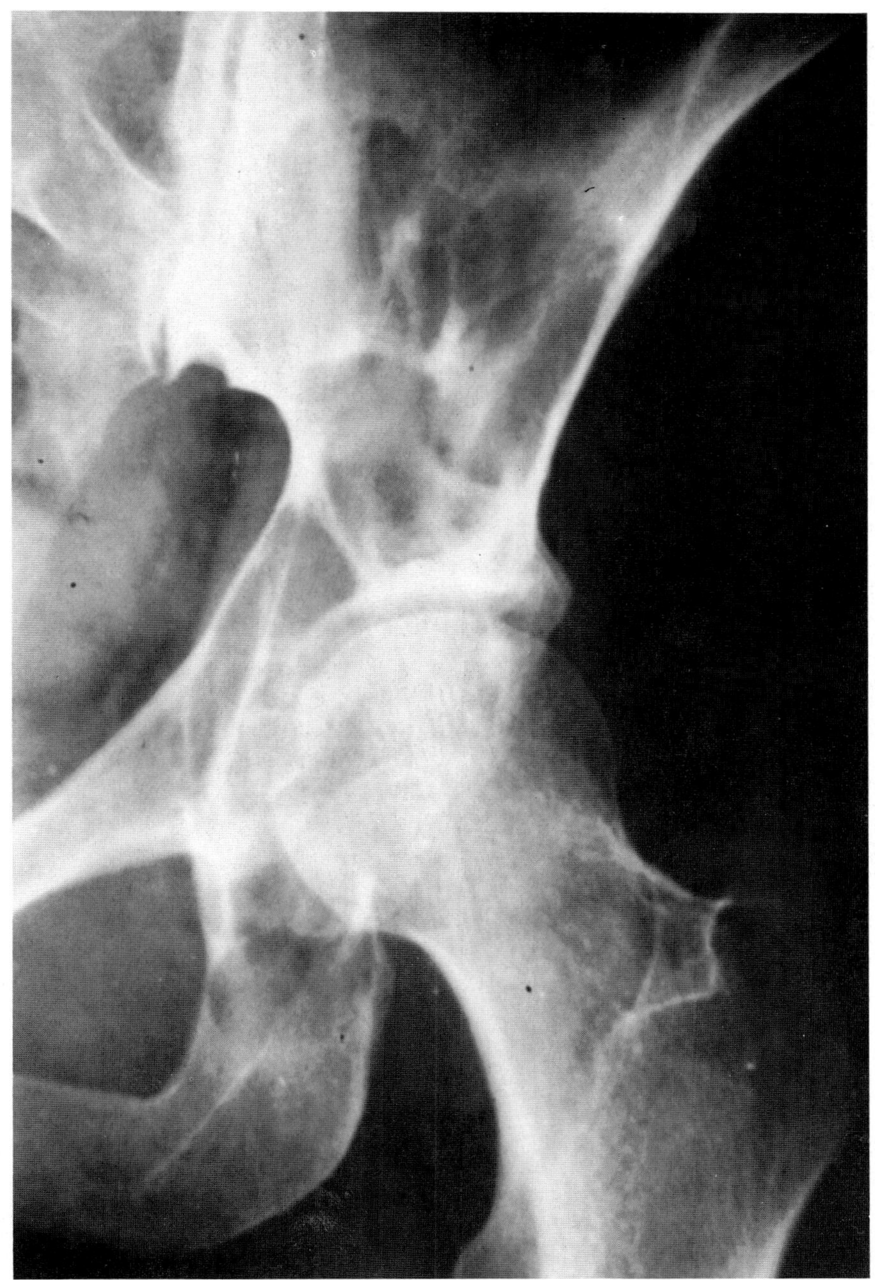

This 42-year-old woman had a two-year history
of hip pain.

- What possible diagnoses would you consider?

- What is the most likely diagnosis?

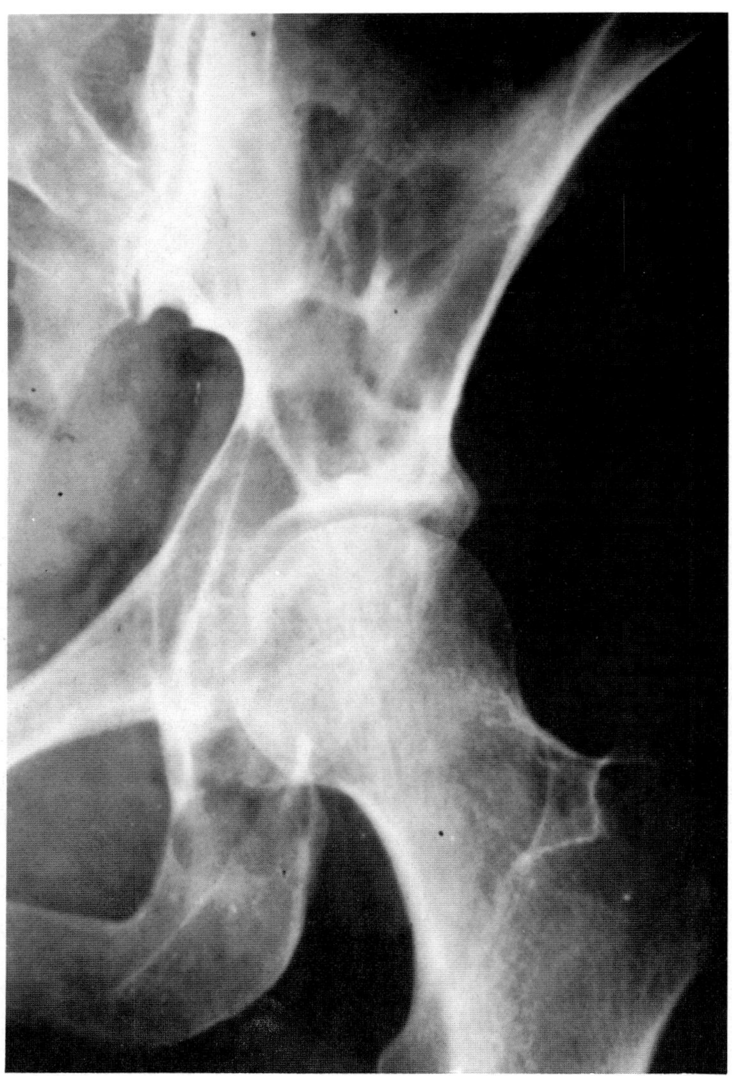

A well-defined lytic lesion is present in the left ilium and ischium and extends to the subarticular margins of the hip and possibly the sacro-iliac joint. Bony trabeculae cross the lesion which is causing minimal expansion of the innominate bone.

The site and appearance in a middle-aged patient presenting with pain suggest a diagnosis of plasmacytoma. However, fibrous dysplasia, a giant-cell tumour, an expansile metastasis, a brown tumour of hyperparathyroidism and a low-grade bone sarcoma could each produce a similar appearance; a definitive diagnosis can only be made at biopsy, which was performed in this case.

Plasmacytomas occur most frequently in the spine, pelvis and ribs. Pain is a common presenting feature and pathological fractures may occur. Such lesions are often accompanied by tumoural extension into the soft tissues; some suggestion of this complication is present in this case and could be confirmed by CT examination.

As abnormality of plasma protein is proportional to the total mass of the tumour, plasma electrophoresis may be normal at presentation. The majority of plasmacytomas eventually progress to multiple myeloma.

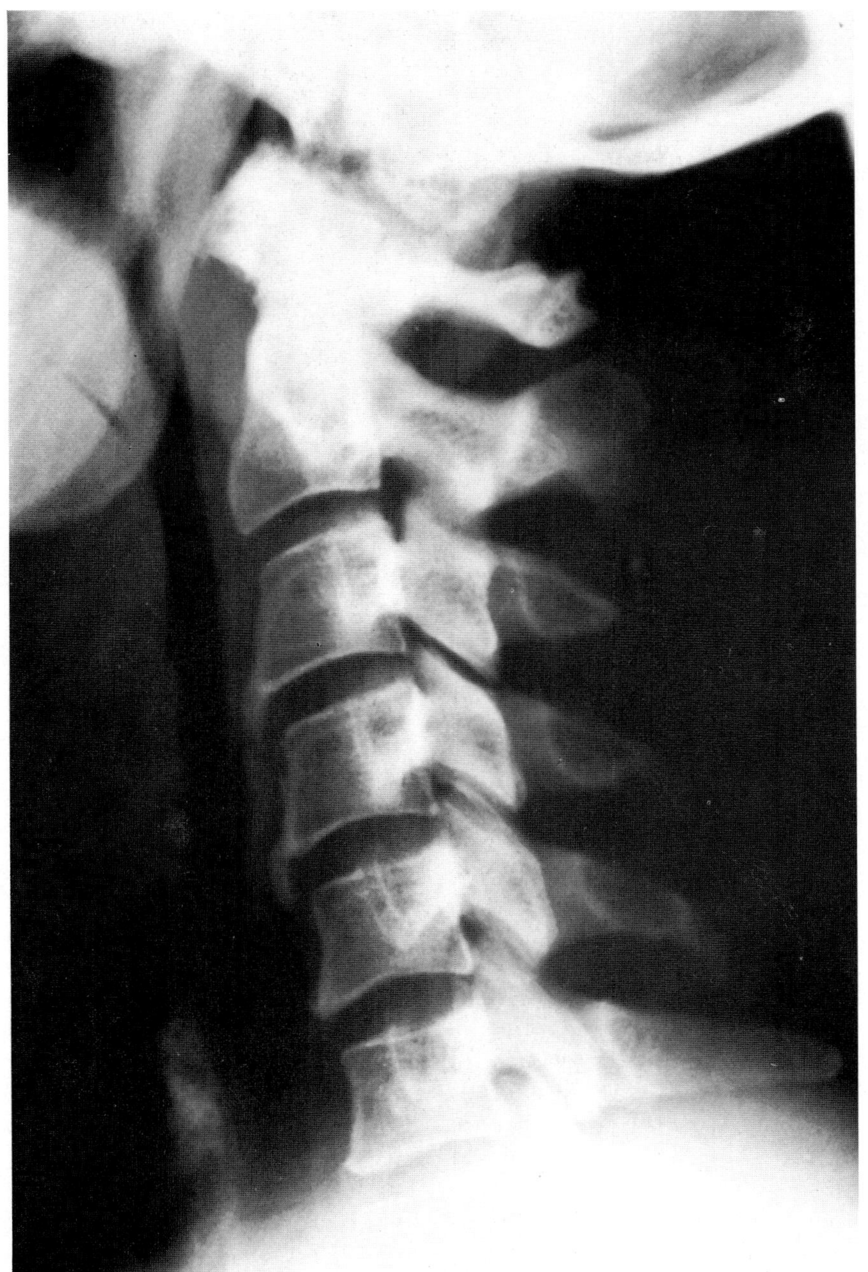

This 53-year-old man complained of pain in the neck, of acute onset and radiating to the left shoulder. No history of trauma was obtained.

- Comment on the radiograph.

- What is the most likely diagnosis and how might you confirm the clinical suspicion radiologically?

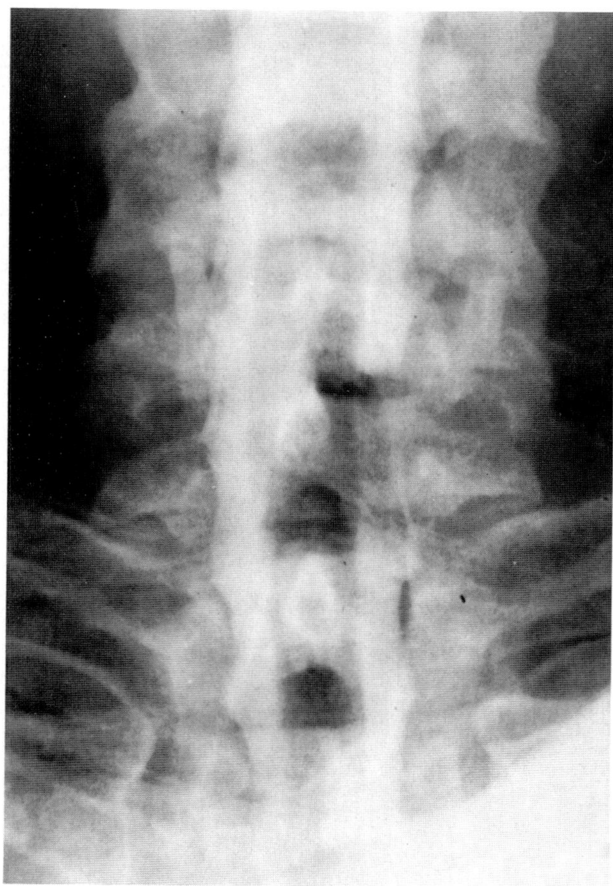

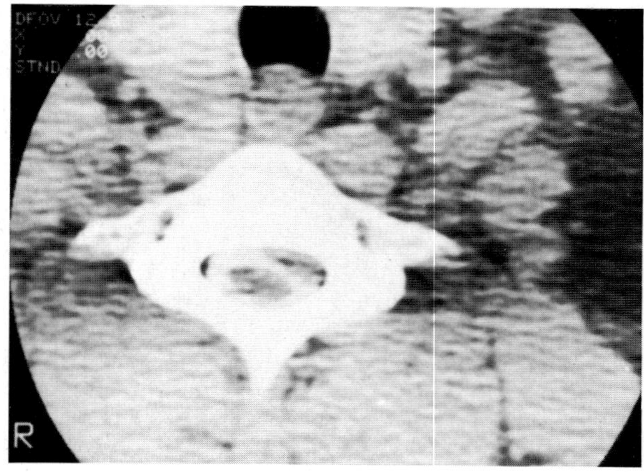

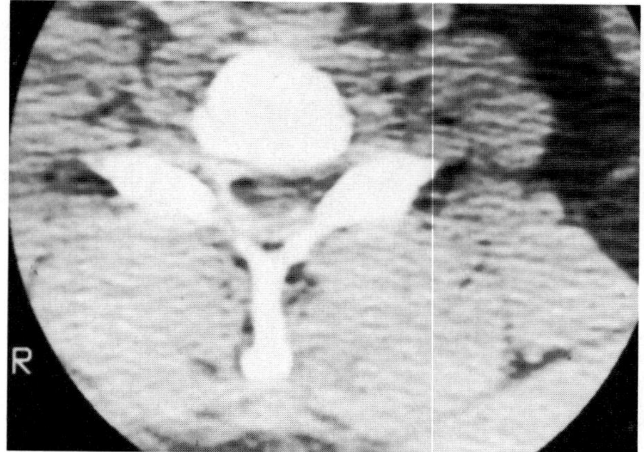

The lateral view of the cervical spine shows loss of the normal cervical lordosis (a non-specific finding related to pain and muscle spasm) and narrowing of the C6/7 disc. In the absence of bony degenerative changes, the appearances are probably due to an acute protrusion of an intervertebral disc.

The diagnosis was confirmed by the cervical myelogram which shows thecal indentation at the C6/7 level on the left and compression of the left C7 nerve root.

Acute protrusion of the normal cervical disc is rare and associated with severe injury in the young. In older patients acute protrusion of a degenerative disc may occur spontaneously. Frequently, no associated bony degenerative change is found.

The spinal cord occupies most of the vertebral canal in the cervical spine and cord compression may result from even a small midline protrusion. CT examination is often more useful than myelography in detecting the smaller protrusions, although the lack of epidural fat may make differentiation between disc and thecal sac difficult without intrathecal contrast.

The scans performed following myelography in this patient demonstrate how the herniated disc is causing not only compression of the nerve root but also encroachment on the subarachnoid space and displacement of the spinal cord.

Discectomy was performed with relief of symptoms.

Reference

Daniels, D. L., Grogan, J. P., Johansen, J. G. et al. (1984) Cervical radiculopathy: computed tomography and myelography compared. *Radiology*. **151**, 109-113.

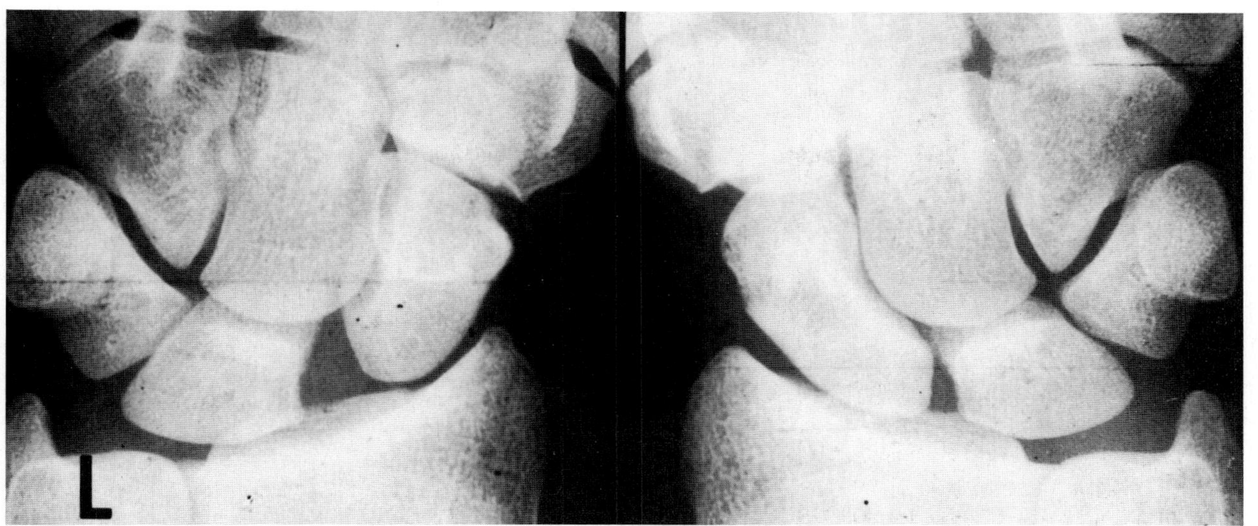

This man fell and injured his left wrist. The right wrist is shown for comparison.

- What abnormality is present in the left wrist?

- How is this appearance caused?

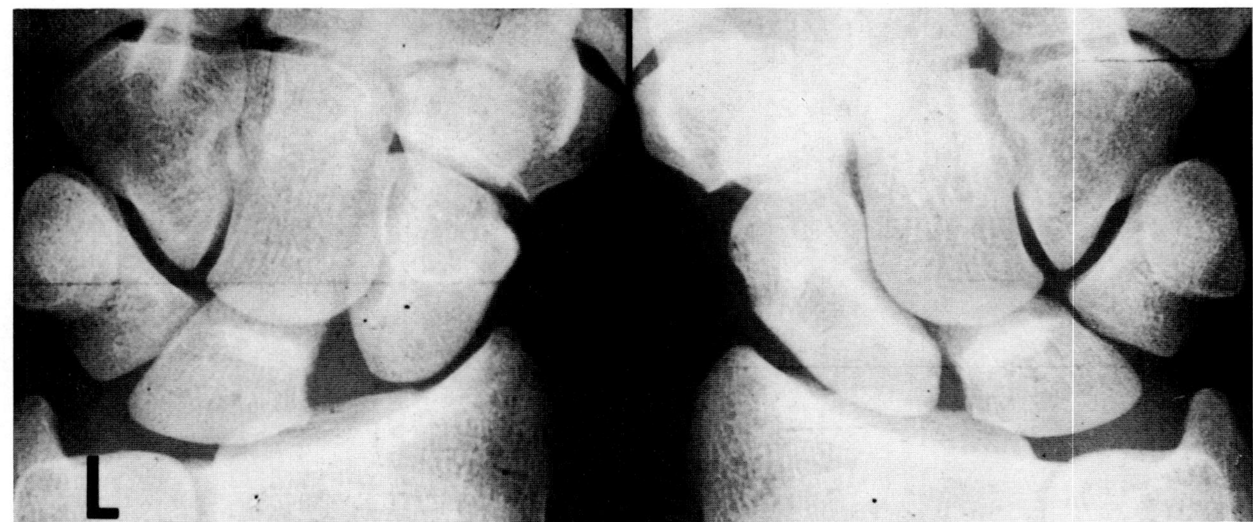

The PA view of the left wrist shows an abnormally wide space between the scaphoid and lunate bones—the 'Terry Thomas' sign (recalling the central upper incisors of that comedian)—foreshortening of the scaphoid and a cortical 'ring' at the distal pole of the scaphoid. The appearances are those of a rotational subluxation or dislocation of the scaphoid.

This injury follows acute dorsiflexion of the wrist and is due to rupture of the dorsal radiocarpal ligament and the ligaments joining the scaphoid, lunate and capitate. The patient presents with wrist pain or a poor grip.

A definite diagnosis may be made if the scapholunate distance is at least 4 mm; a distance of 2 mm is suspicious. The scaphoid foreshortening and the ring sign are due to rotation of its distal pole.

Reference

Hudson, T. M. et al. (1976) Isolated rotatory subluxation of the carpal navicular. *Amer. J. Roentgenol.*, **126**, 601-611.

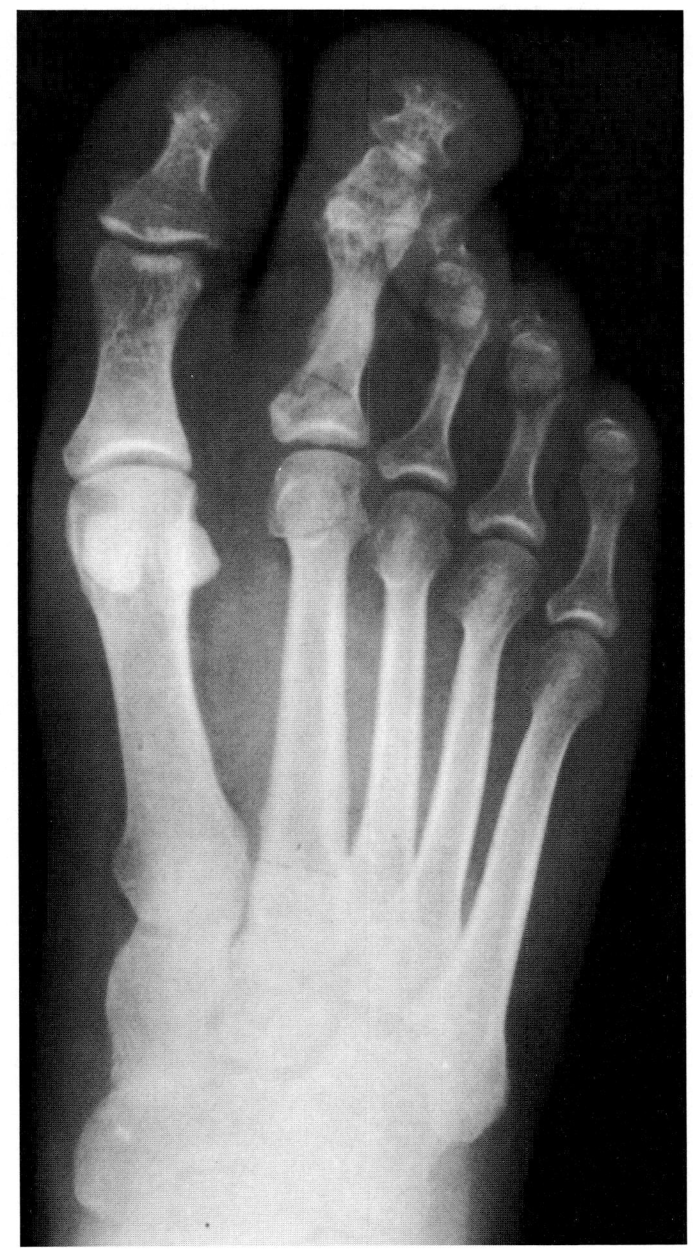

This 34-year-old woman sought treatment following difficulty in buying shoes.

- What is the diagnosis?

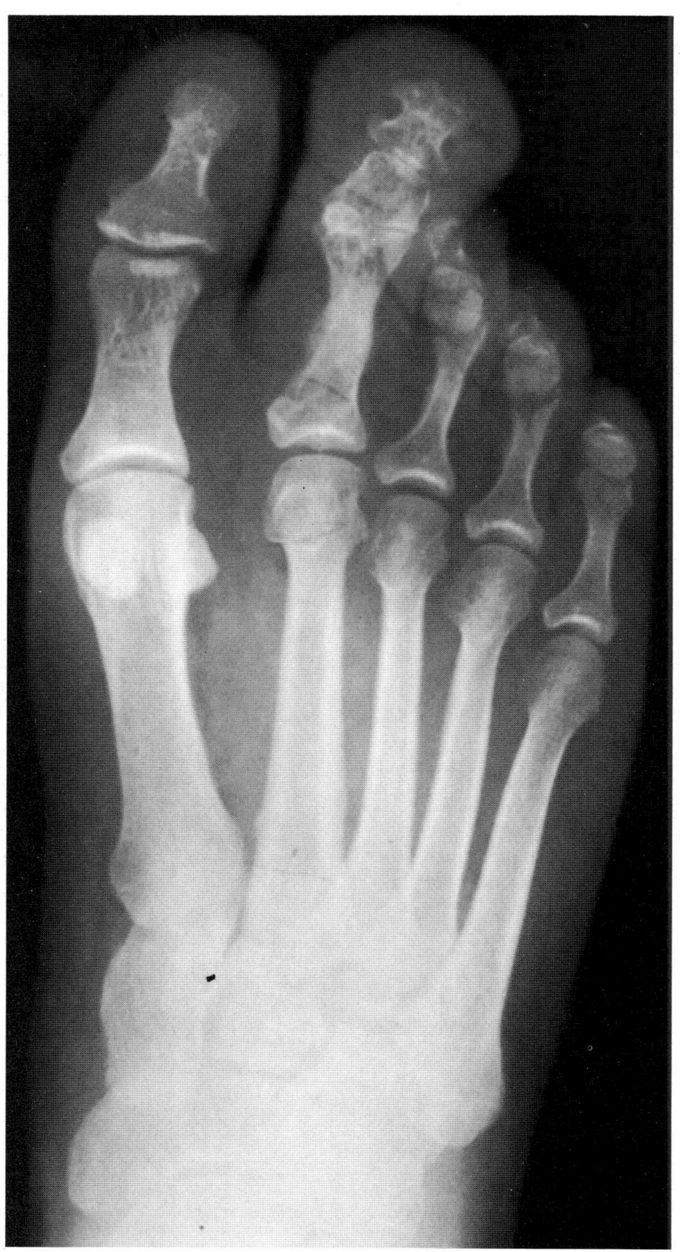

The bony and soft tissue hypertrophy of the second toe are characteristic of macrodystrophia lipomatosa. Although not apparent radiologically in this patient, an increased amount of fatty tissue is typically present and may be associated with lipomas more proximally in the limb.

This congenital anomaly has an equal sex incidence and predominantly affects the hands. It is often unilateral but may involve more than one digit. Bony overgrowth, with formation of osteophytes and exostoses, becomes more prominent with age.

Following partial amputation of the toe the patient was able to wear normal shoes.

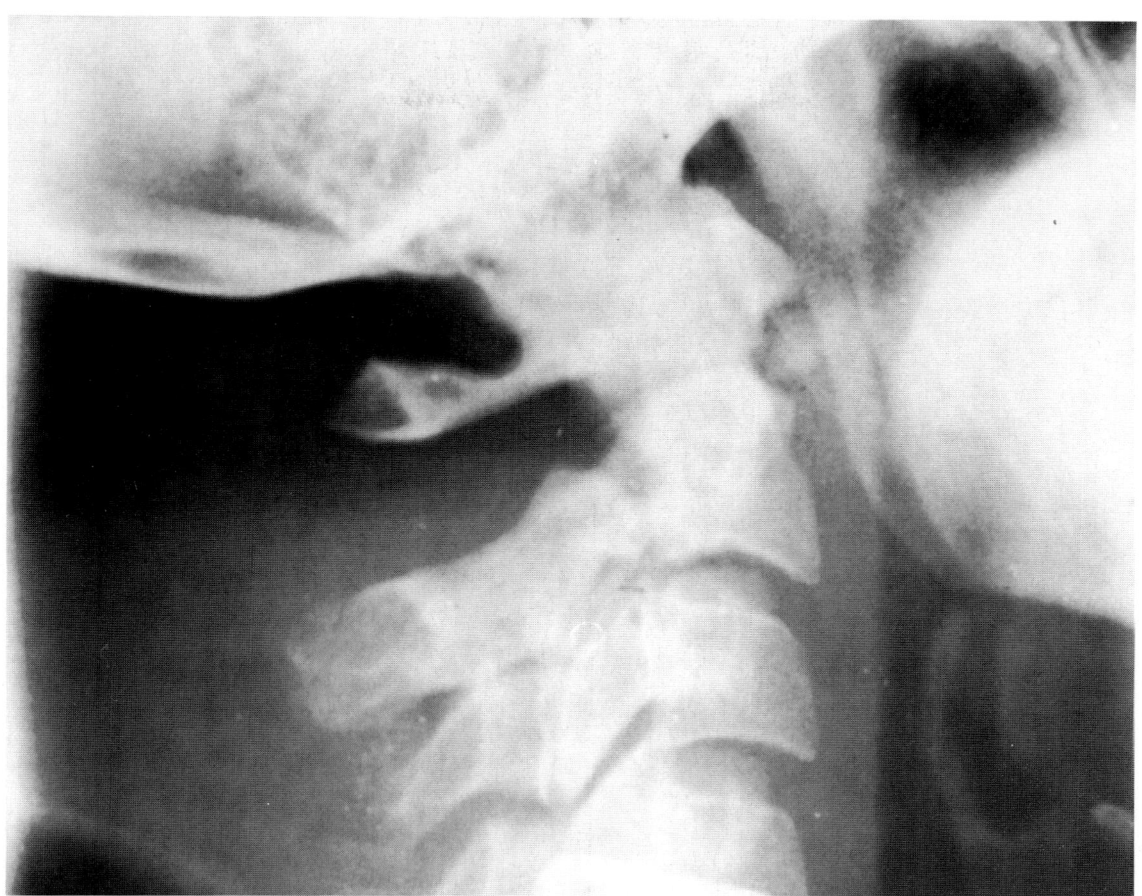

This woman was a front seat passenger in a car involved in a road traffic accident. She struck her head on the dashboard and subsequently complained of pain and limited movement in her neck.

Neurological examination was normal.

- What is the mechanism of injury?

- How does the injury derive its name?

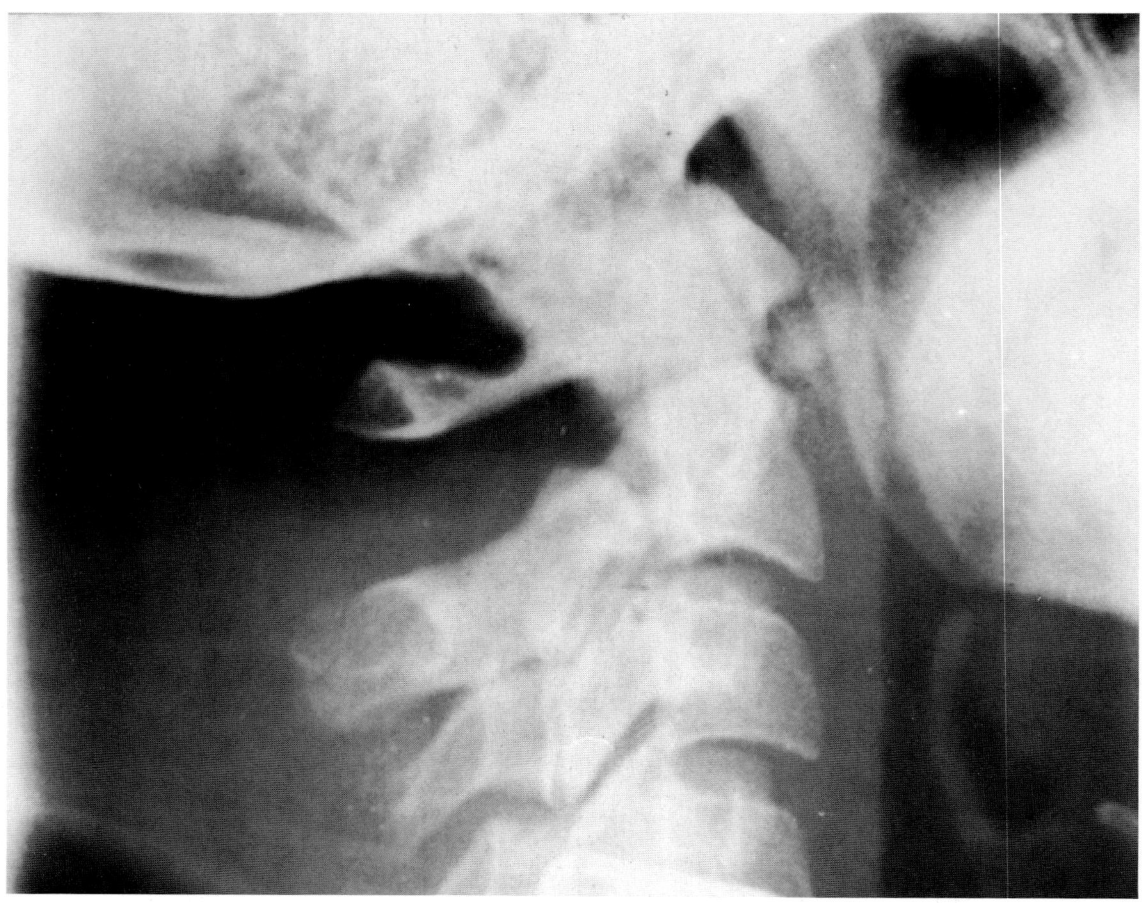

The lateral view of the upper cervical spine shows an oblique fracture through the pedicle of C2 with a minor degree of forward subluxation of the body of C2 on C3.

This is a 'hangman's' fracture caused by acute hyperextension of the neck. The commonest mode of injury is an RTA where sudden deceleration causes the face to strike the steering wheel or windscreen, forcing the head backwards in relationship to the cervical spine. The full force of the hyperextension is transmitted through the pedicles of C2 on to the apophyseal joints. The pedicles are relatively weak and are liable to fracture while the anterior longitudinal ligament usually ruptures. This allows forward subluxation of the body of C2 on C3. Note that the spinolaminar junction at the base of the spinous process of C2 is displaced backwards so that the spinolaminar line from C1 to C4 is broken at the C2 level.

If the hyperextension is transient, the fracture may cause relatively little neurological damage. If the force is sustained, the cord will be transected. The injury is known as a hangman's fracture because, in a judicial hanging, it causes sudden death by respiratory paralysis, thus avoiding death by strangulation. It is of course the hanged prisoner who suffers the injury and not the hangman, so that the fracture is misnamed.

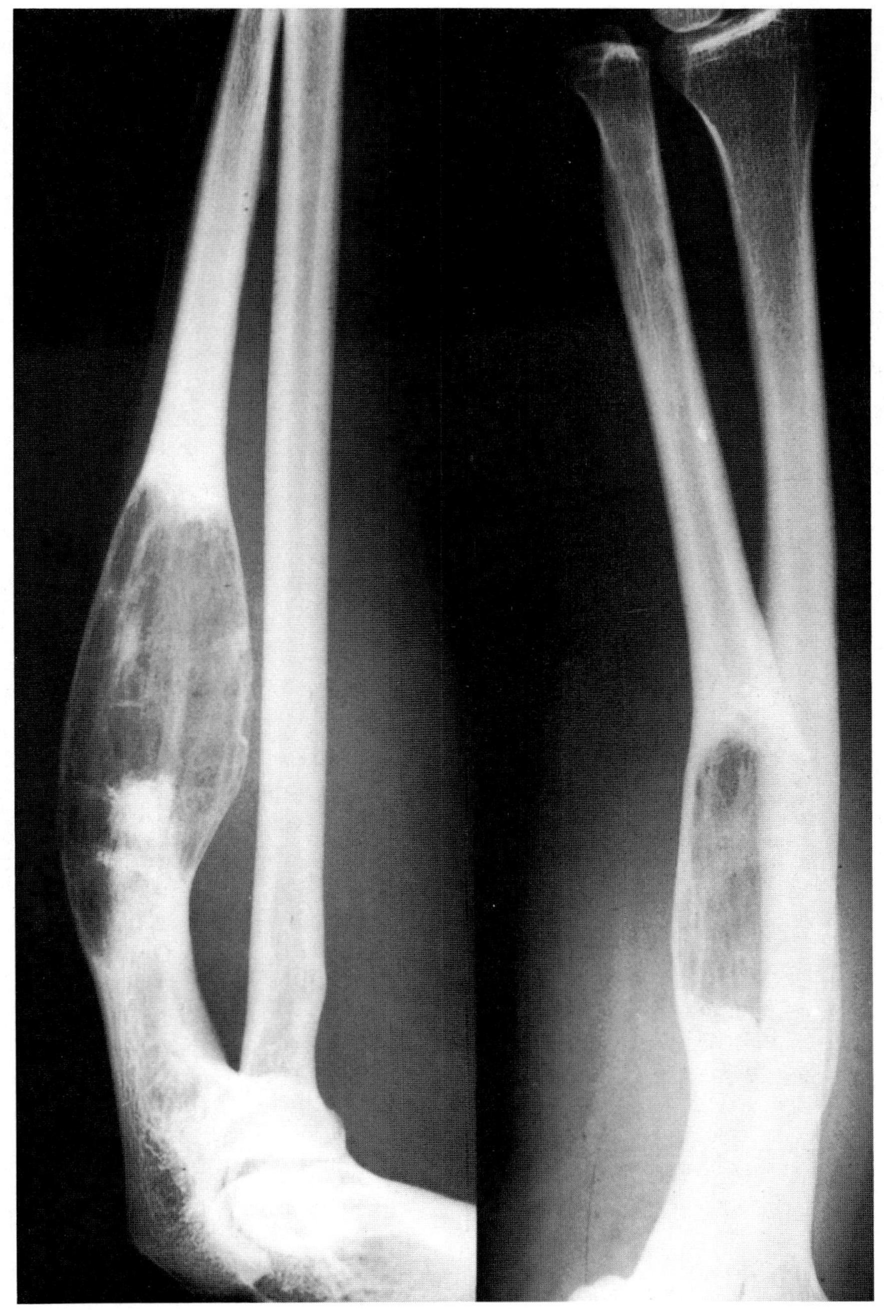

This woman aged 35 complained of long-standing deformity of her forearm.

- Describe the radiographs and suggest a diagnosis.

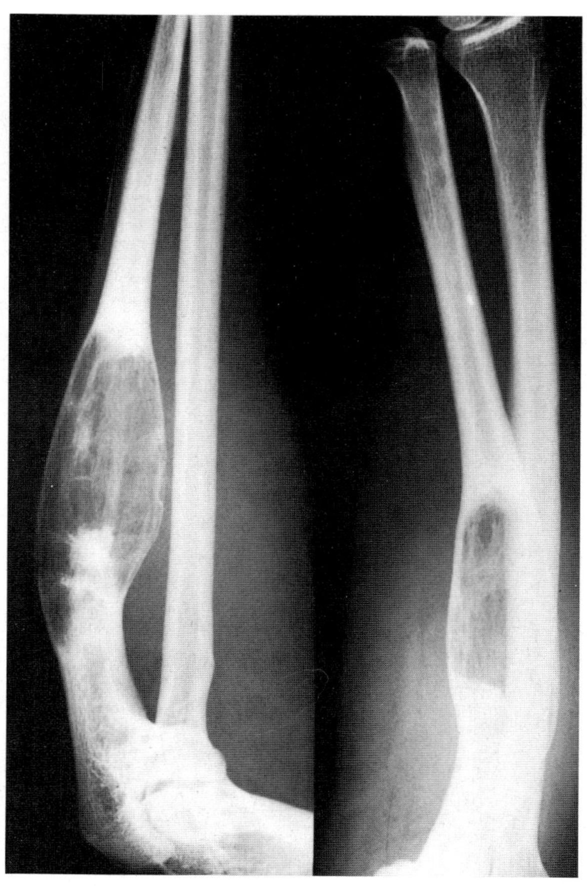

AP and lateral views of the forearm show bowing and deformity of the ulna. An expanded, relatively radiolucent lesion is present in the diaphysis and has thinned the intact cortex. Fine irregular bony trabeculae traverse the lesion and flecks of calcification are seen within it on the lateral view. A band of dense bone separates the lesion from the rest of the diaphysis.

The appearances are those of a benign lesion and are most consistent with fibrous dysplasia. Other possibilities include a brown tumour (no other evidence of hyperparathyroidism) and an enchondroma (which would not tend to produce such a bony deformity). As the lesion is not completely lucent and the adjoining bone is sclerotic, a bone cyst should not be considered.

Monostotic fibrous dysplasia is the most common variety of this dysostosis. Sites involved include the skull, facial bones and long bones, and it is the commonest cause of a solitary expanded lesion of a rib. Fibrous dysplasia may exist in most age groups, but often presents in the second and third decades with localised pain and/or deformity due to overgrowth of bone, as in this case. Pathological fractures can occur.

The radiological appearances depend on the site and maturity of the lesion. In the long bones fibrous dysplasia is found in the diaphyseal or diametaphyseal regions. It is predominantly radiolucent with either a 'ground glass' or trabeculated appearance. Cortical thinning, a sclerotic rim and flecks of calcification, as shown in this case, are all typical findings.

Reference

Gibson, M. J. and Middlemiss, J. H. (1971) Fibrous dysplasia of bone. *Brit. J. Radiol.*, **44**, 1-13.

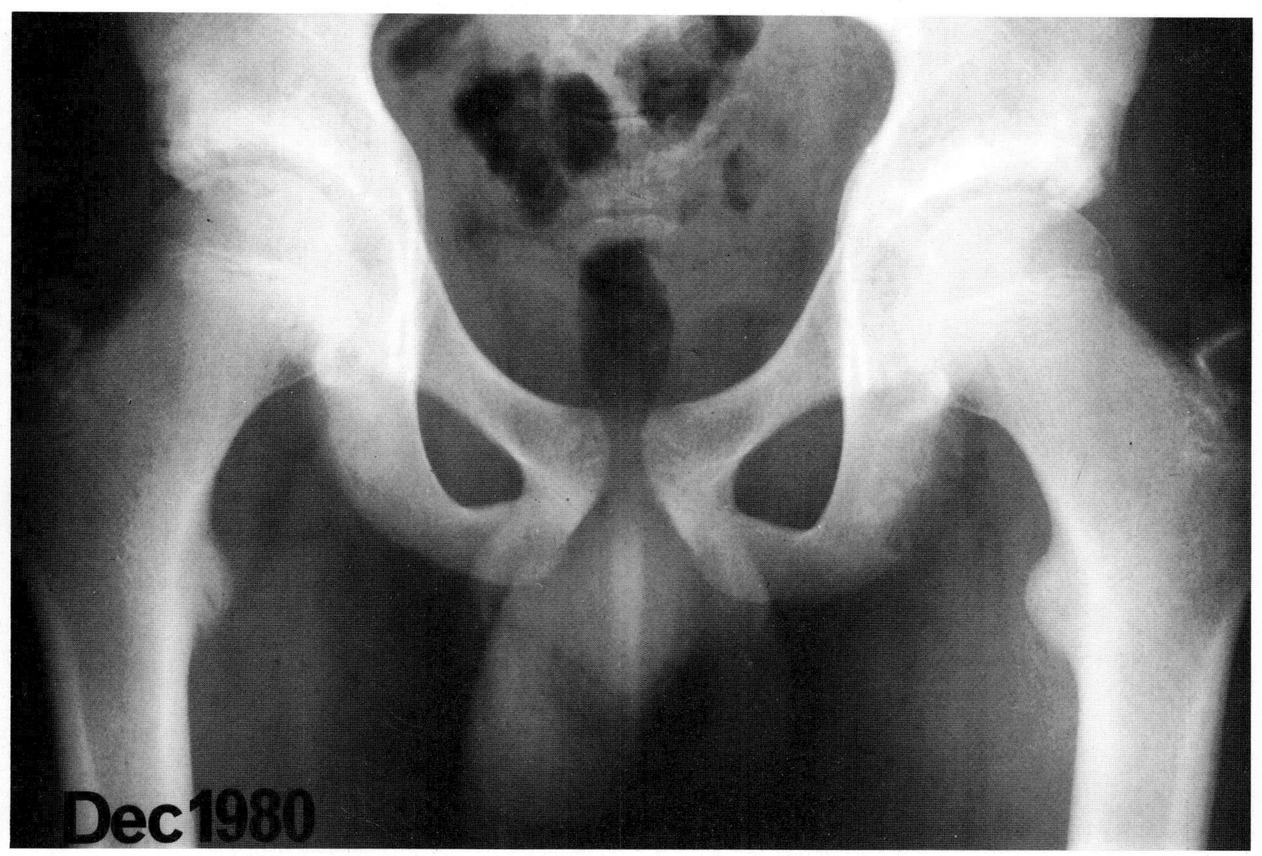

This teenager developed a painful limp while at a school sports day. On examination there was marked tenderness over the left ischial tuberosity.

- What is the aetiology of this condition?

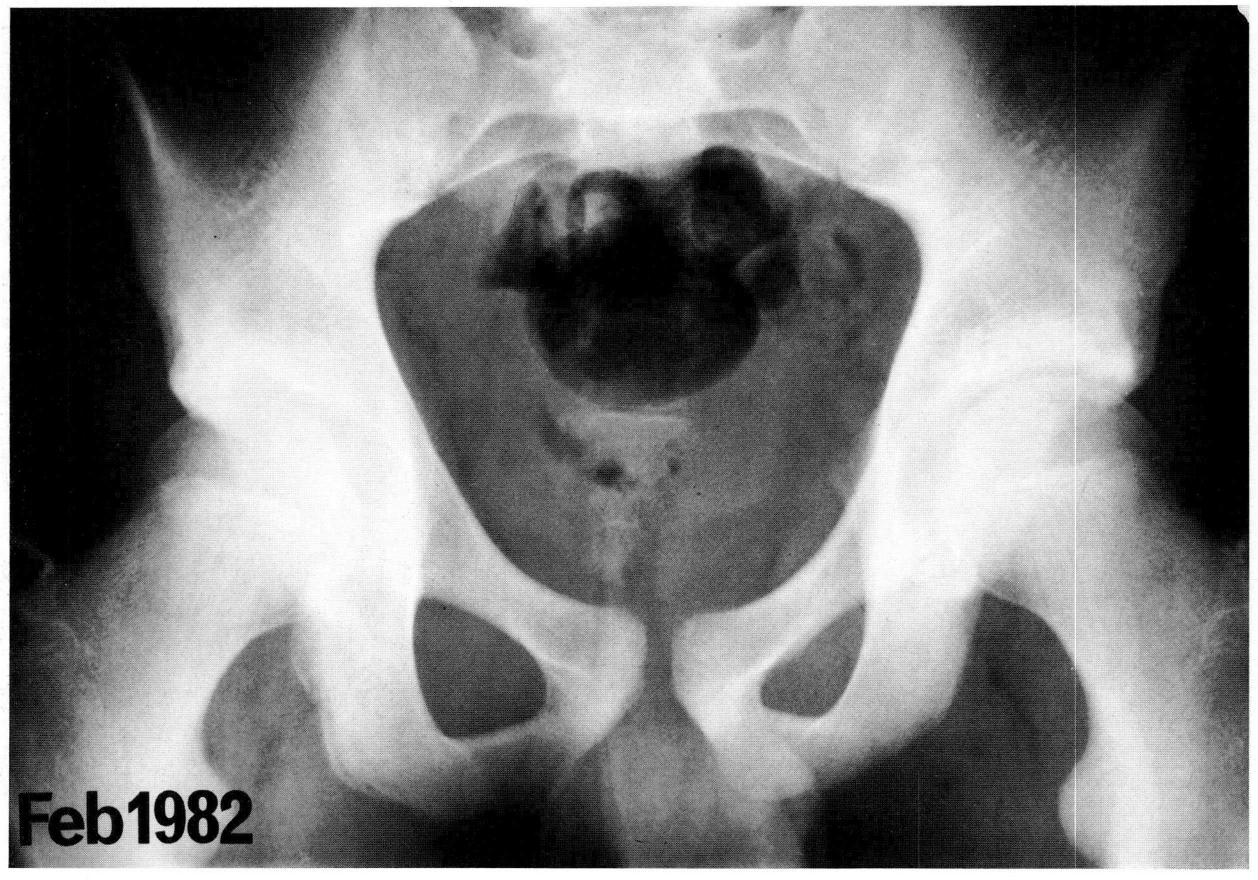

The non-united ossification centre or apophysis of the left ischial tuberosity has been avulsed and has rotated to overlie the ischium. It is important to recognise this injury and not to interpret the appearances as being due to an expanding lesion of the ischium, as this may lead to unneccesary surgical intervention.

The apophysis for the ischial tuberosity appears at puberty and fuses at about 25 years. Avulsion fractures are caused by a strong contraction of the hamstring muscles, which take their origin from the ischial tuberosity, during strenuous activity. Patients are usually participants in sports such as hurdling and long jump, and this boy had been running at the time of onset of pain.

Other pelvic apophyses which may be avulsed include the anterior superior iliac spine (sartorius), the anterior inferior iliac spine (rectus femoris) and the iliac crest (anterior abdominal muscles). Management is conservative and, with healing, bony union usually occurs. A radiograph obtained 15 months later in this patient (see above) shows that the ischium and apophysis have fused on the left with cessation of growth. Normal growth has continued on the right where the apophysis has remained unfused.

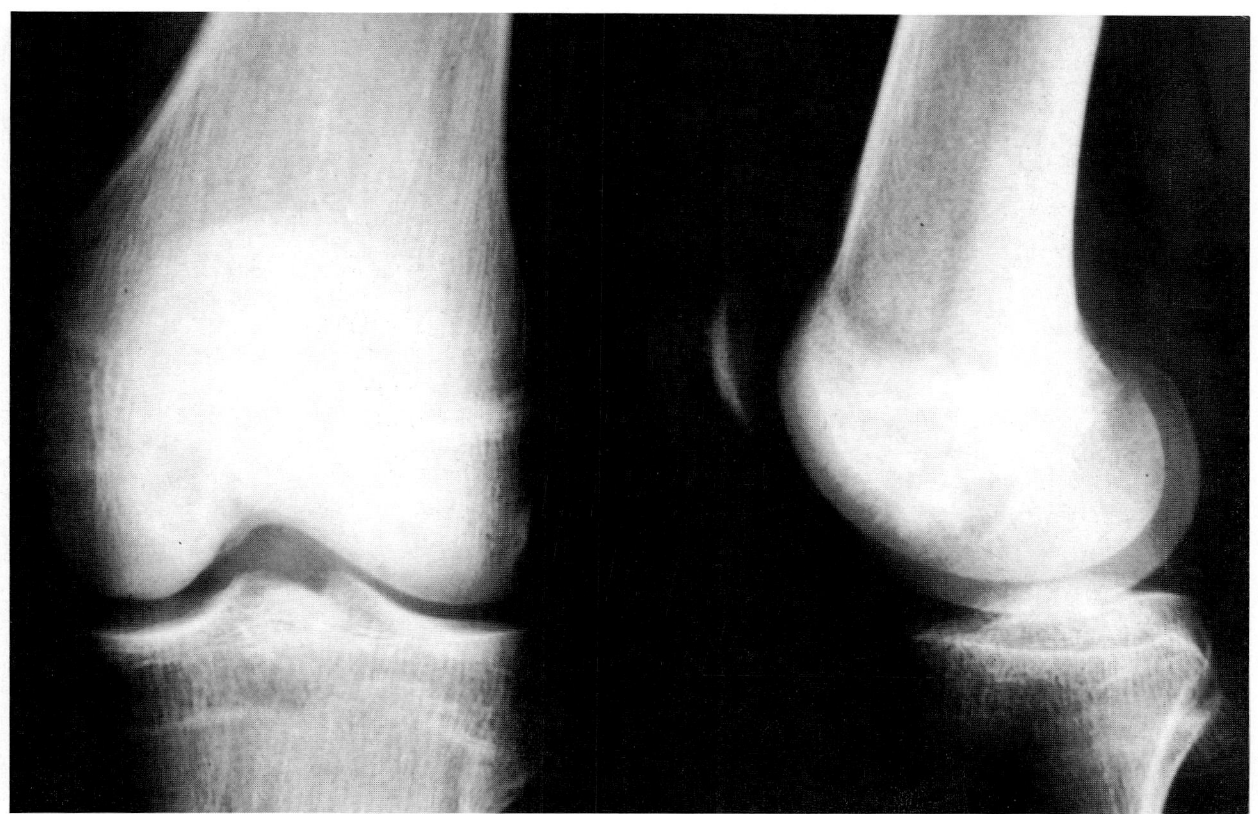

This boy aged 13 complained of a painful knee and, on examination, had a localised area of tenderness over the medial femoral condyle.

- Describe the radiographic appearance and suggest a diagnosis.

- What other radiographic technique would be useful in confirming your diagnosis?

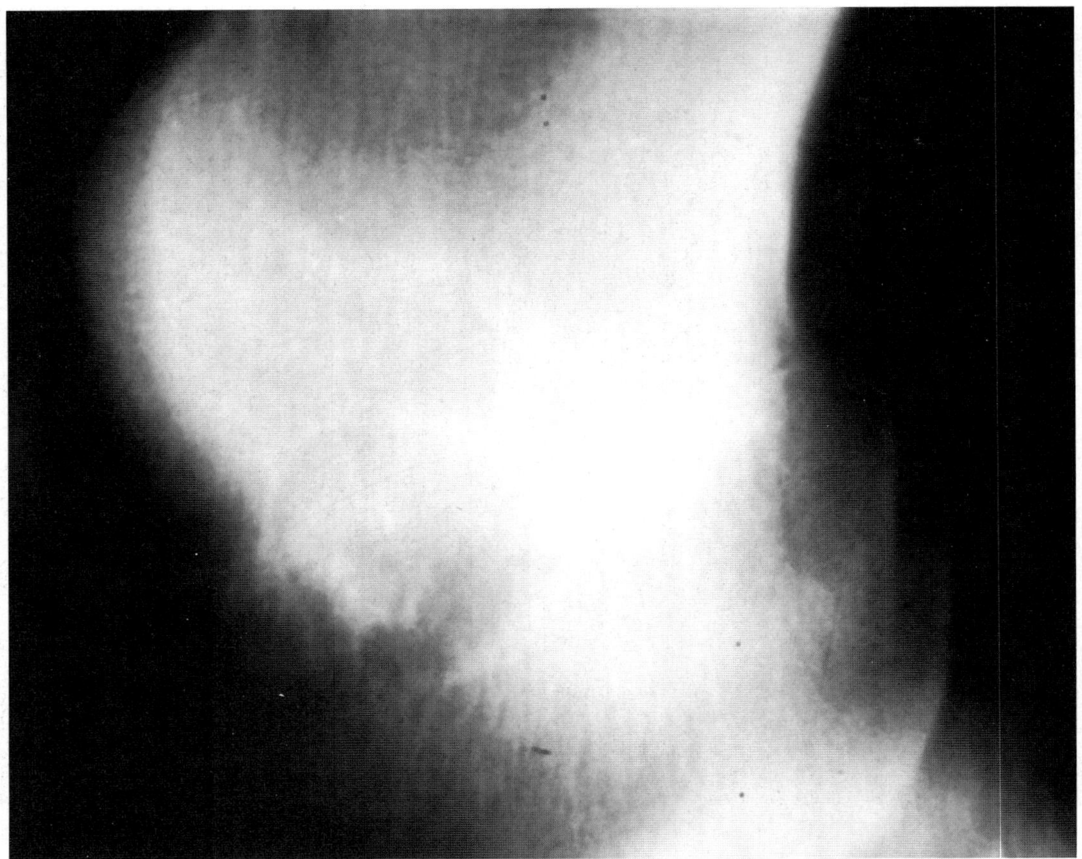

These views of the left knee show a rounded lucency in the medial femoral condyle which appears to be surrounded by ill-defined sclerosis. The bone is not expanded and the lesion is apparently confined to the epiphyseal region.

With tomography the abnormality is shown more clearly. It comprises a well-defined lucency with a fine sclerotic rim and central calcification, and does not extend across the closing growth plate.

The age of the patient and the site and appearance of the lesion are characteristic of a chondroblastoma. These benign tumours occur in the epiphyses and apophyses of the immature skeleton and are twice as common in males as in females. Presentation is usually with localised pain and swelling and limitation of movement.

Pathological fractures have been reported. Chondroblastomas are found most frequently in the proximal humerus, femur, proximal tibia and pelvis; 50 per cent occur in the lower limbs. Although they may be confined to an epiphysis or apophysis, they may extend across the growth plate. When this occurs, the greater part of the tumour lies on the epiphyseal aspect. Calcification of the matrix occurs radiologically in less than 50 per cent of cases; if this is very marked, the lesion may be mistaken for an osteoblastoma.

Reference

Bloem, J. L. and Mulder, J. D. (1985) Chondroblastoma: a clinical and radiological study of 104 cases. *Skeletal Radiol.*, 14, 1-9.

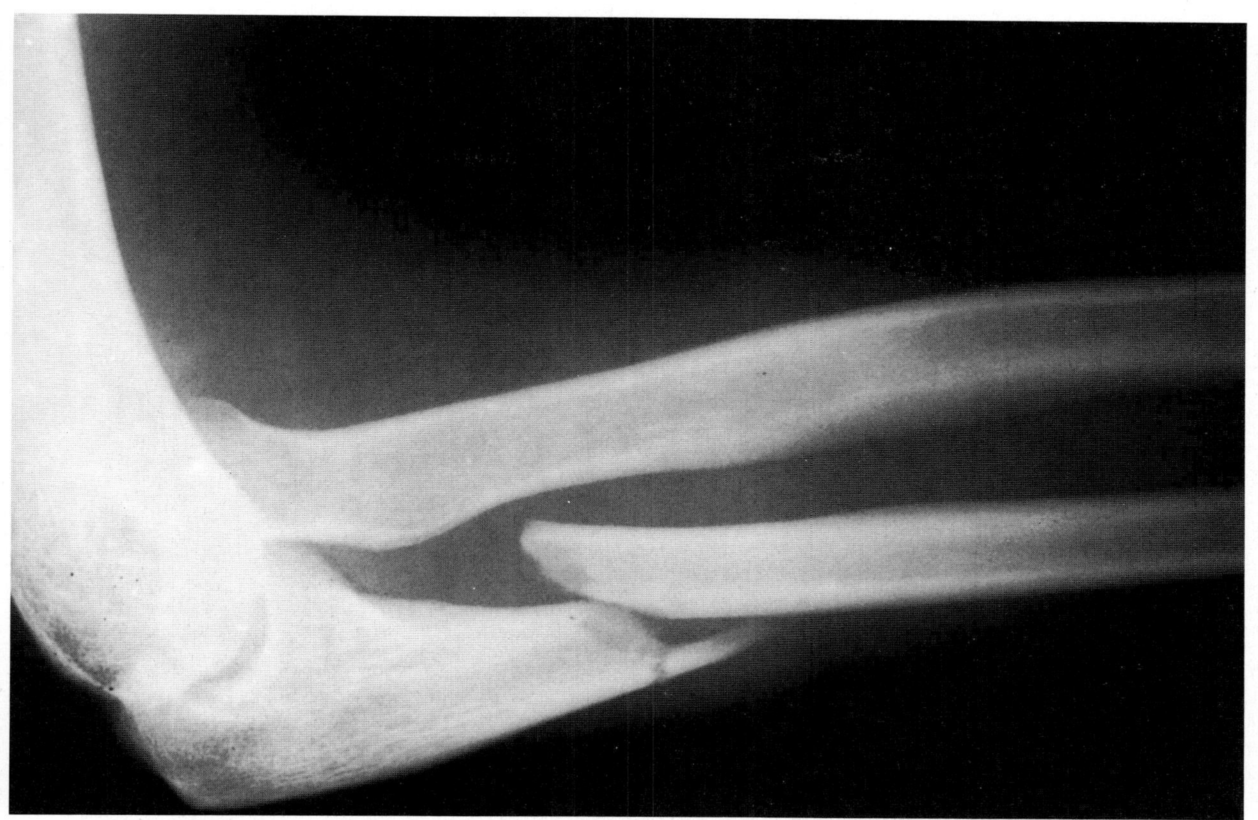

This radiograph was obtained following an RTA.

- What are the features of this injury and what is the name given to it?

- What is the importance of detecting it?

A95

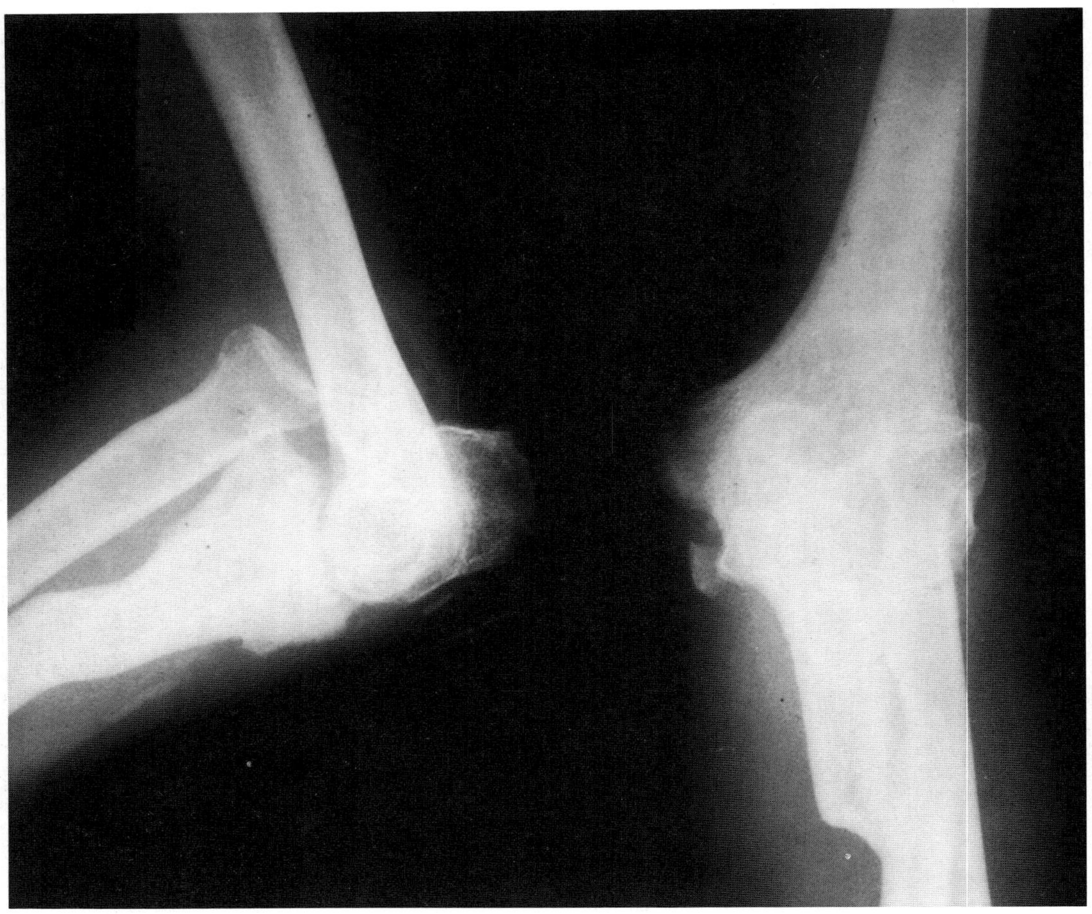

The lateral view of the elbow shows a fracture through the proximal shaft of the ulna with overlap of the fragments and consequent anterior dislocation of the radial head. This is a Monteggia fracture-dislocation.

Fracture, caused by indirect injury, through the shaft of only one of the paired forearm bones will almost always result in proximal or distal dislocation of the other bone. The radial dislocation may be difficult to recognise in a Monteggia injury but if undetected may cause damage to vessels and the radial nerve, and can result in new bone formation around the elbow (as in another untreated patient shown above) and limitation of motion due to persistent dislocation of the radial head.

Dislocation is confirmed if the normal alignment between the radius and capitulum is lost in any plane. Anterior dislocation of the radius is most common, being present in 65 per cent of Monteggia injuries.

Giovanni Battista Monteggia (1762-1815) was Professor of Anatomy and Surgery in Milan and described the fracture-dislocation in 1814, the same year as Abraham Colles described his fracture.

Reference

Bruce, H. E., Harvey, J. P., Jr. and Wilson, J. C., Jr. (1974) Monteggia fracture. *J. Bone Joint Surg.*, **56-A**, 1563-1576.

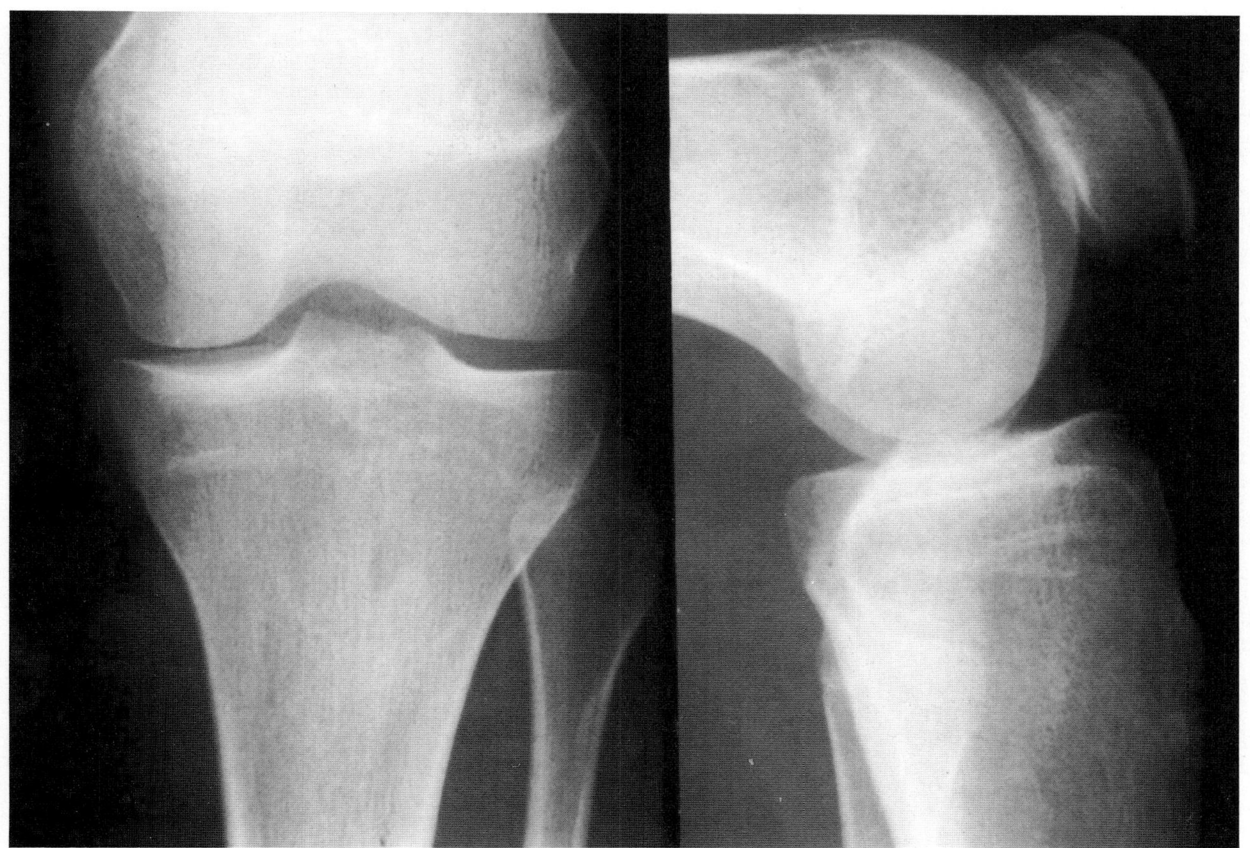

This 14-year-old girl gave a one-year history of leg pain which had been attributed to a lipoma.

- Suggest two possible diagnoses.

- How would you distinguish between them?

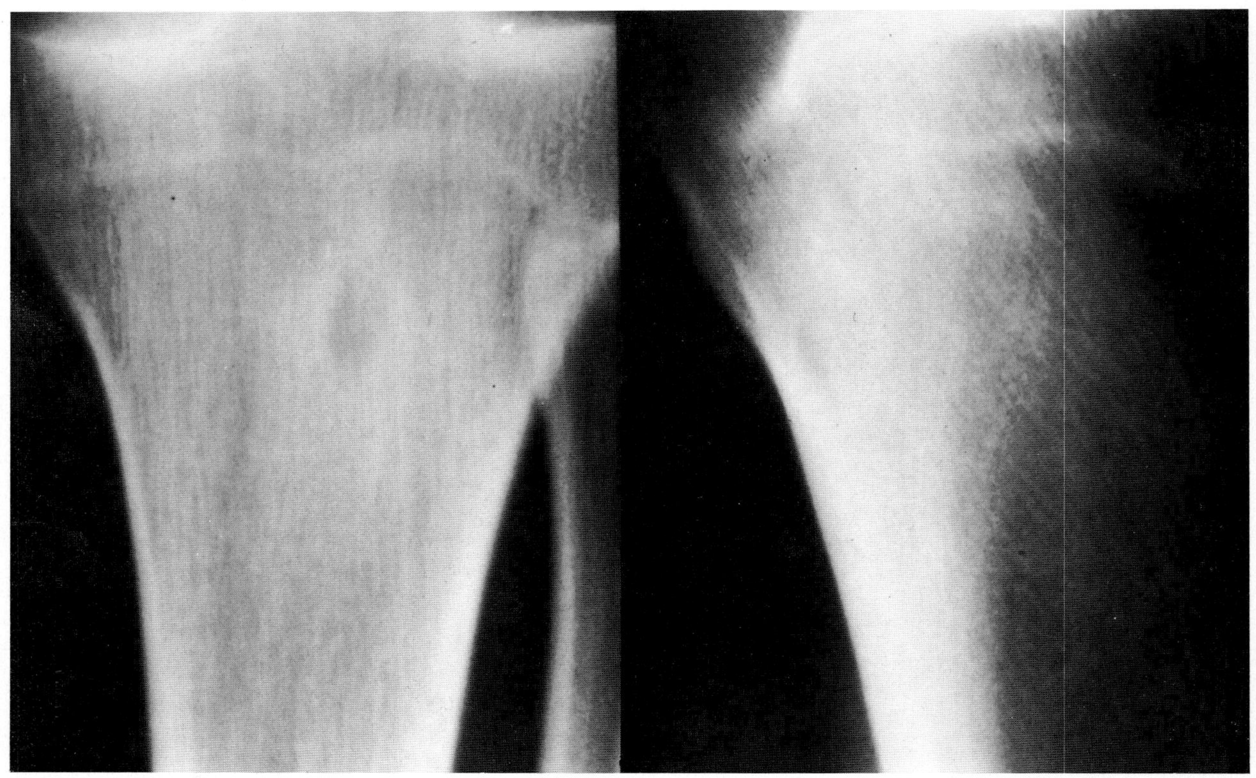

A small lucency with surrounding sclerosis lies subcortically in the posterior part of the metaphyseal region of the proximal tibia. The site and radiological appearances would be equally consistent with an osteoid osteoma and a Brodie's abscess, but the patient's pain was relieved by aspirin and this is the typical response of an osteoid osteoma.

The two may sometimes be distinguished with a radionuclide bone scan, as an osteoid osteoma is a vascular tumour and may show an uptake of isotope greater than a subacute abscess. This case not only demonstrates the increased uptake in the osteoma but also the normal high uptake in the growth plates around the knee. Tomography of the lesion clearly shows the lucent nidus which, in osteoid osteoma, is generally accepted to be less than 1 cm in diameter, and may contain a central density. These benign lesions usually present with severe pain, which is worse at night and relieved by aspirin. The pain will persist unless the entire nidus is removed at surgery. The specific pain is probably due to the containment of the vascular lesion, which contains neural axons, within a rigid bony shell.

Reference

Omojola, M. F., Cockshott, W. P. and Beatty, E. G. (1981) Osteoid osteoma: an evaluation of diagnostic modalities. *Clin. Radiol.*, 32, 199-204.

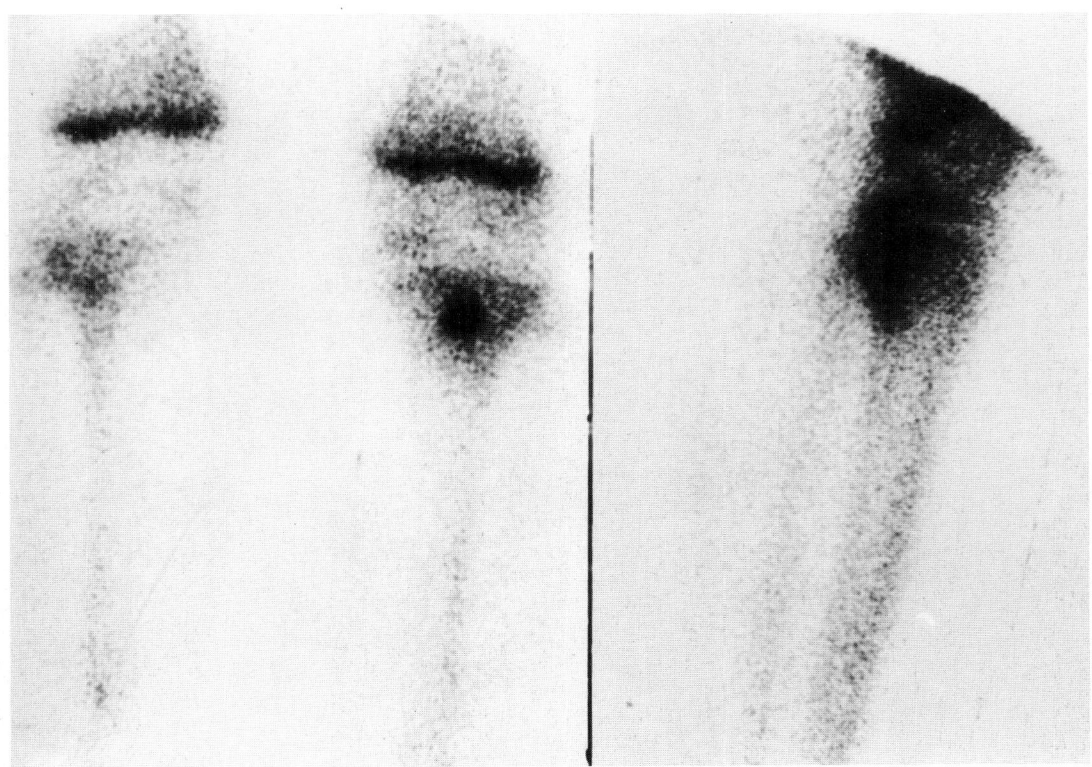

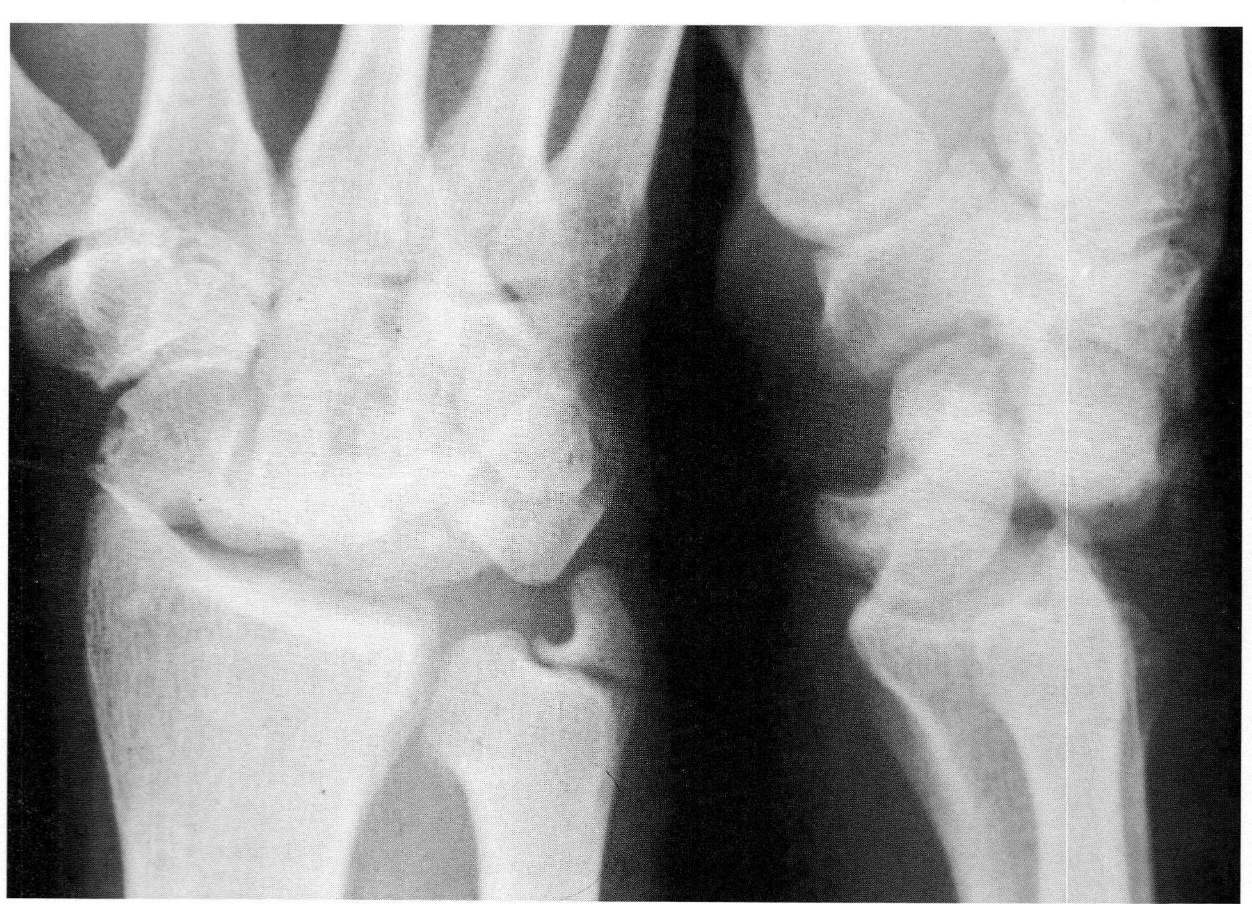

A 20-year-old motorcycle scrambling enthusiast was seen after falling off his motorcycle and injuring his wrist.

- Identify the injuries.

- How may the post-reduction film help?

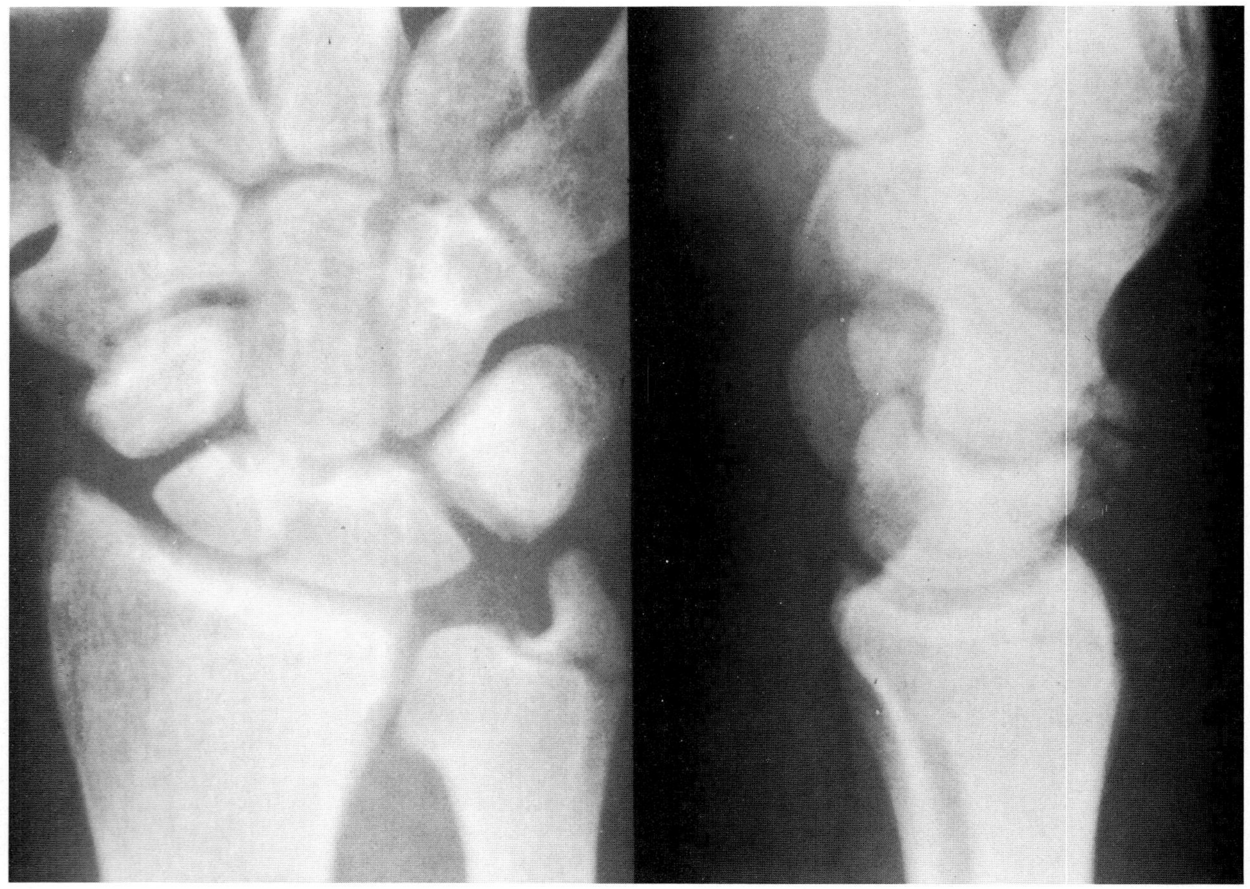

In the lateral projection of the wrist the proximal articular surface of the lunate has almost maintained its normal congruent relationship with the radius and the capitate has been displaced dorsally. This is termed a perilunate dislocation.

An associated fracture of the ulnar styloid is present; an old non-united fracture of the scaphoid is only clearly visible on the post-reduction film shown above.

Perilunate and lunate dislocations comprise ten per cent of carpal injuries and the former are twice as common as the latter. Seventy-five per cent of perilunate dislocations have an associated scaphoid fracture; fractures of other carpal bones and of the radius and ulna are also found. Fractures are often shown better on the post-reduction film, when the anatomy approaches the normal.

Further Reading

Grainger, R. and Allison, D. (1987) *Diagnostic Radiology*. pp. 1221-1522. Churchill Livingstone, Edinburgh & London.

Murray, R.O. and Jacobson, H.G. (1977) *The Radiology of Skeletal Disorders*. Second edition. Churchill Livingstone, Edinburgh & London.

Park, W. M. and Hughes, S.P.F. (1987) *Orthopaedic Radiology*. Blackwell Scientific Publications, Oxford.

Rogers, L.F. (1982) *Radiology of Skeletal Trauma*. Churchill Livingstone, New York & Edinburgh.

Sutton, D. (1987) *A Textbook of Radiology and Imaging*. Fourth Edition. pp. 2-323. Churchill Livingstone, Edinburgh & London.

Index

(References are to case numbers)